COOK THIS NOT THAT!™

KITCHEN SURVIVAL GUIDE

The No-Diet Weight Loss Solution

BY DAVID ZINCZENKO
AND MATT GOULDING

RODALE

Eat This, Not That! is a registered trademark of Rodale Inc.
© 2010 by Rodale Inc.

All rights reserved. No part of this publication may be reproduced or transmitted in any form
or by any means, electronic or mechanical, including photocopying, recording, or any other information
storage and retrieval system, without the written permission of the publisher.

Rodale books may be purchased for business or promotional use or for special sales. For information,
please write to: Special Markets Department, Rodale Inc., 733 Third Avenue, New York, NY 10017.

Printed in the United States of America
Rodale Inc. makes every effort to use acid-free ∞, recycled paper ♻.

Book design by George Karabotsos

Photo editing by Tara Long

Cover photographs by Thomas MacDonald/Rodale Images.
Food styling by Diane Simone Vezza and Melissa Reiss

All interior photos by Mitch Mandel and Thomas MacDonald/Rodale Images,
and food styling by Diane Simone Vezza and Melissa Reiss,
with the exception of the following: pages 50, 140, 216, 278 © Ray Kachatorian;
page 166 © Olivier Pojzmon-Zuma/Corbis; page 290 © Nikolai Golovonoff; page 291 © Food Pix

Library of Congress Cataloging-in-Publication Data is on file with the publisher
ISBN-13: 978–1–60529–442–1 paperback

Distributed to the trade by Macmillan
12   14   16   18   20   19   17   15   13   11   paperback

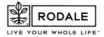

We inspire and enable people to improve their lives and the world around them

For more of our products visit **rodalestore.com** or call 800-848-4735

DEDICATION

To anyone who has ever burned a casserole,
scorched a steak, or suffered any other defeat,
big or small, in the kitchen. We've done
the same too many times to count,
and yet we keep coming back for more.

—Dave and Matt

ACKNOWLEDGMENTS

Cook This, Not That! was an ambitious project that presented many unique challenges that would have vanquished most other teams. But we're fortunate enough to work with people well versed in the ways of making the impossible possible. Thanks to all of those who made this book a reality, especially:

To Maria Rodale and the Rodale family, who have done as much to improve the way Americans eat as any other family in this country.

To George Karabotsos and his crew of ace designers, including Laura White, Mark Michaelson, Courtney Eltringham, Elizabeth Neal, and Rob Campos. Your collective ability to bring our words to life exceeds any and all expectations.

To Clint Carter, a jack of all food trades who helps make these books tick. Also, to Carolyn Kylstra, Anna Maltby, Sophie Fitzgerald, and Kelly and Katie Kennedy— your willingness to tackle any issue is more impressive than ever.

To Tara Long, whose preternatural ability to make food look beautiful and delicious has kept us all in a state of perpetual hunger throughout the production of this book.

To the immensely talented Rodale book team: Steve Perrine, Karen Rinaldi, Chris Krogermeier, Debbie McHugh, Nancy Bailey, Sara Cox, Mitch Mandel, Tom MacDonald, Troy Schnyder, Melissa Reiss, Nikki Weber, Diane Vezza, Joan Parkin, Jennifer Giandomenico, Wendy Gable, Keith Biery, Liz Krenos, Brooke Myers, Sean Sabo, and Caroline McCall. There aren't enough words on this page to properly express our gratitude for all that you do to make these books what they are. Thank you.

And to our friends, family, and loved ones: There's no one we'd rather cook for.

—Dave and Matt

Check out the other informative books in the *EAT THIS, NOT THAT!*® series:

Eat This,
Not That!
(2007)

Eat This,
Not That!
for Kids!
(2008)

Eat This,
Not That!
Supermarket
Survival Guide
(2009)

Eat This,
Not That!
The Best (& Worst!)
Foods in America!
(2009)

Eat This,
Not That!
2010
(2009)

Eat This,
Not That!
Restaurant
Survival Guide
(2009)

CONTENTS

Come with us to a magical place.

It's a place of comfort and ease, a place where you're in control and no one can tell you what to do. It's a place where you can be as inventive, creative, and wacky as you want, and everything you do is perfectly all right. And best of all, it's a place where you can eat all your favorite foods and still lose all the weight you want.

Indeed, this place is so magical, you can not only lose weight and eat great but also grow wealthier and healthier, just by spending more time there.

So, what is this magic place?

It's your kitchen.

Let's Get Cooking!

It's a terrible time to become a chef. But it's a great time to become a cook.

Ever since the American economy hit a giant RESET button back in September 2008, things have changed—a lot. We've grown wiser with our money, and we're determined to spend it smartly. Whereas once we aspired to drive the biggest, broadest, hungriest SUV on the block, today Humvees look as outdated as bell-bottoms. Whereas once we admired the men and women boasting power suits and toting briefcases, today most kids whose parents work on Wall Street lie to their friends to save face. "My dad? He's, um, he's . . . in jail!"

And while the TV seems to bring us nothing but celebrity chefs—and wannabes who are willing to be humiliated by celebrity chefs—in the real world, we're starting to take a second look at our restaurant culture as well. In 2008, 28 percent of Americans said they had visited a fine dining restaurant in the past month. In 2009, that figure dropped to just 19 percent. And 52 percent of respondents in a poll by Mintel said that they are spending less at restaurants than they did the year before. Sorry, Gordon Ramsay, but it's suddenly a cold day in Hell's Kitchen.

And that's a good thing, for our wallets, our waistlines, and our overall health. It's not a huge leap to look at all the drive-thrus and quickie sandwich shops and prepackaged take-out meals, then look at our growing bellies and thinning wallets and think—hmm, maybe there's a connection here.

And there is.

The Better Way to Eat

Forget dieting. Forget joining a gym. Forget the ads for the Ab-inator device you saw on QVC. If you really, truly want to lose weight, there is no quicker way to shave pounds off your body—and dollars off your food bill—than to cook more at home. That's what *Cook This, Not That!* will teach you to do.

Now, we don't mean to say you should avoid restaurants and prepared supermarket foods like the plague. The *Eat This, Not That!* series is designed to help you make smart swaps at all your favorite restaurants and in choosing all your favorite supermarket foods.

But in many cases, the very smartest swap you can make . . . is to make it yourself. Just check out this sampling of restaurant and prepared supermarket foods and see how many calories you can save if you simply learn to cook these very basic dishes at home.

Who Blew up the Food?

	Restaurant	Supermarket	Home-Cooked
PIZZA (per slice)	210 calories 11 g fat (4 g saturated)	510 calories 22 g fat (10 g saturated)	187 calories 5.5 g fat (2 g saturated)
HAMBURGER (regular)	830 calories 50 g fat (16 g saturated)	350 calories 16 g fat (6.5 g saturated)*	329 calories 12 g fat (4.5 g saturated)
STEAK	655 calories 47.5 g fat (21 g saturated)	360 calories 14 g fat (6 g saturated)	243 calories 8 g fat (2.5 g saturated)
WAFFLES (no syrup)	547 calories 8 g fat (4 g saturated)	170 calories 2.5 g fat (0 g saturated)	218 calories 10.5 g fat (2 g saturated)
PIE	533 calories 30 g fat (11 g saturated)	355 calories 21.5 g fat (10 g saturated)	355 calories 17 g fat (5 g saturated)
GRILLED CHEESE	430 calories 26.5 g fat (8 g saturated)	590 calories 22 g fat (7 g saturated)	270 calories 15.5 g fat (9.5 g saturated)
PASTA	867 calories 34 g fat (15 g saturated)	840 calories 42 g fat (16 g saturated)	422 calories 10.5 g fat (2.5 g saturated)
ENCHILADA	1,315 calories 65 g fat (25 g saturated)	380 calories 9 g fat (2 g saturated)	304 calories 10 g fat (3 g saturated)
ROAST BEEF SANDWICH	571 calories 25 g fat (11 g saturated)	700 calories 29 g fat (11 g saturated)	245 calories 8.5 g fat (1 g saturated)

Burgers sold premade but not prepared in store

Imagine that, over the course of a week, you cooked these nine foods instead of going out to eat them. You'd save a whopping 3,385 calories just in that 1 week alone—essentially, a pound's worth of flab. Cooking just these nine foods at home instead of letting the pimply-faced grease purveyor at your local chain restaurant do it for you would shave an unbelievable 50 pounds of fat off your body in just 1 year.

Why the dramatic discrepancy? In part, it has to do with the ingredients—restaurants want to mess with your taste buds by adding as much fat, salt, and sugar as they can to everything they touch. But another issue is serving size. In 2008, the USDA found that people eat an estimated 107 more calories each time they choose to eat out instead of eating at home. And a 2002 study looked at restaurant portion sizes and found that they far exceeded what they should be. By weighing foods, researchers found that, compared with USDA portion sizes, the following foods ballooned considerably.

Pasta: 480 percent oversize
Muffins: 333 percent oversize
Steak: 224 percent oversize
Bagels: 195 percent oversize
Hamburgers: 112 percent oversize

Of course, you'd still save a ton of calories and money by buying prepared foods in the supermarket—just under 1,700 calories a week. But why lose only half the weight you want to? And why spend more than you have to? And why settle for something that was cooked by a stranger yesterday (or last week or maybe even months ago)?

It's so easy to shave off the pounds, just by mastering a few simple cooking skills. So why don't we all do it? That's the mystery.

Let's solve it.

Who Moved My Cheeseburger?

Here's an experiment: Think of the term "family dinner." Now, close your eyes and imagine what that looks like. Can you see it, smell it, taste it? Yes?

Can you? And more important, how can you still be reading this if your eyes are closed? What are you, superhuman?

Seriously, when we think of the term "family dinner," we almost always think of a family sitting around the dining room table. It's an image that's been carved into our brains over decades by books, magazines, TV shows, and movies. And maybe we remember those dinners from our own past because our parents or grandparents hosted family meals in just that way.

But today's "family dinner" doesn't look like the family dinners we see in movies or read about in books or even conjure up in our own minds. Family dinner cooked at home is rare, after all. We're far more likely to hit the fast-food joint, order a delivery, or heat up something that was prepared in a supermarket than we are to actually cook our own dinner. In 1963, only 28.5 percent of our food dollars were spent on meals prepared outside the home. But by 2006, it was nearly 49 percent—half of our money being sucked away by restaurant- and supermarket-prepared foods. And so, instead of clinking dishware and "Pass the gravy," it's crinkling paper bags and "Who got the Tater Tots?"

And that means we're not in control of our food or our bodies. Sure, you can study that takeout menu like a grad student on Ritalin and pore over the side panels of the packaged food labels like Tom Hanks trying to crack the DaVinci Code, but in the end, no matter how careful you are, you're still not in charge.

That's why we want to take you to the kitchen.

But before we go there, come with us for a moment to your local fast-food restaurant or sit-down joint. Let's say you're hungry for a cheeseburger. Order one.

But before you do, answer a few questions: Does this burger contain lean beef or fatty beef? And just how old is that beef, anyway? (There's no way to tell, since a fast-food burger could contain beef from dozens of different cows. Eww.) Is it properly cooked, or is there some *E. coli* hanging around, as has happened at several burger chains over the past few years? And how many calories are in that burger? If you're ordering the A.1 Peppercorn Burger at Red Robin (nice balloon, kid), you're tackling 1,440 calories—about the amount of calories you should eat, in total, for all three meals, not just one.

And what about the bun? Is it made with whole grains or with refined flour that will create a sugar rush in your bloodstream, helping to increase the odds that you'll join the one in three Americans who develop diabetes in their lifetime? (And is that bun fresh or has it been tanning under a sunlamp since 6 a.m.?) If you ordered the Bacon Cheddar Minis at Ruby Tuesday, you got a whole lot of bun in relation to your burger—and a whole lot of the 1,358 calories those burgers pack are carb calories, rushing sugar into your bloodstream.

And the condiments—are they exactly what you want, or are they exactly what the penny-pinchers at the big multinational corporation have decided is best for their profit margins? If condiments include ketchup, mayonnaise, even relish, then they also contain high-fructose corn syrup, which has been shown to interfere with your body's ability to process the hormone leptin—the hormone that tells you when you're full. Oops!

Oh, wait, sorry . . . you wanted fries with that? Okay, but are those fries cooked lightly with a coating of heart-healthy olive oil? Or do they get a bath of trans-fatty acids, which have been shown to raise your risk of obesity and heart disease? If you're eating at Jack in the Box, those medium fries come with 7 grams of cholesterol-spiking trans fat—more than you should eat in 3 days!

Wash it down with a shake, okay? Maybe a chocolate one. But if you're at Cold Stone and you order the Gotta Have It PB&C milk shake, you've just slurped down an additional 2,010 calories. That's a whole day's worth of calories for an adult woman *plus* more saturated fat than you should eat in 3 days. And you didn't even eat your burger yet!

What an adventure! And that's just a burger, fries, and a shake!

Now, imagine you could eat the exact same meal at home, except for a few slight differences: You could eliminate more than two-thirds of the calories and most of the harmful fats—and at the same time ensure that the food itself was actually fresh, because you prepared it yourself. Oh, and the cost? A typical burger, shake, and sides at a low-end chain restaurant like T.G.I. Friday's will cost you nearly $35. At home? Less than 6 bucks.

Makes you want to learn how to cook, right?

Good thing you bought this book.

What You'll Gain by Cooking It Yourself

We don't mean to freak you out with gnarly stories about psycho calorie counts, processed-food poisoning scares, and rumors of teenage chefs spitting in the fish sandwiches (that never, ever happens, honest). This is a positive book about positive change. So let's take a look at what you'll gain now that you're ready to make the move to the kitchen.

You'll lose weight and look better.

The foods we recommend in *Cook This, Not That!* are designed predominantly to target belly fat—by keeping your belly full of smart, healthy choices that keep your resting metabolism revving and never let you go hungry. That means you'll be at the top of your game and burning fat all day, every day, even when you sleep!

You'll reshape your body.

Most "diets" force you to cut down on the amount of food you're eating, but that's not your goal, or ours! Instead, by staying full, you'll retain lean muscle while trimming away only flab—so you'll be sculpting the body you've always wanted, effortlessly!

You'll save time and stress.

When you command your own kitchen, everything is under your control. You want zucchini instead of spinach with your steak? Make it so. You like a little cinnamon in your pancake mix? Thy will be done. You hate those little sesame thingies on the sandwich buns? Banish them forever. Most of the recipes in this book take about half as much time as it does to get a pizza delivered, and as you cook more, you'll get into a rhythm that allows you to cook once or twice and eat well for a week, by smartly managing portions and leftovers.

You'll bulk up your wallet, not your waistline.

There's an old saying: Look the part and you'll get the part. Well, research shows that people who are leaner and fitter are viewed as being more competent and successful than those who are overweight. Don't believe me?

A New York University study found that people packing on an extra 40 pounds make 9 percent less than their slimmer colleagues. And when you take control of your meals, you save money, too.

You'll even improve your health.
The list of health problems that come as side orders with our overstuffed restaurant entrées is long and depressing: Diabetes, heart disease, high blood pressure, stroke, cancer, gout, and back pain are just the beginning. But imagine being able to sidestep them all!

The time to take back control of your weight, your health, your wallet, and your life is now.

Fortunately, the only tool you'll ever need is right in your hands!

But Wait—I Don't Have Time to Cook!

Ugh. We knew someone was going to pipe up about the time factor. You, in the back of the class, with your hand raised—what's the problem?

You say you don't have time to cook? That's weird. You have time to get in the car and drive to a restaurant and wait for the kid in the paper hat to fry up your dinner. You have time to go to the store (again) to buy something to pop into the microwave and eat standing up over the sink. You even have time to call the delivery place, then sit around waiting for the bell to ring like one of Pavlov's dogs.

If you have time for all that, then trust us: You have time to cook.

The vast majority of the meals in this book can be executed in 30 minutes or less—less time than it takes to find the delivery menu, wait on hold, give your order, and then spend the next half hour grousing about how long it takes for them to get here. And you'll actually spend less time in the store than you usually do, because you'll shop once and eat for a week, instead of having to pop in every night to find something digestible.

So let's give it a shot. What do you have to lose—except your belly?

Chapter 1

Cook This, Not That!

The Truth About Your Food

When we were little kids, having dinner was a simple three-part process:
1. Eat the meat and potatoes.
2. Take all the green stuff and feed it to the dog.
3. Ask for dessert.

This system worked great for generations of kids—although not so great for generations of dogs. We grew up pretty happy and pretty healthy, and Mom and Dad were right; when we got older, we actually tried, and liked, some of the green stuff.

But then, a couple of things happened:
1. A lot of people in our neighborhood started to get fat.
2. A lot of people in the government developed an opinion about why all the people were getting fat.

And suddenly, food got really complicated (for the dog, too, thanks to scares over tainted dog food from China). Something that ought to be easy as pie—literally—became fraught with challenges, shrouded in myth, and obscured by a combination of complicated government regulation, marketing mystique, and dietary hysteria.

How Something Easy Got So Complicated

There's an old saying that "A little bit of knowledge is a dangerous thing." And nowhere can that point be illustrated more clearly than in Americans' dietary attitudes—in particular, our attitudes toward fat.

In an effort to help its citizens eat more healthfully, the USDA issued guidelines back in the 1970s that recommended against eating too much saturated fat because saturated fat can raise cholesterol, and high cholesterol can lead to heart disease. Pretty simple, right?

But as journalist Michael Pollan outlines in his book *In Defense of Food,* this was a very simple approach to a very complicated issue, and it's probably done a lot of damage to our public health. The USDA's recommendation drove people to abandon saturated fat like, say, butter and substitute something that seemed pretty harmless: trans fat, like what you find in many margarines.

Indeed, food marketers scrambled to take advantage of the healthy properties of trans fat—and what a coup that was! Unlike normal fats, trans fat stays solid at room temperature, so you can turn it into cookies, muffins, cupcakes, and hundreds of other supermarket staples and it'll never leak grease onto the cardboard box. Genius! And because trans fat was good for us and so adept at carrying delicious flavors along on its tributaries of tallow, marketers had no reason not to load our foods with it at every possible turn.

But the case was closed before all the evidence was in. Turns out that saturated fat isn't quite as bad for you as the government "experts" decided: While it raises bad cholesterol, it also raises good cholesterol. So the link between saturated fat and heart disease is less clear-cut than one might think. There's still a case against saturated fat—it doesn't do a whole lot for your body, nutritionally, and it's easily stored in your belly, in your butt, or in the handbags where your triceps used to be. But it's not the time bomb for your ticker that it's been made out to be. What can really damage your heart, raise your cholesterol, increase your risk of stroke?

Trans fat

Oh. Hmm. Sorry, American population. Turns out trans fat—the stuff the government wanted you to eat, the stuff that margarine commercials for several decades touted as the cure for heart disease—is, in fact, the deadliest fat known to man. It's not even natural—it's a substance concocted, marketed, and consumed by people, and it's caused a lot of damage.

Today, the USDA recommends limiting trans fat to less than 2 grams per day. So it makes a lot of sense to scour the supermarket shelves for goods that say "no trans fat" on the label. Phew! That makes eating much simpler, because . . .

Oops. Stop. Hold up.

Here's trouble: The US government, ever understanding toward poor, defenseless multinational food corporations, was loath to ban trans fat altogether, since it had become such a ubiquitous part of our nutritional landscape. So the government did, yet again, a bad, bad thing: They ruled that a convenience food can claim "no trans fat" on its label if it carries less than 0.5 gram of the stuff.

In other words, you could eat four servings of supermarket convenience foods that say "no trans fat" on the label and still come close to exceeding your daily value of trans fat! Even if you ate nothing else all day!

Wow. Did we get shafted or what?

Here's the actual good news: So much of the confusion about what to eat and how to eat surrounds the stuff that's prepackaged or cooked up in a restaurant. Cook at home, for example, and you'll automatically put a damper on your trans fat consumption. That's because, whereas it's tough to discern which fast-food burgers and sit-down steaks carry it, it's easy to banish trans fat from your kitchen. Try this simple test: Put a stick of margarine and a stick of butter on the kitchen counter. Wait an hour. Now look: The butter is runny, which is what natural fat is supposed to look like at room temperature. The margarine looks like Tori Spelling's bust—unnaturally firm. (Or just read the ingredients on the back label: Anything with partially hydrogenated oil or shortening is cursed with the stuff.)

The point is, at home, in the comfort of your kitchen, you're in full control. No secret fats, no hidden sugars, no misleading menu descriptions. Just you and the simple building blocks for your next meal.

Here's a quick look at some of the other staples that you'll be playing with as you hone your emerging culinary skills. Understand them—and how most of them are actually your friends—and you'll be able to handle any cooking conundrum with confidence.

Best Foods Index

Eating well isn't just about losing weight—it's about feeling better in every possible way, from fighting off the stress of a bunk economy to maximizing the effects of a serious workout. We've pinpointed 10 foods you'd do well to eat everyday and provided you the blueprints for putting each into action.

Best food for your brain: BLUEBERRIES

Anthocyanidin, the antioxidant pigment responsible for the blueberry's hue, has a powerful bolstering effect on learning and memory. Several studies have indicated that cognitive functions increase along with blueberry consumption.
>>> *Blueberry recipes: pages 52, 56, 318*

Best food for all-day energy: QUINOA

Quinoa has higher concentrations of energy-producing B vitamins than any other whole wheat grain.
>>> *Quinoa recipe: page 294*

Best food after a workout: GREEK YOGURT

Not only does Greek yogurt have two to three times the amount of protein of normal yogurt, it also has all the amino acids you need to rebuild your muscles after a trip to the gym.
>>> *Greek yogurt recipes: pages 52, 56, 134, 148, 156, 322*

Best food for boosting your mood: SALMON

Add happiness to the list of perks derived from the omega-3 fats in salmon. Several studies have linked EPA and DHA, the dominant form of omega-3s in fish, to a decreased risk of depression. >>> *Salmon recipes: pages 42, 178, 232*

Best food for healthy skin: ALMONDS

After examining the diets of 453 people, Australian researchers found that monounsaturated fats exhibited protective properties and actually prevented both wrinkles and sun damage. Almonds, avocados, and olive oil all fit the bill.
>>> *Almond recipes: pages 114, 293*

Best food for surviving flu season: RED BELL PEPPER

Vitamin C is essential to your liver's ability to eliminate toxins, and vitamin A increases the efficacy of white blood cells and antibodies. A red bell pepper has twice as much vitamin C as an orange and three times as much A as a tomato.
>>> *Red pepper recipes: pages 136, 184, 188, 234, 246, 258, 260*

Best food to fight cavities: CHEESE

Studies have demonstrated that chewing cheese can increase the concentration of calcium in plaque, which helps to protect your teeth against cavities. Not to mention that following a sugary food with cheese can boost the pH in your mouth back to the safe zone.
>>> *Cheese recipes: pages 52, 60, 92, 104, 108, 130, 136, 230, 318*

Best food for your sexual health: DARK CHOCOLATE

The flavonoids found in cocoa not only improve bloodflow but also trigger a feel-good endorphin release that follows chocolate consumption, giving it the potential to light up the bedroom.
>>> *Dark chocolate recipes: pages 242, 262, 312, 320, 324, 328*

Best food to keep your joints greased: SPINACH

Vitamin E has been shown to reduce the pain in arthritic subjects, while the Boston University Medical Center found that those with the highest intakes of vitamin C were three times less likely to strain or injure joints than those with the lowest intakes. Spinach packs both C and E in abundance.
>>> *Spinach recipes: pages 68, 106, 240, 280, 295*

Best food to squash stress: STRAWBERRIES

Strawberries pack a ton of serotonin-inducing natural sugars, plus a single cup of the fruit boasts 160 percent of your day's vitamin C. A German study found that vitamin C helped clear out cortisol, the hormone responsible for stress-related symptoms like high blood pressure and hazy thinking.
>>> *Strawberry recipes: pages 56, 314, 328*

The Fat Scorecard

Rule number 1 (as well as rule numbers 2 through 78): Don't be afraid to use fat in your cooking.

Your body needs fat to perform metabolic functions that range from keeping brain cells firing (your gray matter is 70 percent fat) to healing scrapes to breaking down other nutrients. In fact, some of the healthiest foods we can eat—including omega-3 fatty acids (the stuff you get in fish oil tablets) and mono-unsaturated fatty acids (which come from avocados and walnuts and the like)—are out-and-out fats.

That's why we've created this scorecard, to lift the fog from the fats and help you decide which to use in your kitchen. For each fat we looked at the balance of omega-3s to omega-6 fatty acids—another kind of fat that's essential but that Americans eat too much of. (Omega-6s come from seeds and nuts, while 3s come from leaves.) We looked at the overall percentage of monounsatu-rated (good) fats. Then we considered whether a fat was high in saturated or—in the case of margarine—trans fat. What we came up with was a list of fats ranked from best to worst based on these criteria. The ones lightest in color should be the first ones you grab when preparing food at home, and the ones at the bottom should be pretty much banned from your kitchen. Get this down and you'll be set to lose weight and stay healthy while preparing restaurant-worthy meals in your own home.

Canola oil

Calories perTbsp: 124

Fat Stats:

Total Saturated: 7 percent	
Total Monounsaturated: 63 percent	
Total Polyunsaturated: 28 percent	
Omega-6 to Omega-3 Ratio: 2.5:1	

What You Need to Know: Canola tops our list with its near-perfect ratio of omega-6 to omega-3 fats. According to a study review published last year in *Experimental Biology and Medicine*, people who have lowered this ratio have been able to battle cancer, arthritis, and asthma more effectively. **When to Use:** Often. This is the best option for common cooking situations. Canola oil can withstand relatively high levels of heat, and its flavor is fairly neutral, so it won't dominate a dish.

Soybean oil

Calories perTbsp: 120

Fat Stats:

Total Saturated: 16 percent	
Total Monounsaturated: 23 percent	
Total Polyunsaturated: 58 percent	
Omega-6 to Omega-3 Ratio: 7.5:1	

What You Need to Know: Soybean oil is the invisible fat. It's the one you're eating when you don't have any clue what you're eating. The typical American eats 27.6 times more soy-bean oil than olive oil, and much of that comes from generic bottles labeled as "vegetable oil." It's the main reason why our omega-6 to omega-3 ratios are so out of whack. **When to Use:** Soybean oil is cheap and versatile (hence its ubiquity), but you're better off with canola or peanut oil.

Olive oil

Calories perTbsp: 119

Fat Stats:

Total Saturated: 14 percent	
Total Monounsaturated: 73 percent	
Total Polyunsaturated: 11 percent	
Omega-6 to Omega-3 Ratio: 13:1	

What You Need to Know: Olive oil is loaded with polyphenols, antioxidants that help battle many diseases such as cancer, osteoporosis, and brain deterioration. To get the full effect, though, you need to choose an oil of the extra-virgin variety; it has the highest polyphenol concentration.
When to Use: Expensive extra-virgin, with its robust flavor, should be saved to dress salads, vegetables, and cooked dishes. For cooking purposes, regular or light olive oil is sufficient.

Peanut oil

Calories perTbsp: 119

Fat Stats:

Total Saturated: 17 percent	
Total Monounsaturated: 46 percent	
Total Polyunsaturated: 32 percent	
Omega-6 to Omega-3 Ratio:	
not enough omega-3 to count	

What You Need to Know: Peanut oil is loaded with a monounsaturated fat called oleic acid (OEA). New research at the University of California, Irvine, has found that this particular fat functions to bolster memory; OEAs also appear to help reduce appetite to promote weight loss.
When to Use: Because of its high smoke point, peanut oil should be your go-to oil for frying and many high-heat tasks like wok-cooking stir-fries and pan-searing pieces of meat and fish.

Sesame oil

Calories perTbsp: 120

Fat Stats:

Total Saturated: 14 percent	
Total Monounsaturated: 40 percent	
Total Polyunsaturated: 42 percent	
Omega-6 to Omega-3 Ratio: 138:1	

What You Need to Know: Sesame oil comes stacked with sesamol. A study published in the academic journal *Pharmacological Research* showed that during a 20-week treatment, this potent antioxidant was able to reduce skin tumors on mice by 50 percent.
When to Use: There are two different varieties of sesame oil—a light cooking oil good for high-heat cooking and a dark oil made from toasted seeds that's best used like a condiment, added to sauces or drizzled over noodle dishes.

Lard

Calories perTbsp: 115

Fat Stats:

Total Saturated: 39 percent	
Total Monounsaturated: 45 percent	
Total Polyunsaturated: 11 percent	
Omega-6 to Omega-3 Ratio: 10:1	

What You Need to Know: Lard's gotten a bad rap. Not only does the pig blubber carry a third less saturated fat than butter, it also has as much oleic acid as peanut oil. Problem is most supermarket varieties are hydrogenated to increase shelf life, which means they're packing trans fat. But getting lard at home is easy—just save your bacon drippings.
When to Use: Many swear by lard for pie crusts and frying chicken. If you find a trans fat-free variety, use it sparingly.

Butter

Calories perTbsp: 102

Fat Stats:

Total Saturated: 63 percent	
Total Monounsaturated: 26 percent	
Total Polyunsaturated: 4 percent	
Omega-6 to Omega-3 Ratio: 8.7:1	

What You Need to Know: Butter is an excellent source of conjugated linoleic acid, which actually functions as a cancer-fighting mechanism in your body. That doesn't mean you want to move healthy oils out to make room for more butter, just realize modest use in the kitchen is totally acceptable.
When to Use: It's a logical choice for baked goods and adds a rich note to certain sautés and sauces. When it comes to buttering toast, whipped butter cuts your fat and calories in half.

Margarine

Calories perTbsp: 100

Fat Stats:

Total Saturated: 19 percent	
Total Trans: 18 percent	
Total Monounsaturated: 48 percent	
Total Polyunsaturated: 30 percent*	
Omega-6 to Omega-3 Ratio: 11.5:1	

What You Need to Know: To truly be considered margarine, sticks and tubs must contain at least 80 percent vegetable oil, and generally that oil is of the trans fatty, partially hydrogenated variety. If you really want to get away from butter, opt for a spread made with healthy fats. We like Smart Balance Buttery Spread with Flax Oil.
When to Use: Never use margarine that contains trans fat, but find a healthier version for occassional use.

*Numbers add up to more than 100 because the trans fats are also counted among the monounsaturated and polyunsaturated fats.

The Meat Scorecard

Mother Nature, ever one to go about following Her own whims without taking our needs into consideration, has yet to get hip to the nutritional program. Hence, until we can convince You-Know-Who to amend Her ways, cows, chickens, and pigs will continue to be born without nutrition labels.

Because there's no easy labeling on meat, no cartoon characters to sell us pigs and cows, most of us view the choice between, say, beef and pork loin as one that's as arbitrary as choosing between Aquafina and Dasani. Except that when it comes to choosing a protein source, there can be

a huge difference: Meat can be either a powerful weight-loss tool—or a truckload of tummy-maxing trouble.

On the plus side, between 10 percent and 30 percent of the calories you burn every day get burned by the simple act of eating and digesting your food. And your body uses almost twice as many calories digesting protein as it does fats and carbohydrates. (Pretty cool, huh? That's like making a third of your money by shopping.) Plus, meats have wildly different amounts of various nutrients—minerals like zinc and iron and a range of B vitamins.

On the negative side, meat can carry a lot of fat—some of it healthy fat and some of it not so healthy. But how can you tell which cut of which animal is going to boost your muscles and help strip away fat, and which will just bloat your middle like a snake that swallowed an ostrich egg?

To help you differentiate one choice of meat from another,

we've created a protein scoring system that takes into account all the relevant nutritional considerations. We began by looking at the ratio of protein to fat. (Because meat is comprised entirely of these two macronutrients, finding a high protein-to-fat ratio is essential to the character of the cut.) Next we factored in the density of 10 essential micronutrients. Finally, we rounded out our analysis with saturated fat and cholesterol levels. What you get is a scorecard that removes the mystery from the meat by letting you pit pork chops against ground beef and T-bones against dark meat turkey.

Oh, and one more note: Whenever possible, look for free-range or grass-fed versions of your favorite meats. They may cost a bit more, but you'll find not only a richer flavor but also a higher protein-to-fat ratio, more micronutrients, and no residual hormones and antibiotics. And, hey, it's still cheaper than restaurant food!

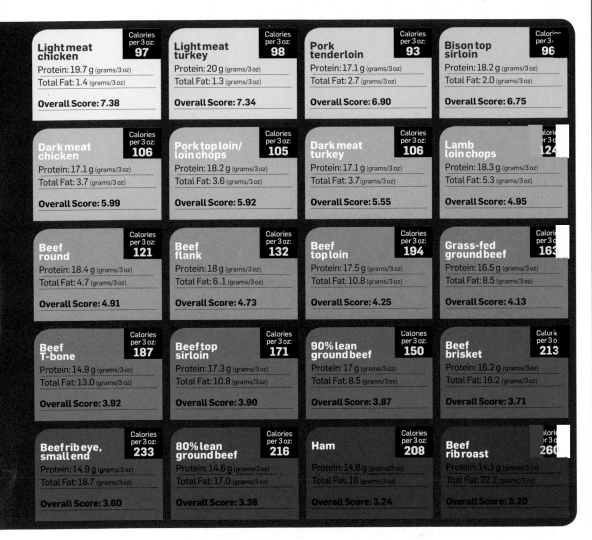

Light meat chicken
Calories per 3 oz: 97
Protein: 19.7 g (grams/3 oz)
Total Fat: 1.4 (grams/3 oz)
Overall Score: 7.38

Light meat turkey
Calories per 3 oz: 98
Protein: 20 g (grams/3 oz)
Total Fat: 1.3 (grams/3 oz)
Overall Score: 7.34

Pork tenderloin
Calories per 3 oz: 93
Protein: 17.1 g (grams/3 oz)
Total Fat: 2.7 (grams/3 oz)
Overall Score: 6.90

Bison top sirloin
Calories per 3 oz: 96
Protein: 18.2 g (grams/3 oz)
Total Fat: 2.0 (grams/3 oz)
Overall Score: 6.75

Dark meat chicken
Calories per 3 oz: 106
Protein: 17.1 g (grams/3 oz)
Total Fat: 3.7 (grams/3 oz)
Overall Score: 5.99

Pork top loin/loin chops
Calories per 3 oz: 105
Protein: 18.2 g (grams/3 oz)
Total Fat: 3.6 (grams/3 oz)
Overall Score: 5.92

Dark meat turkey
Calories per 3 oz: 106
Protein: 17.1 g (grams/3 oz)
Total Fat: 3.7 (grams/3 oz)
Overall Score: 5.55

Lamb loin chops
Calories per 3 oz: 124
Protein: 18.3 g (grams/3 oz)
Total Fat: 5.3 (grams/3 oz)
Overall Score: 4.95

Beef round
Calories per 3 oz: 121
Protein: 18.4 g (grams/3 oz)
Total Fat: 4.7 (grams/3 oz)
Overall Score: 4.91

Beef flank
Calories per 3 oz: 132
Protein: 18 g (grams/3 oz)
Total Fat: 6.1 (grams/3 oz)
Overall Score: 4.73

Beef top loin
Calories per 3 oz: 194
Protein: 17.5 g (grams/3 oz)
Total Fat: 10.8 (grams/3 oz)
Overall Score: 4.25

Grass-fed ground beef
Calories per 3 oz: 163
Protein: 16.5 g (grams/3 oz)
Total Fat: 8.5 (grams/3 oz)
Overall Score: 4.13

Beef T-bone
Calories per 3 oz: 187
Protein: 14.9 g (grams/3 oz)
Total Fat: 13.0 (grams/3 oz)
Overall Score: 3.92

Beef top sirloin
Calories per 3 oz: 171
Protein: 17.3 g (grams/3 oz)
Total Fat: 10.8 (grams/3 oz)
Overall Score: 3.90

90% lean ground beef
Calories per 3 oz: 150
Protein: 17 g (grams/3 oz)
Total Fat: 8.5 (grams/3 oz)
Overall Score: 3.87

Beef brisket
Calories per 3 oz: 213
Protein: 16.2 g (grams/3 oz)
Total Fat: 16.2 (grams/3 oz)
Overall Score: 3.71

Beef rib eye, small end
Calories per 3 oz: 233
Protein: 14.9 g (grams/3 oz)
Total Fat: 18.7 (grams/3 oz)
Overall Score: 3.60

80% lean ground beef
Calories per 3 oz: 216
Protein: 14.6 g (grams/3 oz)
Total Fat: 17.0 (grams/3 oz)
Overall Score: 3.38

Ham
Calories per 3 oz: 208
Protein: 14.8 g (grams/3 oz)
Total Fat: 16 (grams/3 oz)
Overall Score: 3.24

Beef rib roast
Calories per 3 oz: 260
Protein: 14.1 g (grams/3 oz)
Total Fat: 22.2 (grams/3 oz)
Overall Score: 3.20

The Carb Scorecard

Despite the rampant carb-mongering that still exists in nutritional circles, carbohydrates should account for up to 45 percent of calories in a healthy diet. The trick is to be sure that you're getting the bulk of yours from quality sources—something the carb-fearing cabal tends to ignore.

That's where the Carb Scorecard comes in. Think you know barley from bulgur? Or pasta from rice, for that matter? By considering four parameters, we've ranked 10 common carbs from best to worst.

The first and most important parameter in our scoring system is fiber. (Americans are eating only about 14 of the 25 daily grams they need to be healthy.) Then we added and subtracted points for protein-based calories and sugar-based calories, respectively. Finally, we factored in the concentration of a dozen nutrients, among which are iron, magnesium, selenium, and a bundle of B vitamins.

Bulgur

Calories per cup: 151

Carb Stats:
Fiber: 8 g
Protein: 5.5 g

What You Need to Know: Want to incorporate whole wheat into your home cooking? Bulgur's your solution. It's one of the most-fibrous pantry stuffers you can find, and because it has been parboiled before packaging, it cooks in no time.
How to Use: Perfect for putting together nutritious side dishes on the fly. To make a simple tabbouleh—a staple in Mediterranean cooking—simply combine the bulgur with lots of chopped parsley, garlic, diced tomatoes, olive oil, and lemon juice.

Quinoa

Calories per cup: 222

Carb Stats:
Fiber: 5 g
Protein: 8 g

What You Need to Know: This South American grain is loaded with protein, and unlike the protein in wheat, quinoa contains all the amino acids that your body needs to function. That puts this protein on par with the stuff you'd find in eggs, milk, and beef. What's more, quinoa is more nutritionally stacked than any other whole grain on this list.
How to Use: Quinoa cooks like rice and makes an excellent substitute for more common—but less nutritional—grains. Try using it as a bed for grilled chicken or fish, tossing with roasted vegetables for a simple salad, or stir in raisins, brown sugar, and milk for breakfast.

Enriched pasta

Calories per cup: 221

Carb Stats:
Fiber: 2.5 g
Protein: 8 g

What You Need to Know: Of all the refined grain products in your pantry, pasta is the least threatening. The reason? Unlike white bread, which is almost completely devoid of fiber, white pasta is generally prepared with at least a couple of grams still intact. Factor in the slurry of vitamins that get added during the enrichment process and you have a carb source that's not all bad, but calorie-dense nonetheless.
How to Use: Switching to whole-wheat noodles will more than double your fiber load and boost your protein intake. Ronzini Smart Taste and Barilla Plus are both fantastic options.

Brown rice

Calories per cup: 216

Carb Stats:
Fiber: 3.5 g
Protein: 5 g

What You Need to Know: In the competition of grains, rice emerges as one of the weaker options, but it's not a total loser. Not only does the unrefined grain deliver reliable doses of both fiber and protein, but it also carries a healthy spread of nutrients that includes more than a quarter of your day's selenium, an antioxidant that has been shown to hinder the proliferation of cancer cells.
How to Use: Rice's popularity stems in large part from its versatility. Use it as a base for curries and stir-fries; stir it into soups; or wrap it with beans and cheese inside a whole-wheat tortilla for a fiber-loaded burrito.

Oatmeal

Calories per cup: **166**

Carb Stats:
Fiber: 4 g
Protein: 6 g

What You Need to Know: A unique blend of nutrients makes oats one of the heart-healthiest foods in your kitchen. The collaborative efforts of beta-glucan, a powerful class of fibers, and avenanthramide, an antioxidant unique to oats, fuel the cereal grain's winning battle against LDL cholesterol. And get this: A study of satiety published in the *New England Journal of Medicine* showed that oatmeal more than doubled the stomach-filling potential of white bread.
How to Use: Sure oatmeal is great on its own, but also try stirring rolled oats into pancake and muffin recipes.

Whole-wheat bread

Calories per 2 large slices (85g): **210**

Carb Stats:
Fiber: 6 g
Protein: 11 g

What You Need to Know: In theory, wheat bread should always have more fiber and nutrients than white bread, but that's not always the case. In fact, some wheat breads are made with the same refined flour; they're just colored with molasses to make them appear heartier. Look for loaves that say "100 percent whole wheat" on the package, and to be sure, flip them over and look at the ingredient statement. Is the first ingredient whole wheat? Bingo.
How to Use: Develop a taste for the robust flavor of wheat and you'll never go back to white. Also try to sneak in whole wheat buns for burgers and dogs.

Pearled barley

Calories per cup: **193**

Carb Stats:
Fiber: 6 g
Protein: 3.5 g

What You Need to Know: Although ranked fifth on our list, barley is still one of the healthiest grains. What it lacks in protein it makes up for in cholesterol-lowering beta-glucan, the same fiber that allows oatmeal to carry an FDA-approved heart healthy seal. Researchers in Australia recently found that barley could help lower LDL cholesterol levels.
How to Use: Barley takes about an hour to cook, so make a big batch and use throughout the week. Try it with berries and warm milk in the morning, stirred into winter soups, or as a vegetable-strewn pilaf for dinner.

Couscous

Calories per cup: **176**

Carb Stats:
Fiber: 2 g
Protein: 6 g

What You Need to Know: Couscous is nothing more than wheat fashioned into tiny pasta granules. Problem is, few couscous manufacturers add back the nutrients they strip out. That means the extra boost of iron and B vitamins that you expect to find in pasta is all but absent. Here's some advice: If you like the consistency of couscous, try replacing it with quinoa. Similar shape and size, but the quinoa will earn you extra nutrients and more than twice the amount of fiber.
How to Use: Opt for whole-wheat couscous and lace it with toasted pine nuts, golden raisins, and cilantro.

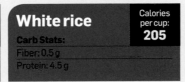

White rice

Calories per cup: **205**

Carb Stats:
Fiber: 0.5 g
Protein: 4.5 g

What You Need to Know: White rice, like most refined grains in America, must have certain missing nutrients stuffed back into it before it's sold to consumers. The problem is that what goes back in represents a mere drop in the bucket compared with what's taken out. Compared with brown, white rice has drastically lower concentrations of magnesium, potassium, copper, and selenium, to name a few. Furthermore, the grain is pathetically devoid of fiber.
How to Use: If ever you choose white over brown rice, make sure you boost your plate with other sources of fiber and vitamins—namely, vegetables.

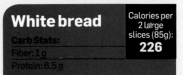

White bread

Calories per 2 large slices (85g): **226**

Carb Stats:
Fiber: 1 g
Protein: 6.5 g

What You Need to Know: Generally speaking, you want to avoid white foods. Cauliflower is an exception, but white bread certainly is not. To strip it of its natural earth tone, manufacturers remove about 40 percent of the grain, and in the process they eliminate a load of healthy fats, vitamin E, and fiber. So not only are you losing essential nutrients, but you're also digesting your food faster. That means your blood sugar rises higher, your mood shifts easier, and your stomach gets empty quicker.
How to Use: Sparingly.

The Dairy Scorecard

Milk is the most versatile food in the world, no doubt about it. It arrives fresh from the cow as a homogenous white liquid but quickly becomes separated into any number of yogurts, cheeses, and spreads. Some of the fat becomes butter; some becomes cream. It's frozen into ice cream or allowed to curdle into cottage cheese, the protein extracted for use as a supplement. It's like *Night of the Living Dead,* except instead of zombies, we have dairy farmers, walking around with jugs of lactose and milk fat. Okay, maybe it's not that severe, but with the prevalence

of diary in our diets, it's best to know the good from the evil.

To help clue you in, we've devised a scoring system that allows you to easily see the relative nutritional content of 13 common dairy foods. In it we consider five variables. The top two, protein and fat, were the most heavily weighted. Dairy protein is loaded with amino acids, putting it among the best protein sources in the food supply. Dairy fat, on the other hand, is highly saturated, so it's best in moderation.

Next we considered nutrient density. Some dairy products, like yogurt and cheese, carry heavier loads of calcium and B_{12} than others, such as butter and cream, so they were rewarded accordingly. Finally, we docked points for two naturally occurring nutrients, sodium and sugar. The result is a totem pole of dairy products. The ones darkest in color should be relegated to a tiny role in your diet, but the lightly colored ones are all-star health foods.

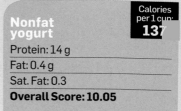

Nonfat yogurt

Calories per 1 cup: 137

Protein: 14 g
Fat: 0.4 g
Sat. Fat: 0.3
Overall Score: 10.05

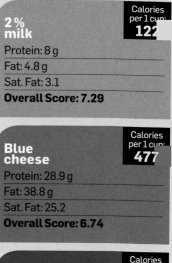

2% milk

Calories per 1 cup: 122

Protein: 8 g
Fat: 4.8 g
Sat. Fat: 3.1
Overall Score: 7.29

Blue cheese

Calories per 1 cup: 477

Protein: 28.9 g
Fat: 38.8 g
Sat. Fat: 25.2
Overall Score: 6.74

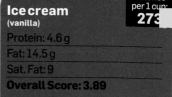

Ice cream
(vanilla)

Calories per 1 cup: 273

Protein: 4.6 g
Fat: 14.5 g
Sat. Fat: 9
Overall Score: 3.89

2% cottage cheese
Calories per 1 cup: 194
Protein: 26.74 g
Fat: 5.5 g
Sat. Fat: 2.2
Overall Score: 9.55

Fat-free milk
Calories per 1 cup: 83
Protein: 8.3 g
Fat: 0.2 g
Sat. Fat: 0.1
Overall Score: 9.45

Low fat 1% milk
Calories per 1 cup: 102
Protein: 8.2 g
Fat: 2.4 g
Sat. Fat: 1.5
Overall Score: 8.22

Whole yogurt
Calories per 1 cup: 149
Protein: 8.5 g
Fat: 8 g
Sat. Fat: 5.1
Overall Score: 6.93

Swiss cheese
Calories per 1 cup: 410
Protein: 29.1 g
Fat: 30 g
Sat. Fat: 19.2
Overall Score: 6.83

Whole milk mozzarella cheese (shredded)
Calories per 1 cup: 336
Protein: 24.8 g
Fat: 25 g
Sat. Fat: 14.7
Overall Score: 6.79

Whole milk
Calories per 1 cup: 149
Protein: 7.7 g
Fat: 8 g
Sat. Fat: 4.6
Overall Score: 6.46

Cheddar cheese (shredded)
Calories per 1 cup: 455
Protein: 28.1 g
Fat: 37.5 g
Sat. Fat: 23.8
Overall Score: 6.16

Half-and-half
Calories per 1 cup: 315
Protein: 7.2 g
Fat: 27.8 g
Sat. Fat: 17.3
Overall Score: 4.43

Sour cream
Calories per 1 cup: 444
Protein: 4.8 g
Fat: 45.4 g
Sat. Fat: 26.4
Overall Score: 3.39

Cream
Calories per 1 cup: 414
Protein: 2.5 g
Fat: 44.4 g
Sat. Fat: 27.6
Overall Score: 1.44

Butter, unsalted
Calories per 1 cup: 1,628
Protein: 1.93 g
Fat: 184 g
Sat. Fat: 116.6
Overall Score: 1.33

Nutrition Nuggets

America has more obese people than overweight people.

1 medium carrot has 340 percent of your daily vitamin A. Wheat flour has 470 percent more fiber than white flour.

45

Percent of people who eat fewer than five home-cooked dinners per week. Seventeen percent don't even eat three.

Almond butter has 79 percent more heart-healthy monounsaturated fats than peanut butter. (It also has close to half as many saturated fats.)

An 8-ounce cup of 2 percent milk has 40 more calories than an 8-ounce cup of fat-free milk.

The number of obese children has tripled since 1980.

Although it has just as much sodium as table salt, sea salt does not contain iodine, an essential mineral that your body needs for metabolic and thyroid functions.

Men
who moderately drink alcohol 3 to 7 days a week are at a 32 percent lower risk of heart attack than men who drink less than once a week.

Frozen peas have up to 4 times as much vitamin C as canned peas.

Organic wine averages a third more antioxidants than conventional wine.

A typical serving of potatoes has nearly 5 times as many antioxidants as a typical serving of broccoli.

Your blood sugar rises 39 percent less if you toast your white bread.

Women
who take a forward-thinking approach to food and cooking (that means they try new recipes, plan meals, and shop with a list) have a higher intake of vegetables.

Frozen produce often has higher nutrient density than fresh. But a study in the *Journal of the Science of Food and Agriculture* found that for some vegetables canning degraded as much as 95 percent of the vitamin C and damaged every B vitamin in the food.

People who eat more than two servings of vegetables a day have a 40 percent slower rate of cognitive decline than those who eat one serving or less.

The average veggie burger contains five times the sodium of the average beef burger.

In an 11-year Japanese study, those who drank the most green tea were less likely to die of any cause throughout the course of the study.

Overweight people who weigh themselves at least once a week are 6 times more likely to lose weight.

A third of adolescents eat two or fewer family meals per week.

Wild blueberries have 50 percent more antioxidants than cultivated blueberries.

If you shop at a farmers' market, you're 3.2 times more likely to eat 5 servings of fruits and vegetables a day than if you shop at a supermarket.

Grass-fed beef has up to three times more conjugated linoleic acid, a unique beef-based fat that fights cancer and promotes weight loss.

Drinking 3 glasses of red wine a week decreases your risk of colon cancer by 68 percent.

A cup of store-brand bran flakes cereal has more than twice as much fiber as a cup of Cheerios.

Tuna accounts for 39 percent of the mercury in the US diet. Choosing light over albacore can cut your methylmercury risk by two-thirds.

89 percent of foods marketed to kids provide poor nutrition.

Adding blueberries instead of strawberries to your cereal will more than double your antioxidant intake.

People who eat with napkins in their laps tend to have lower body mass indexes.

Cut out 96 calories from your daily diet and you'll be 10 pounds lighter one year from today.

Compared to iceberg, romaine lettuce has more of just about every nutrient, including 8.5 times more vitamin C.

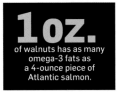
1oz. of walnuts has as many omega-3 fats as a 4-ounce piece of Atlantic salmon.

Compared with an 8-ounce glass of orange juice, a single medium orange has half as much sugar and 3 more grams of fiber.

Coffee is by far the richest source of antioxidants in the American diet. (Cream and sugar turns a 10-calorie cup of coffee into an 80-calorie cup. Do that once a day and gain 7 pounds in a year.)

Chapter

2

Cook This, Not That!

The Eat This, Not That! Kitchen

Cooking first-rate food requires nothing more than a few good staples and a handful of tools.

We know this guy (for the sake of not embarassing him, let's call him Cornelius) who loves food. Cornelius subscribes to all the big cooking magazines and religiously follows every food blog on the ol' interweb. His kitchen could be a showroom for the world's finest cookware and appliance purveyors: Thousands of dollars' worth of gleeming copper pots and pans hang above his Viking range and his knife collection looks like it belongs to John Rambo. His counter is lined with a dozen fancy olive oils and salts and his fridge houses half the cheeses of France. One time we asked Cornelius if he'd mind cooking dinner and he looked at us with a blank stare: "Mind if we order out?"

Getting Back to Basics

When it comes to cooking and eating great, healthy food, you don't need a whole lot: a few sturdy pots and pans and a handful of reliable kitchen staples. You can spend all the cash you want on outfitting your kitchen with the finest equipment and fanciest ingredients known to man, but meals don't cook themselves.

We're all about honest, simple food. And we're not afraid to use the real ingredients delicious food demands. You won't find a lot of light mayonnaise, Splenda, and fat-free half-and-half (really, Land O'Lakes?) in the ingredient lists. You won't find a lot of sneaky tricks like folding pureed broccoli into your brownies, using Fiber One cereal as breading, or replacing butter with applesauce in the chocolate cookies. ("You can't taste the difference!" Yeah, right.) You won't even find a lot of recipes that don't have cheese, butter, or oil of some kind.

What you will find are recipes created with approachable, affordable ingredients combined in a smart, straightforward way. You'll recognize every last piece of food that these recipes call for as being just

that: food, not some crazy science experiment created in a lab. (Fat-free half-and-half, by the way, contains 10 ingredients.) The portion sizes are perfect, which is to say, substantial enough to satisfy a hearty appetite, but modest enough to stave off the food comas that typically accompany dining-out misadventures. You will find some cool tips and tricks on every page but never at the expense of delicious food.

Just remember: These aren't diet recipes, but they are recipes that will help you lose weight if you commit to cooking them a few times or more a week. Case in point: As we committed ourselves to the kitchen to produce this book, we tested up to 10 recipes a day, which meant eating our way through dish after dish in the name of scrupulous culinary research. (Plus, we wouldn't want to waste food, would we?) After 6 weeks of what felt like over-the-top indulgence, we expected to blow up like beach balls on a hot August afternoon. Between the two of us, we lost 2 pounds. Not a lot, but that happened eating seven or more meals a day. Imagine if you eat just three?

The $331 Kitchen

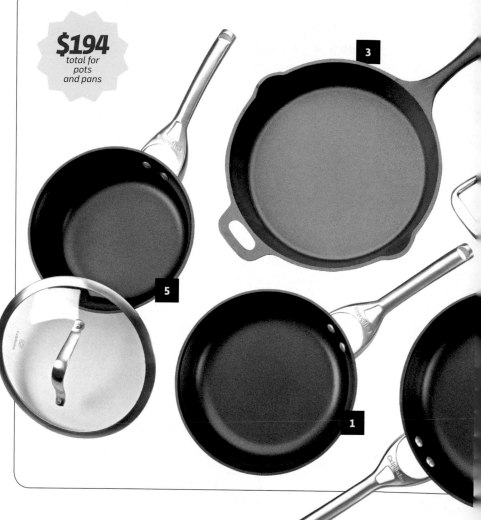

$194
total for pots and pans

Saunter down to Williams-Sonoma and pick up a 15-piece All-Clad stainless steel cookware set and you'll drop $1,100. Tack on a set of Henckels knives, a 15-piece tool set, and a few gadgets and you're out over 2 grand before you chop the first onion. Truth is, you need only a few all-purpose pots, pans, and tools to turn out four-star food from your kitchen every night, and quality and price don't always correlate in the kitchen. We've highlighted the essentials and our favorite affordable picks in each category. All told, we'll have your kitchen fully outfitted for less than the cost of a fancy meal out.

Nonstick skillets 1 2

Calphalon Contemporary Nonstick 10" and 12" Omelette Pans ($50)

In his memoir, *Kitchen Confidential*, Anthony Bourdain detailed the most important test of all when choosing a good pan: Imagine cracking someone's head with the pan, he says. "If you have any doubts about which will dent—the victim's head or your pan—then throw that pan right in the trash." Not only would these skillets crack a hard skull, the slick, durable nonstick coating will last for years. Retail price is $135 if sold separately, but at Bed, Bath & Beyond, you'll find these two sold together for a quarter of the price of a single All-Clad nonstick skillet.
Best for: Scrambles, omelets, sautéed vegetables, and fish

Cast-iron skillet 3

Lodge Logic 12" Skillet ($34)

It's what our moms used, and our moms' moms, and their moms' moms... After all these years, a better cooking implement simply does not exist. Cast iron holds heat extremely well, making it perfect for developing the type of crust on a thick steak or burger that only a grill could match. A seasoned skillet develops a natural nonstick layer, making it adept at more delicate tasks, too, like frying eggs, cooking fish, and sautéeing vegetables. Lodge has been in the cast-iron game since 1896 and still makes one of the finest skillets you'll ever lay a spatula on.
Best for: Seared steak, burgers, blackened fish, pan-frying

Stockpot 4

Cuisinart Chef's Classic Stainless 12-Quart Stock Pot ($70)

The most expensive stockpots can cost up to $300 or more, but you'll never get your money's worth out of them—after all, that's more than this entire page of cookware for a pot used primarily to boil water. Cuisinart and Calphalon both make excellent cookware for a fraction of the price of the top-tier producers. This pot looks and cooks just like its pricier cousins.
Best for: Soups, stews, homemade stock, mashed potatoes, blanching vegetables, boiling pasta

Medium saucepan 5

Calphalon Contemporary Nonstick 2½-Quart Shallow Saucepan with Cover ($40)

Fancy stainless steel and copper sauciers are worth the money if you spend 8 hours a day in the kitchen. For the rest of us, this sturdy saucepan holds and distributes heat well enough for delicate and aggressive tasks alike.
Best for: Simmering sauces, cooking grains, reheating leftovers

(continued on next page)

The $331 Kitchen

1

Cutting board
1

Oxo Good Grips 21" x 14½" Carving and Cutting Board ($22)

If you have the cash, go ahead and buy a thick, heavyset wooden cutting board for most of your major chopping, slicing, and dicing. But if you want an affordable, all-purpose board, this is it. The polypropylene material is nonporous (preventing bacteria buildup) and won't dull your knives. Plus the surface area is large enough to tackle a few jobs at once. Save one side for produce and herbs and the other for raw meat.

Chef's knife
2

Victorinox Forschner 8" ($30)

While the market for hand-forged $300 Japanese and German chef's knives continues to spiral out of control, the best knife out there may just be this humble blade. Made by the same fine people who brought you the Swiss Army knife, this one blade can handle 90 percent of your cutting. *Cook's Illustrated*, the master of in-depth product tests, has awarded this knife their top seal of approval year after year.
Best for: Most big cutting jobs, including chopping vegetables, meat, and herbs

Serrated knife
3

Victorinox Forschner 10¼" Bread Knife ($27)

It's always good to have one blade on hand that can cut through everything. This is that blade.
Best for: Slicing bread, tomatoes, citrus fruit, and sandwiches

Paring knife
4

Victorinox Forschner 4" Paring Knife ($13)

Whether you're cutting that last piece of meat off the bone or putting a fine mince on that garlic clove, some tasks require a bit of finesse. For those moments, this inexpensive but effective piece of steel is all you need.
Best for: Peeling potatoes and apples, coring tomatoes, and other finer cutting tasks

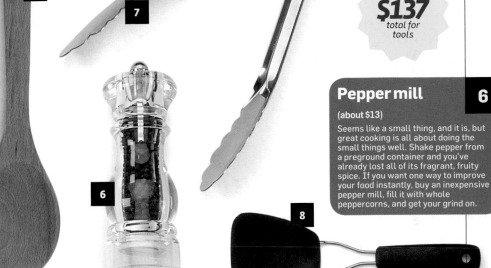

$137
total for
tools

Pepper mill   6

(about $13)

Seems like a small thing, and it is, but great cooking is all about doing the small things well. Shake pepper from a preground container and you've already lost all of its fragrant, fruity spice. If you want one way to improve your food instantly, buy an inexpensive pepper mill, fill it with whole peppercorns, and get your grind on.

Grater   5

Microplane Classic Series Grater/Zester ($13)

Never buy cooking tools that do just one job (we're looking at you, cherry pitter). The Microplane uses hundreds of tiny teeth to make quick work of hard cheese like Parmesan, citrus zest, and whole spices like nutmeg.

Kitchen utensils   7   8   9

Forget the space-wasting, cash-burning 15-piece kitchen tool sets. These are the only three utensils you need.

7. Oneida Stainless Steel Locking 9½" Tongs ($6):
Tongs are the perfect all-purpose kitchen tool, equally adept at turning meat on a grill as they are plucking pasta strings from boiling water to taste for doneness.

8. Oxo Good Grips Nylon Flexible Turner ($7):
One thing tongs are lousy for: handling delicate foods like fish. For that, Oxo's turners are ideal—especially since they won't scratch your nonstick pans.

9. Oxo Good Grips Large Wooden Spoon ($6):
Great for stirring sauces, wok maneuvering, whipping milk and butter into mashed potatoes, and sneaking chili tastes when no one is looking.

The Perfect Pantry

In the real world, not everything can be made from scratch, and having the best packaged building blocks is essential for top-notch healthy cooking. Use these 19 classic kitchen swaps to cut calories and boost flavor.

MAYONNAISE

Eat This

**Kraft Mayo
with Olive Oil
(1 Tbsp)**
*45 calories
4 g fat (0 g saturated)
95 mg sodium*

Not That!

**Hellmann's
Real Mayonnaise
(1 Tbsp)**
*90 calories
10 g fat (1.5 g saturated)
90 mg sodium*

Why settle for low-grade soybean oil mayo when you can get one made with heart-healthy olive oil for about the same price? What we really love is that Kraft caps the calories at half the amount found in regular mayo. More flavor, fewer calories: What's not to love?

CHILI SAUCE

Eat This

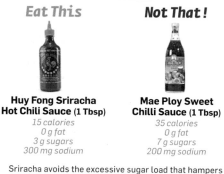

**Huy Fong Sriracha
Hot Chili Sauce (1 Tbsp)**
*15 calories
0 g fat
3 g sugars
300 mg sodium*

Not That!

**Mae Ploy Sweet
Chilli Sauce (1 Tbsp)**
*35 calories
0 g fat
7 g sugars
200 mg sodium*

Sriracha avoids the excessive sugar load that hampers many Asian condiments. The Thai-inspired sauce focuses on a potent blend of chiles, garlic, and vinegar, flavor boosters that are all healthy in their own right, and when combined, comprise one of our favorite condiments.

BARBECUE SAUCE

Eat This

**Stubb's Bar-B-Q Sauce
(2 Tbsp)**
*30 calories
0 g fat
4 g sugars
220 mg sodium*

Not That!

**KC Masterpiece
Original (2 Tbsp)**
*60 calories
0 g fat
12 g sugars
240 mg sodium*

Most popular barbecue sauces carry nearly as much sugar as the sticky goo you pour over your pancakes. Stubb's is a welcome exception, with an impressive line of sauces and marinades that contain less sodium and sugar than any of the other big players in the barbecue aisle.

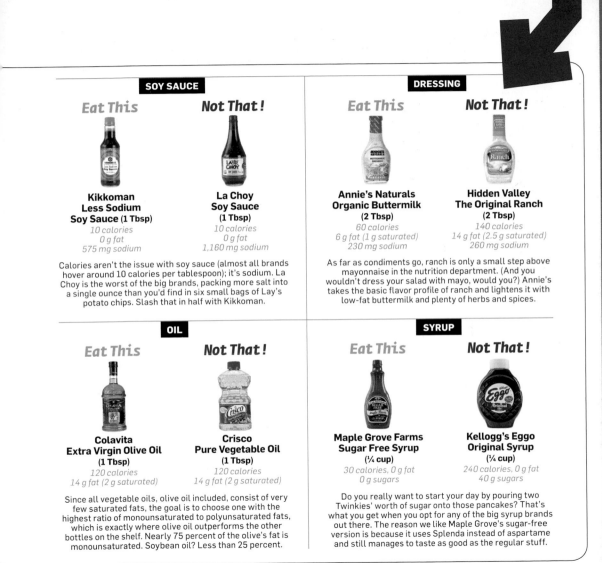

SOY SAUCE

Eat This

**Kikkoman
Less Sodium
Soy Sauce (1 Tbsp)**
10 calories
0 g fat
575 mg sodium

Not That!

**La Choy
Soy Sauce
(1 Tbsp)**
10 calories
0 g fat
1,160 mg sodium

Calories aren't the issue with soy sauce (almost all brands hover around 10 calories per tablespoon); it's sodium. La Choy is the worst of the big brands, packing more salt into a single ounce than you'd find in six small bags of Lay's potato chips. Slash that in half with Kikkoman.

DRESSING

Eat This

**Annie's Naturals
Organic Buttermilk
(2 Tbsp)**
60 calories
6 g fat (1 g saturated)
230 mg sodium

Not That!

**Hidden Valley
The Original Ranch
(2 Tbsp)**
140 calories
14 g fat (2.5 g saturated)
260 mg sodium

As far as condiments go, ranch is only a small step above mayonnaise in the nutrition department. (And you wouldn't dress your salad with mayo, would you?) Annie's takes the basic flavor profile of ranch and lightens it with low-fat buttermilk and plenty of herbs and spices.

OIL

Eat This

**Colavita
Extra Virgin Olive Oil
(1 Tbsp)**
120 calories
14 g fat (2 g saturated)

Not That!

**Crisco
Pure Vegetable Oil
(1 Tbsp)**
120 calories
14 g fat (2 g saturated)

Since all vegetable oils, olive oil included, consist of very few saturated fats, the goal is to choose one with the highest ratio of monounsaturated to polyunsaturated fats, which is exactly where olive oil outperforms the other bottles on the shelf. Nearly 75 percent of the olive's fat is monounsaturated. Soybean oil? Less than 25 percent.

SYRUP

Eat This

**Maple Grove Farms
Sugar Free Syrup
(¼ cup)**
30 calories, 0 g fat
0 g sugars

Not That!

**Kellogg's Eggo
Original Syrup
(¼ cup)**
240 calories, 0 g fat
40 g sugars

Do you really want to start your day by pouring two Twinkies' worth of sugar onto those pancakes? That's what you get when you opt for any of the big syrup brands out there. The reason we like Maple Grove's sugar-free version is because it uses Splenda instead of aspartame and still manages to taste as good as the regular stuff.

(continued on next page)

The Perfect Pantry

BUTTER

Eat This

Land O'Lakes Whipped Butter, unsalted (1 Tbsp)
50 calories
6 g fat (3.5 g saturated)
0 mg sodium

Not That!

Imperial Vegetable Oil Spread (1 Tbsp)
80 calories
8 g fat
(1.5 g saturated, 2 g trans)
105 mg sodium

Nearly every stick margarine in America packs more trans fat in a single tablespoon than you should consume in a full day. Enjoy real butter instead, but opt for the less-dense whipped variety to diffuse the calories.

YOGURT

Eat This

Fage Total 2% Greek Style (6 oz)
90 calories
0 g fat
7 g sugars

Not That!

Yoplait Original 99% Fat Free Strawberry (6 oz)
170 calories
1.5 g fat (1 g saturated)
27 g sugars

Greek yogurt is an *Eat This, Not That!* hall of famer. That's because compared with the regular stuff, it's creamier, it's tastier, and it packs in three times as much protein. Ignore the bells and whistles of fat-free labeling; this Yoplait cup packs nearly as much sugar as a Snickers bar.

ALL-PURPOSE CHEESE

Eat This

Kraft Low-Moisture Part-Skim Mozzarella (¼ cup)
80 calories
6 g fat (3.5 g saturated)
200 mg sodium

Not That!

Kraft Shredded Sharp Cheddar (¼ cup)
110 calories
9 g fat (6 g saturated)
170 mg sodium

Nobody should be deprived of the occasional cheese fix. The key is finding the best possible all-purpose player to keep in the fridge for when the queso-craving is calling. Part-skim mozz is the best candidate for the position, easily beating out Cheddar, Jack, and provolone.

PASTA NOODLE

Eat This

Ronzoni Smart Taste Penne Rigate (56 g)
180 calories
1 g fat (0 g saturated)
6 g fiber

Not That!

Barilla Penne (56 g)
200 calories
1 g fat (0 g saturated)
2 g fiber

Ronzoni's Smart Taste line consists of refined flour fortified with enough fiber to put it on par with the most robust of whole-wheat noodles. It also has as much bone-building calcium as an 8-ounce glass of milk. But here's what makes it the best option at the supermarket: You won't be able to tell them apart from normal noodles.

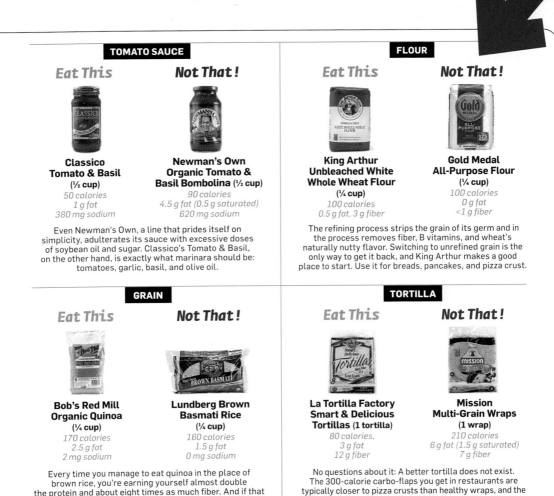

TOMATO SAUCE

Eat This

Classico Tomato & Basil
(½ cup)
50 calories
1 g fat
380 mg sodium

Not That!

Newman's Own Organic Tomato & Basil Bombolina (½ cup)
90 calories
4.5 g fat (0.5 g saturated)
620 mg sodium

Even Newman's Own, a line that prides itself on simplicity, adulterates its sauce with excessive doses of soybean oil and sugar. Classico's Tomato & Basil, on the other hand, is exactly what marinara should be: tomatoes, garlic, basil, and olive oil.

FLOUR

Eat This

King Arthur Unbleached White Whole Wheat Flour
(¼ cup)
100 calories
0.5 g fat, 3 g fiber

Not That!

Gold Medal All-Purpose Flour
(¼ cup)
100 calories
0 g fat
<1 g fiber

The refining process strips the grain of its germ and in the process removes fiber, B vitamins, and wheat's naturally nutty flavor. Switching to unrefined grain is the only way to get it back, and King Arthur makes a good place to start. Use it for breads, pancakes, and pizza crust.

GRAIN

Eat This

Bob's Red Mill Organic Quinoa
(¼ cup)
170 calories
2.5 g fat
2 mg sodium

Not That!

Lundberg Brown Basmati Rice
(¼ cup)
160 calories
1.5 g fat
0 mg sodium

Every time you manage to eat quinoa in the place of brown rice, you're earning yourself almost double the protein and about eight times as much fiber. And if that doesn't do it for you, consider that this wonder grain also delivers more flavor and cooks about twice as fast.

TORTILLA

Eat This

La Tortilla Factory Smart & Delicious Tortillas (1 tortilla)
80 calories,
3 g fat
12 g fiber

Not That!

Mission Multi-Grain Wraps
(1 wrap)
210 calories
6 g fat (1.5 g saturated)
7 g fiber

No questions about it: A better tortilla does not exist. The 300-calorie carbo-flaps you get in restaurants are typically closer to pizza crusts than healthy wraps, and the best from the ubiquitous Mission line isn't much better. Make La Tortilla your go-to for all wrap and burrito uses.

(continued on next page)

The Perfect Pantry

BREAD

Eat This

Martin's 100% Whole Wheat Potato Bread
(2 slices)
140 calories
2 g fat (0 g saturated)
8 g fiber

Not That!

Arnold Natural Health Nut
(2 slices)
200 calories
4 g fat (0 g saturated)
6 g fiber

The Health Nut loaf carries a full 100 calories per slice, yet has less fiber than some of its more moderately size counterparts. Your strategy in the bread aisle is to seek out slices with the best ratio of fiber to calories. Martin's has that, plus 12 grams of protein in every two slices.

DELI MEAT

Eat This

Hormel Natural Choice Smoked Deli Turkey
(2 oz)
50 calories
1 g fat
450 mg sodium

Not That!

Buddig Deli Cuts Smoked Turkey
(2 oz)
90 calories
5 g fat (2 g saturated)
600 mg sodium

There are other low-calorie options in the deli case, but few outside Hormel's Natural Choice can boast being free from nitrates, nitrites, and growth hormones. Whether it's deli meat or pasta sauce, we like our staples as free from food additives and preservatives as possible.

PEANUT BUTTER

Eat This

Smucker's Natural Peanut Butter, Creamy (2 Tbsp)
200 calories
16 g fat (2.5 g saturated)
105 mg sodium

Not That!

Jif Reduced Fat
(2 Tbsp)
190 calories
12 g fat (2.5 g saturated)
210 mg sodium

Here's some advice that seems to fly in the face of conventional wisdom: Choose the peanut butter with the most fat. Natural varieties like Smucker's are made from nothing but peanuts and salt. That means you're trading hydrogenated oils and corn syrup for more healthy fat.

FRUIT SPREAD

Eat This

Smucker's Simply Fruit Blueberry
(1 Tbsp)
40 calories
0 g fat
8 g sugars

Not That!

Welch's Concord Grape Jelly
(1 Tbsp)
50 calories
0 g fat
13 g sugars

The hallmark of a good jelly or jam is that it's made with nothing but real fruit, and this one achieves that by using nothing but fruit and concentrated juice for sweetness. Contrast that with the Welch's jelly: The second and third ingredients are corn syrup and high-fructose corn syrup.

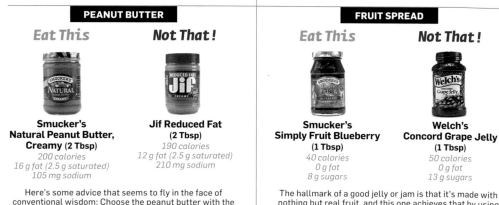

Kitchen Commandments

Eight easy-to-follow rules that will improve your health as much as they'll improve your food

Season to taste.
Very few of the recipes in this book have specific measurements for salt and pepper for a reason: Your mouth is more accurate than a measuring spoon. Taste and adjust as early and often as possible.

Make friends.
Theoretically, you could shop for an entire week's worth of groceries without ever interacting with a store worker. But there's a reason we talk to butchers, bakers, and cheesemongers when we shop: They know their stuff. A great fishmonger will tell you how to cook that snapper fillet, and a friendly butcher will save that last cut of prime beef for his favorite customers. What's that? Your supermarket doesn't have butchers and cheesemongers? Find a new place to shop.

Turn off the GPS.
Recipes aren't immutable laws or edicts handed down from on high by the culinary gods. They're basic road maps, and sometimes the best part of the journey is getting lost and finding your way back.

Adapt at will.
Ingredients aren't set in stone. If you have a bag of unused mushrooms in the fridge but the recipe calls for eggplant, chances are the 'shrooms will do just fine. Don't want to spend $3 on a bunch of celery just to use a single rib? Omit it. You like pork chops more than chicken breast? Switch it. The point is, if you understand the basic techniques and have an idea of what tastes good together, the possibility for creation in the kitchen is infinite.

Shop like an Italian grandma.
They are brilliant cooks not just because it's in their blood, but because they believe it's their fundamental right to take home the best apple, the best wedge of cheese, and the best fillet of fish every time they step into the store. Inspect fruit and vegetables carefully, ask workers when certain cuts of meat came in, and ask if you can taste new cheeses and deli meats before buying.

Join the farm team.
Supermarket produce isn't so super compared with what's at a farmers' market, where the pickings are often organic and always fresh, seasonal, and local. (Go to ams.usda.gov/farmersmarkets/map.htm for a state-by-state list of more than 5,700 farmers' markets.) Not only does eating food close to the source taste better, it's likely fresher, and since certain nutrient levels in produce tend to deplete over time, that means it's likely healthier, too.

Shop with the seasons.
In the golden age of the American supermarket, Chilean tomatoes and South African asparagus are an arm's length away when our soil is still blanketed in snow. Sure, sometimes you just need a tomato, but there are three persuasive reasons to shop in season: It's cheaper, it tastes better, and it's better for you (and the planet).

Treat yourself.
Not just when it comes to calories (which is indeed important) but also with the quality of food you buy. Americans spend less of their income on food than any other country in the world, so adding a few dollars to your food budget in order to secure omega-3-rich grass-fed steaks or glistening wild Alaskan salmon fillets is money well spent. If it's something that will help you look, feel, and function better, isn't it worth it to spend a few extra bucks for the best?

Kitchen Wisdom

The best culinary minds know that simple touches can lead to magical meals.
Here are 18 kitchen tips and tricks that'll ensure every dish makes your taste buds happy.

Teflon coatings can deteriorate on high heat, so save your nonstick pans for gentler tasks like cooking omelets and sautéing fish.

Proper seasoning is paramount. First, lose your saltshaker. Pinch kosher salt straight from a dish. The coarse grains and the touch of your fingers give you maximum control. Add a pinch, taste, and repeat if necessary.

Oops

Too much salt? Use a splash of vinegar to provide a counter-balancing punch of acid and sweetness.

For deeply flavored foods, don't overcrowd the pan. Ingredient overload makes a pan's temperature plummet, and foods end up steaming rather than caramelizing. This adds cooking time and subtracts flavor. All ingredients should fit comfortably in one layer, so use a pan that's big enough for the job, and cook in batches if necessary.

Nothing beats crispy chicken skin. Buy a whole chicken the day before you'll cook it, sprinkle on a table-spoon of kosher salt, and leave it uncovered in the fridge. The air and salt will draw out excess water.

Shop for food on Wednesday. Research shows that only 11 percent of people do it, making it the best time to pick out first-rate products without the clamoring masses.

Pat meat and fish dry before cooking. Surface moisture creates steam when it hits a hot pan or grill, impeding caramelization. If your fish has skin, use a sharp knife to squeegee off the water trapped within it.

Think of a broiler as an inverted grill, a source of concentrated, quick-cooking heat. Chicken, pork chops, and steaks take about 10 minutes to broil; just be sure to flip them midway through the cooking process.

Instantly improve your next TV dinner. After cooking, add fresh herbs, a squeeze of citrus, and a drizzle of olive oil to transform any frozen entrée.

Never store tomatoes in the refrigerator. And keep peaches, potatoes, onions, bread, garlic, and coffee out of there, too. Cold temperatures compromise the flavor and texture of these staples.

Overcooked meat? Salvage dinner: Slice the meat thinly, put it on a plate, and top it with chopped tomato, onion, and jalapeño. Add olive oil and fresh lime juice (or a few spoonfuls of vinaigrette). The acid and oil will restore much-needed moisture and fat to the mistreated meat.

If you slice into your meat right after it comes off the grill, those precious juices, still circulating with residual heat, will bleed out onto your plate. Let the meat rest: Wait 5 minutes before biting into burgers or grilled chicken, 7 minutes before cutting into steaks, and at least 15 minutes before carving a turkey or a larger roast.

Warm food served on a cold plate is a rookie mistake. Heat your dishes in a 150°F oven for 10 minutes before plating a meal. On the flip side, lightly chilled plates (use your freezer) boost the freshness of cold dishes like summer salads.

Try cooking with a 50:50 mixture of butter and olive oil. Butter brings big rich flavors, while oil protects the butter from burning over high heat.

More pucker for the price! Zap lemons, limes, or oranges for 15 seconds in the microwave before squeezing them. The fruit will yield twice as much juice.

Avoid a visit to the E.R. Place a damp kitchen towel underneath your cutting board to prevent it from rocking or slipping while you're chopping or slicing foods.

Freshen up limp vegetables: Drop your aging produce into ice water before cooking. Plants wilt due to water loss; ice water penetrates their cells to restore crispness.

Don't dice a digit. Cut awkward-to-slice vegetables—such as mushrooms, carrots, and peppers—by first cleaving them in half. Then rest the flat parts on the cutting board.

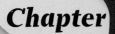

3

Chapter

Cook This, Not That!

Breakfast

The adage is true:
The first meal is the most important.
Let us show you how to get it right every time.

Remember that famous Bill Cosby skit, the one where he begrudingly had to make breakfast for his kids, but then discovers a chocolate cake in his kitchen so he serves them that instead? His kids, veins coursing with sugary sweetness, begin singing his praises: "Dad is great! Give us the chocolate cake!" Then his wife comes downstairs. She is considerably less pleased with his choice of breakfast. Cue laugh track.

No Laughing Matter

This skit was a riot in the early '80s, but it probably wouldn't have much impact today. The thought of chocolate cake for breakfast doesn't carry the shock value it once did. "Chocolate cake for breakfast?" today's audience might say. "What's so funny 'bout chocolate cake for breakfast?" That's because we've become a culture of time crunchers, and as our lives have become filled with weekend chores, long days at work, and new episodes of *Modern Family,* we've let our guard down with our most basic food choices. This is conspicuously more true for breakfast than it is for any other meal of the day. Who among us hasn't dipped our greedy hands into the break-room doughnut box? Or, having skipped breakfast, ducked into a café or gas station to grab a muffin, cinnamon roll, or honey bun? And what do these foods have in common? They're all iterations of Bill's chocolate cake, nutritional black holes that rely on sugar, starch, and fat to suck the energy out of your body and store it in the form of flab around your waist.

Clichéd but undeniably true, breakfast *is* the most important meal of your day. You've spent all night fasting and your stomach is as hollow as a beach ball.

What you choose to eat now will affect the rest of your day; in other words, eat cake and you'll feel like garbage. Studies indicate that a good breakfast—one that involves protein and fiber—can boost your metabolism, improve your performance at work, and influence your eating habits throughout the day. With a good breakfast you can, in essence, lose weight eating more food—and you'll feel great in the process. And here's the best news: This requires neither the knowledge of a chef nor long hours in the kitchen. Just lay out a game plan before you go to bed (scrambled eggs, wheat toast, fresh juice, for example), and then allow yourself a few extra minutes the next day to make it happen. Lucky for you, we have more than a dozen simple, delicious ways to get the job done in the morning hour (see page 38).

We've provided you with the most vital stats for all of the recipes in this book: calories, fat, saturated fat, sodium, and in the cases of desserts, sugars. Unfortunately, not all restaurants are so forthcoming. On the right is a list of the country's largest restaurants that still refuse to provide full nutritional information for their dishes.

Applebee's
California Pizza Kitchen
Carrabba's
Cheesecake Factory
Friendly's
Hooters
IHOP
T.G.I. Friday's

The Great Cereal Spec

While we don't accept excuses for not taking the time to get breakfast right, we do realize every one of you will fall back on a bowl of cereal at some point this year. In fact, the average American consumes more than 160 bowls of cereal annually, so picking the right box could mean knocking 15 pounds off your waistline yearly and infusing your diet with massive doses of vital nutrients. Use our bowl-by-bowl breakdown to find the perfect cereal for you. Our criteria: the highest ratio of fiber to sugar, along with a respectable calorie count. Sidle up and grab a spoon!

Figures are based on 30 grams of cereal.

General Mills Fiber One Original

60 calories
1 g fat
(0 g saturated)
14 g fiber
0 g sugars

The gold standard in cereal. Add sweetness with a bit of fresh fruit.

BEST CHOICE

Nature's Path Organic Smart Bran

90 calories
1 g fat
(0 g saturated)
13 g fiber
6 g sugars

You're getting 52 percent of your daily fiber in every bowl.

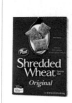

Post Shredded Wheat Original
(spoon size)

170 calories
<1 g fat
(0 g saturated)
6 g fiber
0 g sugars

This one-ingredient cereal (whole wheat!) is the real breakfast of champions.

Kashi Autumn Wheat

105 calories
0.5 g fat (0 g saturated)
3 g fiber
4 g sugars

A semisweet bowl without the risk of a sugar spike.

General Mills Wheaties

111 calories
0.5 g fat
(0 g saturated)
3 g fiber
4 g sugars

Falls just below the 1:1 fiber-to-sugar ratio you want. Still, you could do a lot worse.

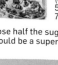

Kashi Go Lean Crunch! Honey Almond Flax

113 calories
3 g fat
(0 g saturated)
5 g fiber
7 g sugars

Lose half the sugar and this would be a superlative cereal.

Kellogg's Smart Start

114 calories
0 g fat
(0 g saturated)
2 g fiber
8 g sugars

Don't be lured in by the buzzwords. This is anything but an intelligent start to your day.

Quaker Natural Granola Oats, Honey & Raisins

123.5 calories
3.5 g fat
(2 g saturated)
2 g fiber
9 g sugars

Most granolas are only a small step above sugary kids' cereals.

Kellogg's Reduced Sugar Frosted Flakes

116 calories
0 g fat
<1 g fiber
8 g sugars

The sugar decrease is minimal and the fiber offering is abysmal.

trum

Kashi GoLean

80 calories
0.5 g fat
(0 g saturated)
6 g fiber
3 g sugars

Low-cal, high-fiber, and a reasonable amount of sugar.

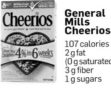

Post Grape-Nuts

103 calories
0.5 g fat
(0 g saturated)
4 g fiber
2 g sugars

A small serving of these breakfast pellets should carry you until lunch.

General Mills Cheerios

107 calories
2 g fat
(0 g saturated)
3 g fiber
1 g sugars

It's hard to beat the ubiquitous yellow box and its admirable balance of fiber and sugar.

General Mills Kix

110 calories
1 g fat
(0 g saturated)
3 g fiber
3 g sugars

As far as the sweet cereals go, this is about as good as it gets. Keep this around for the kids.

Kellogg's Corn Flakes

107 calories
0 g fat
1 g fiber
2 g sugars

The calorie count is okay, but the second ingredient is sugar.

Quaker Life Cereal Original

112.5 calories
1 g fat
(0 g saturated)
2 g fiber
6 g sugars

Seemingly harmless, but Life could do without the Yellow #5.

Kellogg's Raisin Bran

96 calories
0.7 g fat
(0 g saturated)
3.5 g fiber
10 g sugars

Raisins are sweet enough naturally, so why coat them in sugar?

Kellogg's Rice Krispies

118 calories
0 g fat
0 g fiber
4 g sugars

Fiber is cereal's one true virtue, so why start your day with a bowl utterly devoid of it?

General Mills Trix

112 calories
1 g fat
(0 g saturated)
<1 g fiber
11 g sugars

Let the rabbit have them for you; they're no good.

Kellogg's Froot Loops

113 calories
1 g fat
(0.5 g saturated)
<1 g fiber
12 g sugars

The sugar rush will throw you for a loop.

General Mills Lucky Charms

122 calories
1 g fat
(0 g saturated)
1 g fiber
12 g sugars

A rainbow of artificial colors with a pot of sugar at the end.

Post Golden Crisp

122 calories
0 g fat
<1 g fiber
15.5 g sugars

Sugar is the first ingredient. That's all you need to know.

WORST CHOICE

13 Instant Breakfasts

The no-time-for-breakfast excuse is no longer valid—not with these wallet-saving, waist-trimming morning meals at your fingertips.

1 Smear toasted whole-grain bread with whipped cream cheese and top with smoked salmon, sliced tomato, sliced red onion, and capers. (Why not make an extra one for lunch, too?)

2 **Simmer a few cups of your favorite tomato sauce in a skillet. Crack eggs directly into the sauce and swirl in the whites, while leaving the yolks untouched. Cook until the whites are firm and the yolk is set, but still runny. Top with lots of cracked black pepper and fresh parsley, if you like. Eat with crusty bread.**

3 Cook polenta or grits according to package instructions. Top with two poached or fried eggs, chopped scallions, salsa, and a bit of crumbled bacon.

4 **Spread toasted English muffin halves with a spoonful of pesto. Top with scrambled eggs and shredded mozzarella cheese. Place under the broiler until the cheese melts and bubbles.**

5 Simmer half a can of black beans with a cup of chicken stock. Crack two eggs directly into the mixture and cook until the whites are set. Hit it with plenty of hot sauce.

6 *Combine cooked quinoa in a pan with a half cup of milk, a pad of butter, golden raisins, a touch of brown sugar, and toasted walnuts. Heat until hot and creamy.*

7 Add salsa and grated cheese to a small oven-safe bowl or ramekin. Crack two eggs over the top and bake in a 400°F oven until the whites are just set, about 10 to 12 minutes. Eat with whole-wheat toast or corn tortillas.

8 Toast two whole-grain waffles until crispy. Spread one with a thick layer of peanut butter, then top with sliced apples and ham. Top with the other waffle and eat it like a sandwich.

9 Cook polenta or grits according to package instructions. Top with a scoop of ricotta or mascarpone cheese and chopped fresh figs.

10 Spread a toasted whole-wheat English muffin with almond butter. Top with sliced bananas, a drizzle of agave syrup, and crushed almonds.

11 Stir a spoonful of peanut butter into a bowl of plain instant oatmeal. Top with diced apples, crushed walnuts, and agave syrup.

12 Breakfast tacos! Scramble eggs with chopped scallions and hunks of chicken sausage. Serve in warm tortillas topped with black beans, sliced avocado, and salsa.

13 Heat a cup of spicy, not-too-chunky salsa in a skillet. Add a few handfuls of tortilla chips and cook until slightly softened, but retaining pockets of crunchiness—about 90 seconds. Top with a fried egg, thinly sliced onion, crumbled cheese, and a squeeze of lime.

Sunrise Sandwich

with Turkey, Cheddar & Guacamole

We are firm believers in the splendors of the original Egg McMuffin, along with many of the other ready-to-eat breakfast sandwiches that have followed in its wake. But not all handheld breakfast bites are so virtuous, many of them being flooded with excessive carbs and fat. And even the McMuffin can be greatly improved upon, which is exactly what we do here, subbing in lean turkey for Canadian bacon, adding lycopene-rich tomato, and crowning it all with a spread of heart-healthy guacamole.

You'll Need:

- 1 tsp canola or olive oil
- 1 egg
- Salt and black pepper to taste
- 2 oz smoked turkey breast
- 1 slice American, Cheddar, or pepper Jack cheese
- 1 thick slice tomato
- 1 whole-wheat English muffin, split and toasted
- 1 Tbsp Guacamole (see page 303) or Wholly Guacamole

How to Make It:

- Heat the oil in a small nonstick skillet or sauté pan over medium heat until hot. Add the egg and gently fry until the white is set but the yolk is still runny, about 5 minutes. Season with salt and pepper.

- Place the turkey on a plate, top with the cheese, and microwave for 30 to 45 seconds, until the turkey is hot and the cheese is melted.

- Place the tomato on the bottom half of the English muffin and season with salt and pepper. Top with the turkey and egg. Slather the guacamole on the top half of the muffin and crown the sandwich.

Makes 1 serving / Cost per serving: $2.34

Smoked meat products can be high in sodium. Look for turkey with fewer than 500 milligrams of sodium per serving.

380 calories
13 g fat
(3.5 g saturated)
980 mg sodium

Not That!

Dunkin' Donuts Sausage, Egg & Cheese on a Bagel
Price: $3.25

660 calories
29 g fat
(11 g saturated)
1,590 mg sodium

Save!
280 calories
and $0.91!

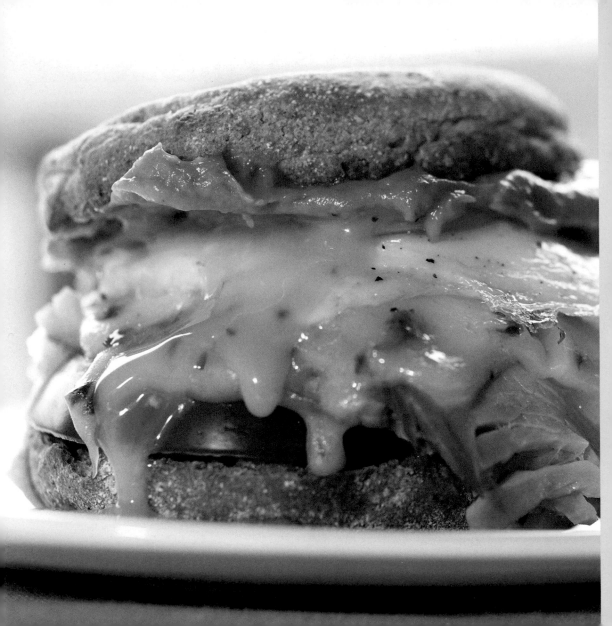

Cook This!
Scrambled Eggs with Smoked Salmon, Asparagus and Goat Cheese

Two eggs scrambled in a pat of butter contain approximately 200 calories. So how does Denny's get from 200 to 1,150 with their Heartland Scramble? And how do so many other restaurants sling together scrambles with more than 1,000 calories? Simple: excessive oil and egregious amounts of cheese. This scramble has all the makings of hearty breakfast fare—butter, cheese, protein—but with healthy fats, fresh vegetables, and a light caloric toll. Serve it with a scoop of roasted potatoes and fresh fruit.

You'll Need:

- 1 Tbsp butter
- 8 stalks asparagus, woody bottoms removed, chopped into 1" pieces
- Salt and black pepper to taste
- 8 eggs
- 2 Tbsp fat-free milk
- ¼ cup crumbled fresh goat cheese
- 4 oz smoked salmon, chopped

Spend the extra dollar or two to buy the highest quality eggs you can find. Free-range farmers' market eggs are best.

How to Make It:

- Heat the butter in a large nonstick skillet or sauté pan over medium heat. When the butter begins to foam, add the asparagus and cook until just tender ("crisp-tender" in kitchen parlance). Season with salt and pepper.
- Crack the eggs into a large bowl and whisk with the milk. Season with a few pinches of salt and pepper and add to the pan with the asparagus. Turn the heat down to low and use a wooden spoon to constantly stir and scrape the eggs until they begin to form soft curds. A minute before they're done, stir in the goat cheese.
- Remove from the heat when the eggs are still creamy and soft (remember, scrambled eggs are like meat—they continue to cook even after you cut the heat) and fold in the smoked salmon.

Makes 4 servings / Cost per serving: $1.43

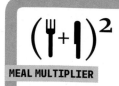

$$\left(\dfrac{\text{\textbf{¶}}}{} + \text{\textbf{|}} \right)^2$$

MEAL MULTIPLIER

There is no shortage of stellar scramble combinations. Invent on the fly, or go with one of these flavor-packed approaches.

- Sautéed mushrooms, zucchini, and caramelized onions
- Chorizo and onion, with diced avocado and chopped cilantro stirred in before serving
- Chunks of chicken or turkey sausage, scallions, and cheddar
- Cherry tomatoes, with a swirl of pesto stirred in at the last moment

320 calories
17 g fat (6 g saturated)
540 mg sodium

1,150 calories
66 g fat
(20 g saturated, 0.5 g trans)
2,800 mg sodium

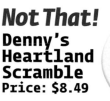

Not That!
Denny's Heartland Scramble
Price: $8.49

Save!
830 calories and $7.06!

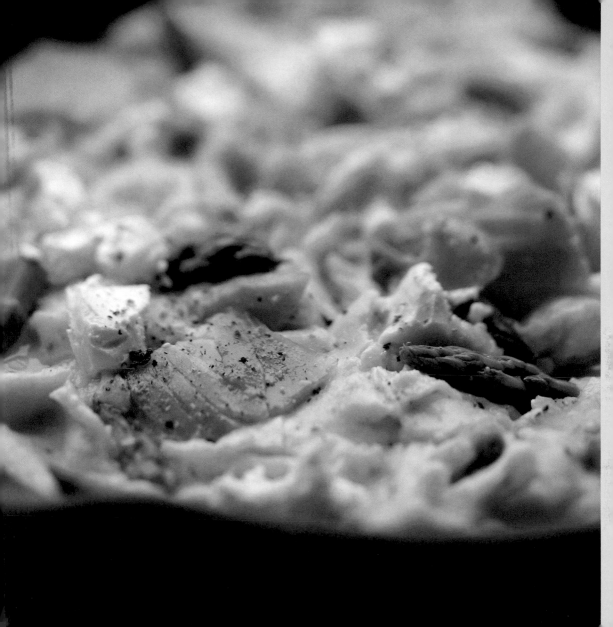

Artichoke-Feta Quiche

Most quiches suffer the burden of excessive amounts of heavy cream and cheese—and often a trans-fat-laden crust. This quiche dispenses with the heavy dose of dairy fat and instead gets its flavor and substance from antioxidant-dense sundried tomatoes, artichoke hearts, and lean chicken sausage. Great for breakfast, or add a small salad and a glass of red wine and call it dinner.

You'll Need:

- 3 extra large eggs
- 1 cup 2% milk
- ½ can (14 oz) artichoke hearts, drained and roughly chopped
- ¼ cup crumbled feta cheese
- 2 Tbsp chopped sundried tomatoes
- 2 links cooked turkey or chicken sausage
- ¾ tsp kosher salt
- Cracked pepper to taste
- 1 frozen piecrust

How to Make It:

- Preheat the oven to 350°F.
- Whisk the eggs until frothy, then stir in the milk, artichoke hearts, feta, tomatoes, sausage, salt, and pepper. Pour into the crust.
- Place in the oven and bake for 45 minutes or until the eggs are completely set (a toothpick inserted into the middle will come out clean) and the top is lightly golden brown. Cool for at least 5 minutes before slicing and serving.

Makes 6 servings / Cost per serving: $2.07

Unless you buy your sundried tomatoes packed in oil, you'll need to soften them in hot water for 10 minutes before cooking.

250 calories
14 g fat (5 g saturated)
890 mg sodium

673 calories
48 g fat (26 g saturated)
1,140 mg sodium

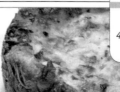

Not That!
Così Quiche Lorraine
Price: $3.49

Save!
423 calories and $1.42!

44

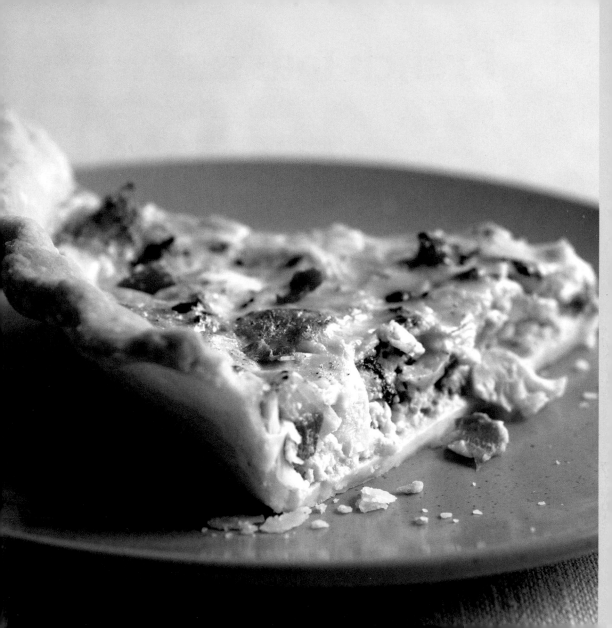

French Toast with Vanilla Bourbon and Caramelized Bananas

The word "stuffed" is never a good sign on a restaurant menu. Case in point: This breakfast calamity from Bob Evans contains a full day's worth of sodium, fat, and saturated fat and nearly 5 days' worth of cholesterol-spiking trans fat! Sweet carb-based breakfasts can never contend with protein-driven dishes, but if you're going to do it, these boozy, banana-topped French toast slices are about as good as it gets.

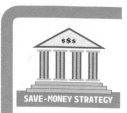

SAVE-MONEY STRATEGY

You'll Need:

- 2 Tbsp unsalted butter
- ¼ cup bourbon, divided
- ¼ cup brown sugar
- ¼ cup crushed walnuts
- 2 ripe but still firm bananas, sliced into ½" coins
- 1 cup 2% milk
- 3 eggs
- 1 tsp ground cinnamon
- 1 Tbsp vanilla extract
- 8 slices sturdy whole-grain bread like sourdough (day-old bread works great)

How to Make It:

- Heat the butter in a medium nonstick pan over medium heat. Add 2 tablespoons of the bourbon and all of the brown sugar and stir to dissolve. Cook for 1 to 2 minutes until bubbly. Add walnuts and cook for an additional 2 minutes; add the bananas and heat through. Stir in ¼ cup milk and keep warm.

- Whisk together the remaining ¾ cup milk, eggs, cinnamon, vanilla, and the remaining 2 tablespoons bourbon. Heat a large cast-iron skillet over medium heat. When the skillet is warm, spray with a light coating of nonstick cooking spray. Working 2 pieces at a time, dip the bread into the bourbon-egg mixture. Let soak for 30 seconds. Flip each piece over and soak the other side for 30 seconds.

- Add the bread to the hot skillet. Cook until golden brown on the bottom, about 3 minutes. Flip and cook for an additional 2 to 3 minutes, until both sides are golden brown and slightly crispy. Serve with the warm banana topping.

Makes 4 servings / Cost per serving: $1.34

Don't have bourbon at the ready in your wet bar? Try dark rum. Don't have rum? Skip the booze entirely and replace with another ½ cup of milk. Like all the recipes in this book, the ingredients can be altered to fit your pantry and your budget. So if you won't otherwise use the booze, don't bother dropping $25 just for this recipe. Cut it entirely from the egg mixture and add a splash of OJ to the bananas instead. Recipes are road maps, not immutable edicts.

490 calories
18 g fat
(4 g saturated)
800 mg sodium

1,493 calories
70 g fat
(21 g saturated, 9 g trans)
2,265 mg sodium

Not That!
Bob Evans Stacked & Stuffed Caramel Banana Pecan Hotcakes
Price: $5.99

Save!
1,003 calories and $4.65!

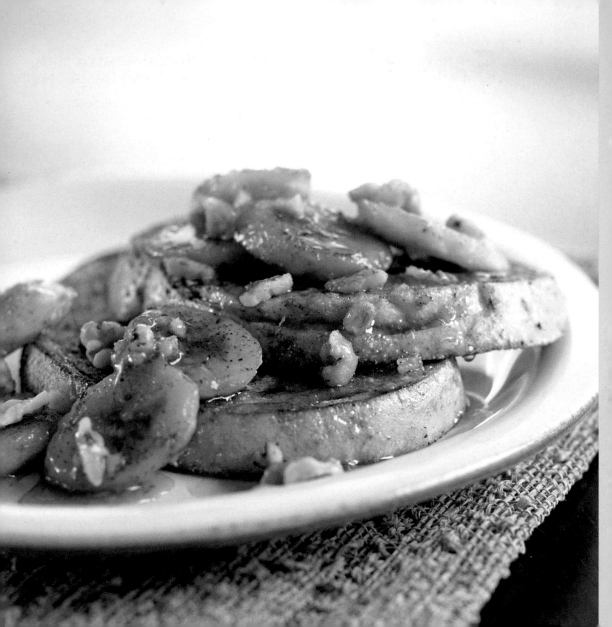

Cook This!
Sausage Frittata with Mushrooms

The more a restaurant manipulates an egg, the less healthy it's likely to be. Omelets rarely contain fewer than 800 calories, and ambitious concoctions like Panera's soufflé will swallow up an entire day's worth of saturated fat. Frittatas, however, give us hope. These Italian open-face omelets are lighter than their American cousins since they're less likely to be loaded with cheese and more likely to be stuffed with vegetables.

You'll Need:

- 1 Tbsp olive oil
- 1 red onion, thinly sliced
- 1 link cooked andouille sausage, diced
- 8 oz mushrooms (any variety—creminis work nicely), stems removed, sliced
- Salt and black pepper to taste
- 8 eggs
- ¼ cup crumbled goat cheese
- 12 chives or 3 scallions, chopped (optional)

How to Make It:

- Preheat the oven to 375°F.
- Place a large oven-safe skillet or sauté pan over medium heat. When the pan is hot, add the oil and onion; cook until translucent, about 3 minutes. Add the andouille and mushrooms and continue sautéing, about 5 minutes. Season with salt and pepper.
- Beat the eggs vigorously with a fork or whisk, then add to the skillet, along with the goat cheese and chives, if using. Place in the oven and bake until the eggs have fully set (a toothpick inserted into the middle will come out clean), about 20 minutes. Let cool and then slice into 4 portions, topping with more chives if you like.

Makes 4 servings / Cost per serving: $2.83

Andouille is a smoked, slightly spicy sausage popular in Cajun cooking. If you can't find it, kielbasa makes a fine substitute.

$$(\uparrow + \textbf{\textsf{I}})^2$$

MEAL MULTIPLIER

Using this recipe as a base, here are four other frittata combinations that work beautifully. Just sub out the mushrooms, sausage, and goat cheese for any of the following:

- 8 spears cooked, chopped asparagus and 2 ounces chopped smoked salmon
- ¼ cup sundried tomatoes, ¼ cup chopped olives, and ½ cup crumbled feta
- 1 cup sautéed spinach, 4 strips crumbled bacon, and ½ cup grated Gruyère
- 1 cup sautéed zucchini, 1 cup low-fat ricotta, and 8 to 10 chopped mint leaves

300 calories
18 g fat (5 g saturated)
450 mg sodium

580 calories
39 g fat
(21 g saturated,
1 g trans)
940 mg sodium

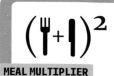

Not That!
Panera Spinach and Bacon Egg Soufflé
Price: $3.49

Save!
280 calories and $0.66!

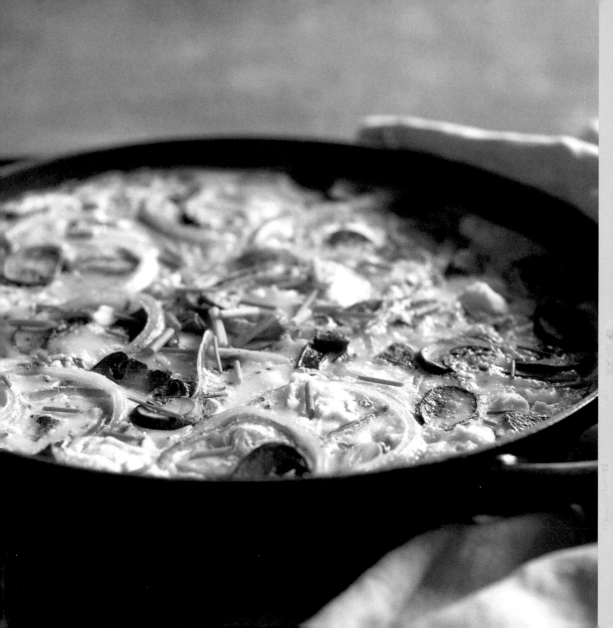

Huevos Rancheros

This is the type of breakfast you want when you really need to deliver on the day. Not only are huevos rancheros intensely flavorful and satisfying, but the balance of protein, fiber, and antioxidants is designed to optimize performance all day long.

You'll Need:

- 1 can (16 oz) whole peeled tomatoes, with juice
- ½ small onion, chopped
- 1 clove garlic, chopped
- 1 Tbsp chopped chipotle pepper
- ¼ cup chopped fresh cilantro
- Juice of 1 lime
- Salt and black pepper to taste
- 1 can (16 oz) black beans
- Pinch of ground cumin
- 8 eggs
- 8 corn tortillas

How to Make It:

- Combine the tomatoes, onion, garlic, chipotle, cilantro, and half of the lime juice in a food processor and pulse until well blended but still slightly chunky. Season with salt and pepper.
- Mix the black beans, cumin, and remaining lime juice in a bowl; season with salt and pepper. Use the back of a fork to lightly mash up the beans, adding a splash of warm water if necessary.
- Coat a large nonstick skillet or sauté pan with nonstick cooking spray and heat over medium heat. Break the eggs into the skillet; cook until the whites have set but the yolks are still loose and runny.
- On a separate burner, heat a medium skillet over medium heat and add the tortillas, 2 at a time; cook for 1 minute on each side, until lightly toasted.
- To assemble the dish, spread the tortillas with the beans, top with the eggs, and top the eggs with the salsa. Garnish with more cilantro, if you like, and serve immediately.

Makes 4 servings /
Cost per serving: $1.77

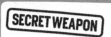

SECRET WEAPON

Chipotle pepper

We admit to having an overwhelming infatuation with these canned chiles, but once you recognize their potential for adding instant flavor to a dish, you will, too. Chipotles are smoked jalapeños, and they come canned with a spicy, vinegary tomato sauce called adobo. You'll see a lot of recipes in this book that call for chipotles, so here's what you do: Buy a can, dump the whole thing into a blender or food processor, and pulse. Use a spoonful to spike salsas, marinades, mashed potatoes, and soups. Beyond being insanely delicious, the capsaicin in chipotle has been shown to boost metabolism.

480 calories
15 g fat (3 g saturated)
680 mg sodium

Not That!
IHOP Huevos Rancheros
Price: $10.54

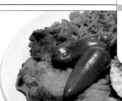

1,150 calories
19 g saturated fat
2,420 mg sodium

Save!
670 calories
and $8.77!

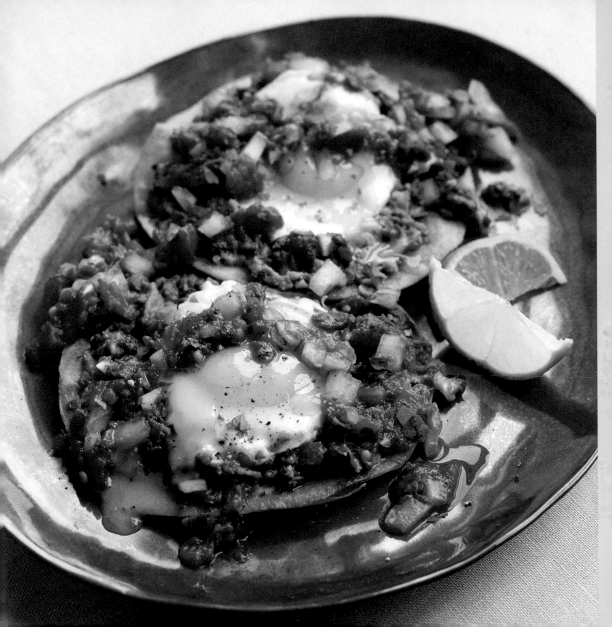

Blueberry Pancakes

Using yogurt and cottage cheese to make these pancakes does two things: It brings extra protein to the breakfast table, and it helps produce the lightest, moistest pancakes you've ever tasted. And once you try this simple blueberry compote, you'll never go back to lackluster syrup again.

Upgrade

You'll Need:

- 2 **cups frozen wild blueberries**
- ½ **cup water**
- ¼ **cup sugar**
- 1 **cup plain Greek-style yogurt (such as Fage 0%)**
- 1 **cup low-fat cottage cheese or ricotta**
- 3 **eggs**
- Juice of 1 lemon
- 1 **cup white whole-wheat flour (we like King Arthur's)**
- ½ **tsp baking soda**
- Pinch of salt

How to Make It:

- Mix the blueberries, water, and sugar in a saucepan. Cook over low heat, stirring often, for 10 minutes or until the blueberries begin to break apart. Whisk together the yogurt, cottage cheese, eggs, and lemon juice in a bowl.

- Mix the flour, baking soda, and salt in another bowl. Add the flour to the yogurt mixture and stir just until blended.

- Heat a large skillet or sauté pan over medium-low heat. Coat with nonstick cooking spray and add batter in large spoonfuls (about ¼ cup each). Flip the pancakes when the tops begin to bubble, 3 to 5 minutes, and cook the second side until browned. Serve with the warm blueberries.

Makes 4 servings / Cost per serving: $2.23

These can be just as easily made with white flour; you'll just sacrifice a few grams of fiber.

NUTRITIONAL

Most supermarket syrups are junk, made almost entirely from high-fructose corn syrup and chemical additives designed to approximate a maple flavor. But real maple syrup can be prohibitively expensive. Solution? Fruit compote. Take a bag of frozen fruit (blueberries, strawberries, mixed berries), dump into a saucepan with ½ cup water and ¼ cup sugar, and simmer for 10 minutes, until the fruit is warm and the mixture has thickened. It's not just cheaper than real maple syrup, it's also better for you than anything else you might top your pancakes or waffles with.

310 calories
8 g fat (3.5 g saturated)
500 mg sodium

Not That!
IHOP Blueberry Pancakes
Price: $7.99

710 calories

Save!
400 calories and $5.76!

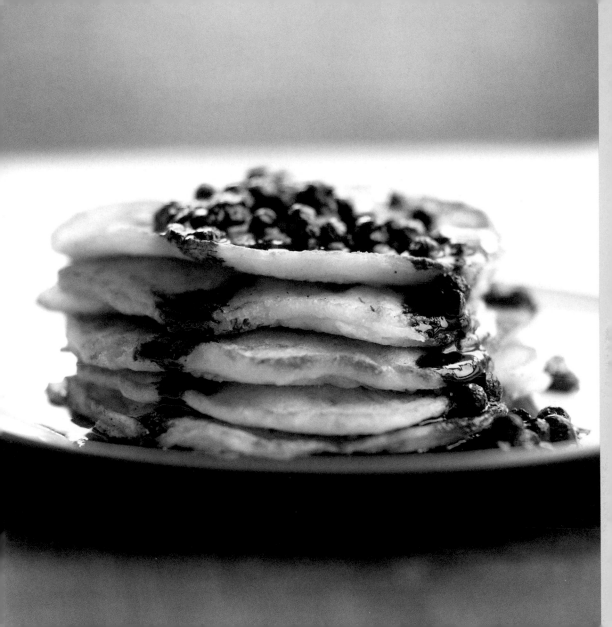

Waffles with Ham & Egg

Waffle and pancake plates are bad enough at most restaurants and diners, but throw in a side of eggs and breakfast meats and you're bound to start your day with the caloric equivalent of a triple cheeseburger. We've made our own version of Denny's superpopular (and supercaloric) Slam by building an open-faced sandwich with a toasted waffle. The ingredients may sound like a strange combination, but the flavors are nicely balanced, the portion size is perfect, and the nutritional profile is just what you want for the most important meal of the day.

You'll Need:

- 4 thick slices Canadian bacon or deli ham
- 4 eggs
- 4 frozen whole-grain waffles
- 2 Tbsp maple syrup
- 4 Tbsp shredded sharp Cheddar cheese
- Salt and black pepper to taste
- Parsley (optional)

How to Make It:

- Heat a nonstick skillet or sauté pan over medium heat. Coat with a bit of olive oil cooking spray and cook the Canadian bacon for a few minutes on each side, until well browned. Remove. Coat the same pan with a bit more spray and cook the eggs (2 at a time, if you must; avoid overcrowding the pan) sunny side up until the whites have set but the yolks are still runny.

- In the meantime, toast the waffles. Top each toasted waffle with a slice of meat, a drizzle of maple syrup, a sprinkle of Cheddar, and the warm fried eggs. Season with salt and pepper and sprinkle with parsley (if using).

Makes 4 servings / Cost per serving: $0.92

We like Van's Gourmet Multi-Grain. Each waffle packs 2.5 grams of fiber and just 95 calories.

$$(\Psi + I)^2$$

MEAL MULTIPLIER

With a whole-wheat waffle as your base, you can build a slew of sweet and savory open-faced breakfast sandwiches. Try one of these.

- Peanut butter, sliced banana, sliced almonds, and a drizzle of honey
- Scrambled eggs, turkey, and guacamole
- Fresh ricotta or mascarpone cheese, sliced strawberries or figs, and agave syrup

270 calories
11 g fat
(3.5 g saturated)
890 mg sodium

940 calories
53 g fat
(17 g saturated)
1,820 mg sodium

Not That!
Denny's Belgian Waffle Slam
Price: $6.79

Save!
670 calories and $5.87!

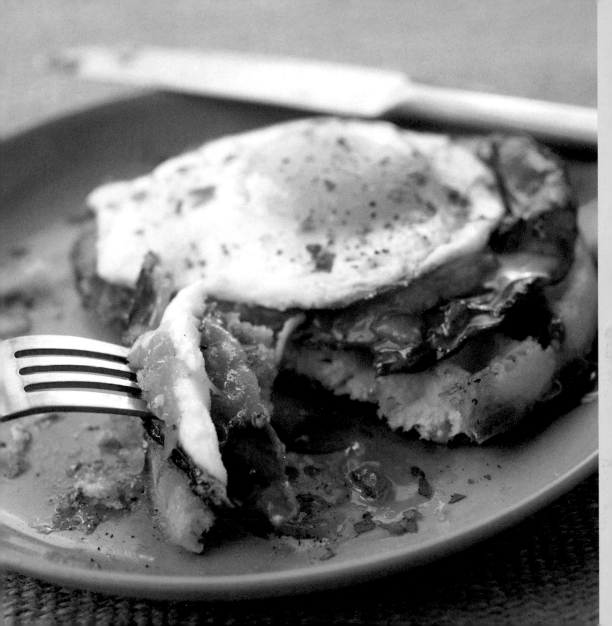

Yogurt Parfait

Fruit-flavored yogurts are essentially glorified ice cream. Read the label of any fruit-on-the-bottom brand and you'll see what we mean: Odds are high-fructose corn syrup is considerably higher on the ingredients list than actual fruit. That's why it's always better to buy plain, protein-rich Greek yogurt and add the real fruit yourself. We do just that here, layering it for visual appeal and tossing in granola for some crunch. Decadent enough to be a dessert but with exactly what you need to start your day: protein and fiber.

You'll Need:

- 1 cup sliced strawberries
- ½ cup blueberries (frozen are good, too)
- 2 tsp sugar
- 4–5 mint leaves, sliced thinly
- 1 container (8 oz) low-fat plain Greek-style yogurt (Fage 2% is our favorite)
- ¼ cup granola

How to Make It:

- Combine the fruit, sugar, and mint in a bowl and allow to sit for 3 to 4 minutes. Spoon half of the yogurt into a bowl or glass, top with half of the fruit and granola, then repeat with the remaining yogurt, fruit, and granola. Pour any accumulated juice from the fruit over the top.

Makes 1 serving / Cost per serving: $2.72

Any juicy fruit will work well here: raspberries, blackberries, kiwi, mangoes.

If you don't dig the thick Greek yogurt, any plain yogurt will work, as long as there are no added sugars.

Master THE TECHNIQUE

Macerating

Don't be put off by the fancy cooking jargon; macerating simply means to soak or steep something in liquid or sugar. Most fruit is sweet enough as it is, but by adding even the barest amount of sugar (in this case, about 30 calories' worth), you'll draw out the natural fructose in the fruit and create a tasty syrup that works beautifully on top of yogurt, pancakes, or even a bowl of ice cream. And fresh mint simply ups the flavor ante and the visual appeal.

330 calories
8 g fat (3.5 g saturated)
34 g sugars

700 calories
13 g fat (4 g saturated)
91 g sugars

Save!

370 calories
and $0.54!

Not That!

Au Bon Pain's Large Blueberry Yogurt with Blueberries and Granola Topping Price: $3.26

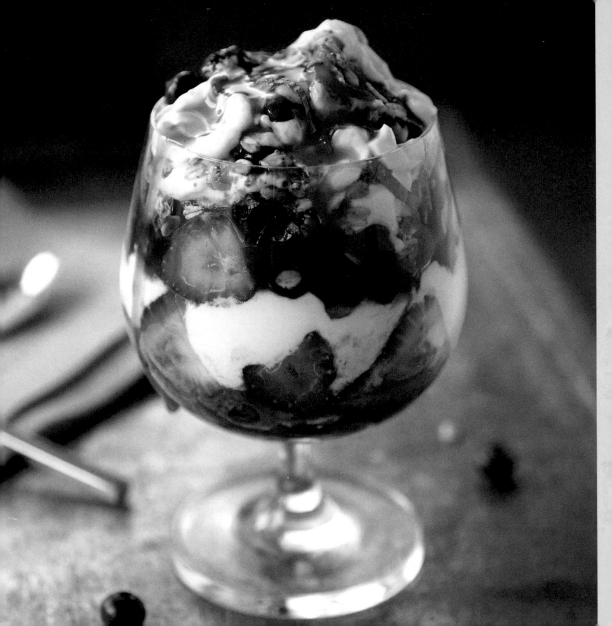

Cook This!
Crispy Ham Omelet with Cheese & Mushrooms

Overstuffed omelets like those at IHOP are eggs at their worst, harboring more calories than a half-dozen doughnuts. Why not spend the 5 minutes at home for a healthier, tastier version?

You'll Need:

2 Tbsp butter

½ lb white or cremini mushrooms, stems removed, sliced

Salt and black pepper to taste

4 slices prosciutto, cut into thin strips

8 eggs

4 Tbsp milk

1 cup shredded Gruyère or other Swiss cheese

Chopped chives or scallions (optional)

How to Make It:

- Heat 2 teaspoons butter in a medium skillet or sauté pan until foaming, then add the mushrooms. Cook until brown and caramelized, 5 to 7 minutes. Season with salt and pepper and remove to a bowl or plate.

- Wipe the pan clean and return to the heat. Add the prosciutto slices (don't crowd) and cook for a minute or two, until the pieces begin to shrink slightly and crisp up. Reserve.

- Heat 1 teaspoon butter in a small nonstick pan set over medium heat. Beat 2 eggs with 1 tablespoon milk and season with salt and pepper.

- Add the eggs to the pan and use a wooden spoon or heat-proof rubber spatula to move them about, as if you were scrambling them. Continue to do this for 30 seconds or so, until about half of the eggs have set, then use your spoon to gently lift the edge of the omelet and swirl the liquid egg around so that it runs underneath to the pan.

- When all but the thinnest film of egg has set, add ¼ cup cheese and a big spoonful of the sautéed mushrooms. Fold the omelet over (either once for a half-moon or twice for a long thin omelet) and gently slide onto a warm plate. Garnish with crispy prosciutto and chives (if using).

- Repeat to make 4 omelets in all.

Makes 4 servings / Cost per serving: $1.87

330 calories
20 g fat (9 g saturated)
570 mg sodium

990 calories

Not That!

IHOP Hearty Ham and Cheese Omelette
Price: $9.56

Save!
660 calories and $7.69!

STEP-BY-STEP

Expert omelets

Learn the art of making silky, light omelets and you can banish the hypercaloric $10 restaurant omelet from your diet for life. Here's how you handle it.

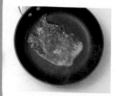

Step 1: *Melt butter over a medium-low flame.*

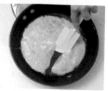

Step 2: *First scramble the eggs, then allow to set.*

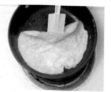

Step 3: *Add toppings and fold over carefully.*

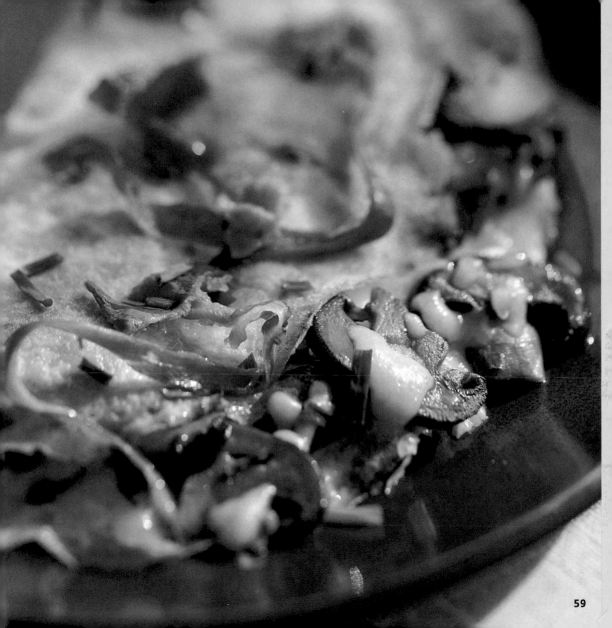

Breakfast Burritos

Take an oversize tortilla and stuff it full of sausage and cheese, and you're in for a rude awakening. By swapping out worthless white tortillas for whole wheat, swapping fatty pork sausage for the lean chicken variety, and adding fiber-rich beans and fresh avocado, we've slashed the calories in half while increasing the overall nutrition (and deliciousness).

You'll Need:

- ½ Tbsp olive oil
- 2 cooked chicken sausage links, diced
- 1 red onion, diced
- 6 eggs, lightly beaten
- Salt and black pepper to taste
- Chopped cilantro
- 4 whole-wheat tortillas (10")
- 1 cup black beans, rinsed, drained, and heated
- ½ cup shredded Cheddar or Jack cheese
- 1 avocado, pitted, peeled, and sliced
- Salsa
- Pickled Jalapeños (see page 304), optional

How to Make It:

- Heat the oil in a large skillet or sauté pan over medium heat. Add the sausage and onion; cook for 5 minutes or until lightly browned. Turn the heat to low.

- Pour the eggs into the skillet. Cook slowly, constantly stirring with a wooden spoon until the eggs are firm but still moist. Remove from the heat, season with salt and pepper, and stir in the cilantro.

- Wrap the tortillas in damp paper towels and heat in the microwave for 45 seconds. (Or heat them individually in a dry pan until warm and lightly toasted.) Divide the eggs, beans, cheese, and avocado among the tortillas. Roll into tight packages and top each burrito with salsa, more cilantro, and jalapeños (if using).

Makes 4 servings / Cost per serving: $2.42

La Tortilla Factory now makes excellent 100-calorie tortillas with 8 grams of fiber. Make them your go-to tortillas for all occasions.

$$\left({\text{\textbf{Y}}} + {\text{\textbf{\textbar}}} \right)^2$$

MEAL MULTIPLIER

Start with a solid tortilla and breakfast wraps and burritos become an incredible portable source of what you need most in the morning: fiber and protein. Try any of these other solid breakfast breakdowns.

- Scrambled eggs with leftover chicken, salsa, and guacamole
- Scrambled eggs with sautéed mushrooms, zucchini, and spinach topped with feta cheese
- Part-skim ricotta topped with sliced bananas, strawberries, and crushed almonds

415 calories
17 g fat (5 g saturated)
625 mg sodium

799 calories
49 g fat
(19 g saturated)
2,427 mg sodium

Not That!
Bob Evans Meat Lovers' BOBurrito
Price: $5.99

Save!
384 calories
and $3.57!

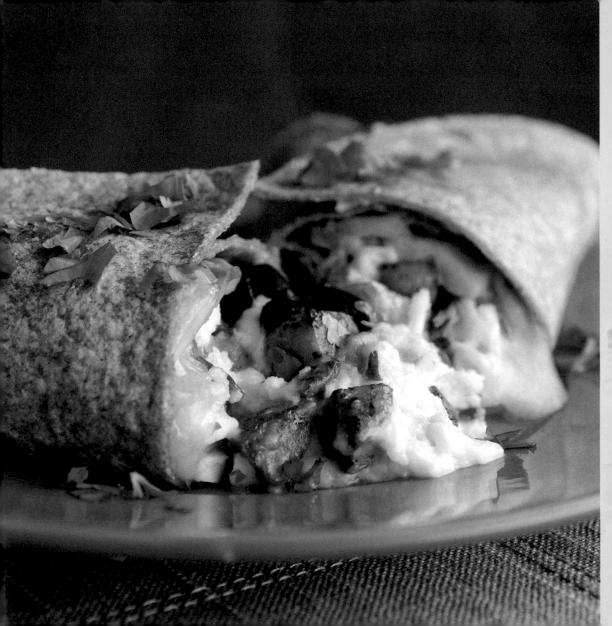

Chapter

4

Cook This, Not That!

Appetizers & Small Bites

The restaurant industry wants to ruin your meal before you start it. We're here to help.

America's appetizer menus are bathed in beige. Let's face it, 90 percent of the appetizers at our favorite restaurants have spent some serious face time with a vat of gurgling oil. Think of the mammoth portions of fried onions, the cheese-bacon-ranch French fries, and the 1,500-calorie "sample platter," which usually comprises some combination of fried cheese, fried chicken, fried calamari, fried shrimp, and fried mushrooms. It's a monochromatic calamity waiting to happen—all before you even sniff an entrée.

Out from the Deep Fryer

Our goal with this book, as with the other *Eat This, Not That!* books, is to help you enjoy the food you eat, and appetizers are the ideal vehicle for culinary appreciation. It's not your fault that the restaurant industry has so badly flogged the idea of the appetizer that it no longer seems congruent with a healthy eating routine. Truth is, a well-played appetizer can completely realign your eating priorities, teaching you to enjoy food while controlling portions and foregoing cheap, processed junk.

That's why, the next time you see a free night on the horizon, you need to seize it. Invite the friends and family, prepare the appetizers, and then let them entertain you with conversation while you work on the entrée. Instead of joylessly scarfing down a 15-minute dinner, you're actually tasting, talking, and moving slowly. You're bonding with loved ones, breaking bread together, and showing them you care enough to prepare real food instead of simply flagging down another waitress to get more chips and salsa.

These next pages are filled with familiar foods, plus a few new faces you may not recognize. We're not eliminating your favorite starters; you'll find wings and skins and melted cheese inside. But we've replaced the breading with savory spice rubs and the soybean oil baths with olive oil drizzles. Wield these creations properly and you'll whet the appetite in all the best possible ways, and believe it or not, you'll also be setting yourself up to consume fewer calories over the course of the meal. Studies show that consuming belly-filling nutrients before a meal, namely protein and healthy fats, can take a serious slice out of your appetite, resulting in smaller portions at mealtime. Use this chapter to realign your relationship with food. Show it that it exists to serve you, and not the other way around.

14 Instant Appetizers

Whether for a crowd of hungry guests or a single rumbling stomach, you're never more than 10 minutes away from a satisfying small bite.

1 Remove the pit from dates, stuff with an almond and blue cheese and warp tightly with half a strip of bacon. Secure with toothpicks and bake at 350°F until the bacon is crisp.

2 Combine sliced garlic, chili flakes, and a few chopped anchovies in a sauce pan with a half-cup of olive oil. Cook for 5 minutes over low heat. Serve with raw radishes, carrots, bell peppers, cauliflower, and sliced fennel.

3 *Sandwich a hunk of mozzarella or Swiss between two olives on toothpicks (pesto drizzle optional).*

4 Fill the bottom of an oven-safe bowl with bean dip or low-fat refried beans. Top with salsa, scallions, and a thin layer of Jack cheese. Bake until the cheese is melted, then crown with chopped pickled jalapeños. Serve with toasted pita or black bean chips.

5 Bloody Mary shrimp cocktail: Mix a few cups of low-sodium V8 with horseradish, Worcestershire, lemon juice, Tabasco, and maybe a bit of vodka. Pour into wine or martini glasses, top with chopped cucumbers and avocadoes, and rim the glass with cooked shrimp.

CHAPTER 4

6

Pop a bag of plain popcorn. Remove from the bag and toss with chopped rosemary, olive oil, and finely grated Parmesan.

7 Roll slices of Swiss cheese around slices of smoked turkey spread with guacamole. Secure with toothpicks.

8 Buy a jar of marinated artichoke hearts, roasted red peppers, and some good marinated olives. Arrange them all on a platter with some chunks of real Parmesan (or Manchego or Gruyère) and thin slices of nice ham.

9 Place 4 ounces of fresh goat cheese in a crock or small glass baking dish. Add some chopped garlic, fresh herbs (if you have any), a drizzle of olive oil, and lots of black pepper. Bake until the cheese is bubbling and serve with warm crusty bread.

10 Stuff Peppadew peppers with tiny balls of mozzarella, called boccoccini.

11 Thread hunks of watermelon, cherry tomatoes, pieces of fresh mozzarella, and leaves of basil on wooden skewers.

12 Peel a mango and cut it into spears. Top with fresh lime juice and chili powder.

13 Wrap slices of melon or cantaloupe with good prosciutto or Spanish ham.

14 Lay out slices of prosciutto or other thinly sliced ham. Mix chopped olives and sundried tomatoes with fresh ricotta, then place a spoonful into the center of the prosciutto slices. Wrap like a burrito.

Artichoke Dip

This classic dip is normally hijacked by a roguish team of full-fat mayo and cream cheese; somewhere, hidden within, lie token amounts of spinach and artichoke. Here, we turn that ratio on its head, plus use a flavorful olive oil–based mayo to cut calories and boost nutrition. Chiles bring some extra heat to the equation, while toasted wheat pitas work as super scoopers. Overall, this reimagined appetizer packs an amazing 14 grams of fiber.

You'll Need:

- 4 large whole-wheat pitas
- ½ Tbsp butter
- 1 onion, finely chopped
- 3 cloves garlic, finely chopped
- 1 jar (12 oz) artichoke hearts in water, drained and chopped
- 1 box (16 oz) chopped frozen spinach, thawed
- 1 can (4 oz) roasted green chiles, drained and chopped
- 2 Tbsp olive oil mayonnaise (made by both Kraft and Hellmann's)
- 2 Tbsp whipped cream cheese

Juice of 1 lemon

Salt and black pepper to taste

How to Make It:

- Cut the pitas into 6 to 8 wedges each and separate the layers. Spread on 2 baking sheets and bake at 400°F for 5 minutes or until crisp.

- Heat the butter in a large skillet or sauté pan over medium heat. Add the onion and garlic and cook for 5 minutes or until softened. Add the artichokes, spinach, chiles, mayonnaise, cream cheese, and lemon juice. Cook, stirring often, for 5 minutes or until hot. Season with salt and pepper. Serve with the pita wedges.

Makes 4 servings / Cost per serving: $2.07

Whipped cream cheese has air beaten into it, making it lighter and easier to spread.

BANK

SAVE-MONEY STRATEGY

Fresh spinach generally runs about $3 a bunch, and because spinach is made up of around 90 percent water, it cooks down to nothing as soon as it touches the pan. Frozen spinach not only costs less than half as much as fresh, but because it's precooked, it yields significantly more actual spinach. Always keep a box in the freezer for this and other recipes that call for cooked spinach.

270 calories
10 g fat
(2.5 g saturated)
520 mg sodium

1,040 calories
85 g fat
(39 g saturated)
3,320 mg sodium

Not That!
Chili's Hot Spinach & Artichoke Dip with Chips
Price: $7.99

Save!
770 calories
and $5.92!

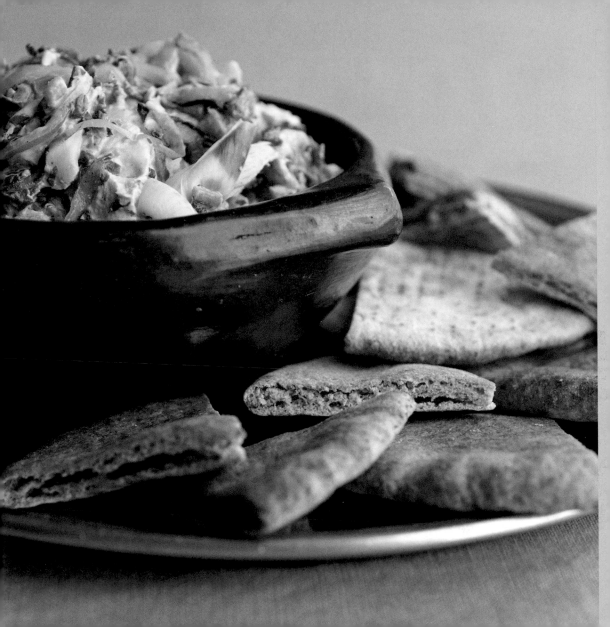

Teriyaki Scallops Wrapped in Bacon

It's a shame that restaurants ignore lean protein like shrimp and scallops in favor of potato skins and fried cheese. What's not to love about a meaty, sweet sea scallop glazed in teriyaki and wrapped in crispy bacon? How about the fact that this one dish will cost you fewer calories than two pieces of wheat toast? Or that it takes about 15 minutes to prepare?

You'll Need:

- 8 large sea scallops
- ¼ cup teriyaki marinade
- 4–8 strips of bacon

Buy "dry" scallops whenever possible, which are wild and natural. "Wet" scallops have been soaked in preservative solution, which decreases quality and increases weight (i.e., cost).

How to Make It:

- Toss the scallops with enough teriyaki marinade to cover and marinate for 30 minutes in the refrigerator.

- Preheat the broiler. Wrap each scallop with just enough bacon to wrap around fully without overlapping (it's best to stretch the bacon fairly thin—it will crisp up easier that way).

- Thread a toothpick through the bacon and scallop to secure. Brush with a bit more of the teriyaki marinade, then place in the oven 6" beneath the broiler. Cook for 10 to 12 minutes, until the scallops are firm and the bacon is fully cooked.

Makes 4 servings / Cost per serving: $3.28

Thin bacon is best here, since it will crisp up quicker, keeping your scallops from overcooking.

110 calories
5 g fat (1.5 g saturated)
650 mg sodium

580 calories
35 g fat (5 g saturated)
1,880 mg sodium

Not That!
Red Lobster Peach-Bourbon BBQ Scallops
Price: $8.99

Save!
470 calories and $5.71!

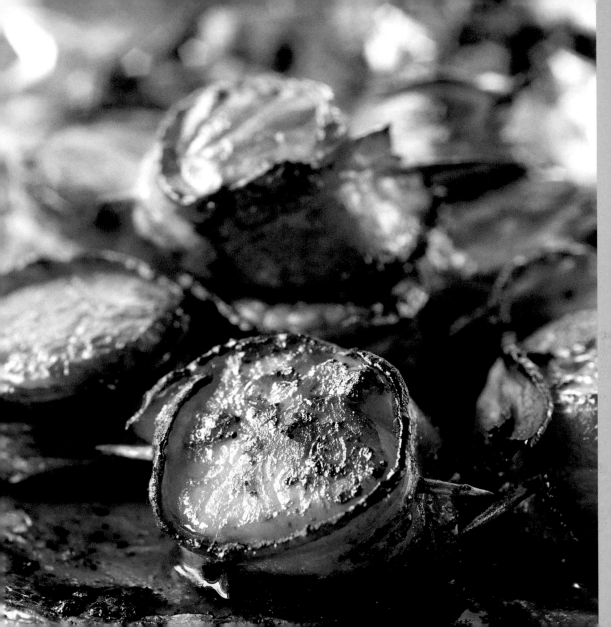

Fiery Buffalo Wings

Americans consume millions of pounds of Buffalo wings each year. Besides being messy, those wings all share one thing: an extended stay in the deep fryer. This method takes an already fatty cut of chicken and doubles the calories. Grilling or oven-roasting your wings, on the other hand, cuts fat significantly; it's also easier, cheaper (no quart of oil for frying), and (especially on the grill) tastier.

You'll Need:

- 2 lb chicken wings (preferably a mix of wing segments and drummettes)
- 1 tsp salt
- 1 tsp black pepper
- 1 tsp chili powder
- 2 Tbsp butter
- 2 Tbsp hot sauce (Frank's Red Hot is best)
- Juice of 1 lemon
- 1 cup plain Greek-style yogurt (we like Fage 2%)
- 2 Tbsp crumbled blue cheese
- Salt and black pepper to taste
- Celery sticks (optional)

How to Make It:

- Preheat the oven to 450°F. Toss the chicken with the salt, pepper, and chili powder and arrange on a baking sheet. Roast until the skin is lightly blistered and the meat is cooked all the way through, about 15 minutes.

- Melt the butter in a large nonstick skillet or sauté pan and add the hot sauce and half of the lemon juice. Remove the wings from the oven and add directly to the hot pan, tossing to thoroughly coat every piece in the sauce.

- Mix the yogurt, blue cheese, and remaining lemon juice. Season with salt and pepper. Serve the wings and the celery (if using) with the blue cheese sauce on the side for dipping.

Makes 8 appetizer servings / Cost per serving: $1.55

Want Asian-style wings? Simply sub in ¼ cup teriyaki sauce for the hot sauce and follow the rest of the recipe.

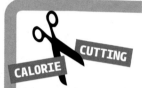

CALORIE CUTTING

Chicken wings have a high fat-to-meat ratio, and although much of that fat is of the same heart-healthy variety you find in olive oil, the calories still add up quickly. To make this dish extra lean, apply the exact same treatment to boneless, skinless chicken tenders, or even peeled and deveined shrimp. Cook them in the oven or on a grill until firm, then toss briefly in the pan with the same hot sauce—spiked butter. You'll cut the calories in half and the fat by about 75 percent.

310 calories
21 g fat (6 g saturated)
680 mg sodium

1,010 calories

Not That!
Hooters 10 piece Buffalo Wings
Price: $9.99

Save!
700 calories and $8.44!

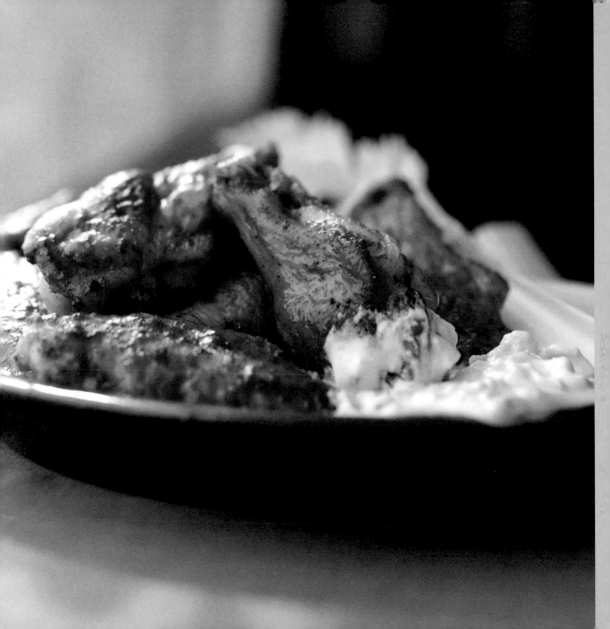

Crispy Quesadillas with Guacamole

Next to nachos, quesadillas are the most perilous food to be found on a Mexican restaurant menu. Overstuffed with cheese and teeming with greasy toppings, quesadillas are all but guaranteed to pack quadruple-digit calories. Tussle with Chili's rendition and you'll take in 35 bacon strips' worth of saturated fat. Our quesadilla reverses the cheese-to-filling ratio, going long on the nutrient-dense vegetables and using just enough chorizo and cheese to make it feel like an indulgence.

You'll Need:

- ½ Tbsp canola oil
- 4 oz chorizo, casing removed
- 1 small red onion, sliced
- 4 oz white button mushrooms, stems removed, sliced
- 1 large poblano pepper, seeded, sliced into thin strips
- Salt and black pepper to taste
- 1½ cups shredded Monterey Jack cheese
- 4 medium whole-wheat tortillas
- Guacamole (see page 303)

How to Make It:

- Heat a large skillet or sauté pan over medium-high heat. Add the oil and chorizo; cook until browned, using a wooden spoon to break up the meat into smaller pieces. Remove from the pan and drain all but a thin film of the fat. Return to the heat and add the onion, mushrooms, and pepper; sauté, stirring occasionally, until the vegetables are brown— 5 to 7 minutes. Season with salt and pepper.

- Divide the cheese between 2 tortillas and top each with half of the vegetable mixture. Top with the remaining tortillas.

- Heat a large cast-iron skillet over medium heat. Spray the pan with nonstick cooking spray and cook each quesadilla individually, until the tortillas are brown and crispy and the cheese is fully melted. Cut into 4 or 6 wedges and serve with the guacamole.

Makes 4 servings / Cost per serving: $3.11

SAVVY SHORTCUT

Individually toasting the quesadillas in a cast-iron skillet yields the crispest, tastiest results imaginable. But if you're making a round for the whole family and want to save time, try the broiler or even the grill (which adds delicious smoky notes to the quesadilla). Simply preheat either, assemble all of your quesadillas, and cook 6" under the broiler or directly on the grill grates for 3 to 4 minutes on one side. Carefully flip, then continue cooking for another 3 to 4 minutes, until toasted on the outside and melted in the middle.

310 calories
16 g fat (5 g saturated)
730 mg sodium

1,480 calories
96 g fat (35 g saturated)
3,510 mg sodium

Not That!
Chili's Fire Grilled Chicken Fajita Quesadilla
Price: $8.99

Save!
1,170 calories and $5.88!

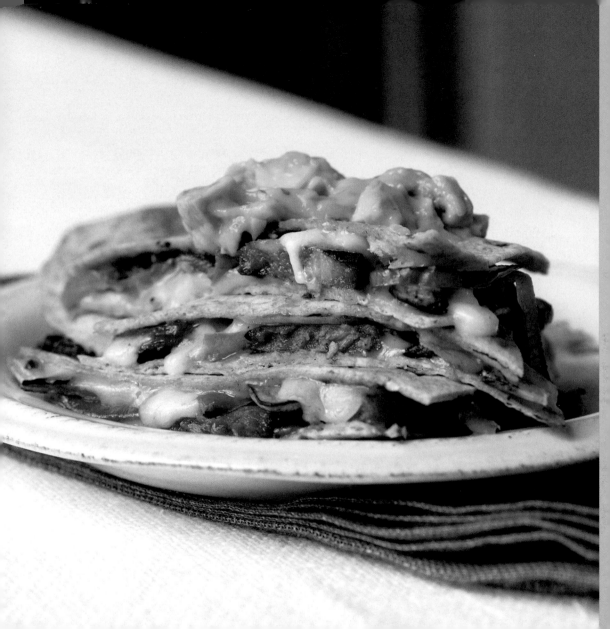

Sliders, 2 Ways

Unless it's dessert, never order anything on a restaurant menu with the word "mini" in it. Sounds counterintuitive, but so-called mini bites come with maximum fat saturation. These tasty burger bites, however, deliver huge flavor for a truly mini caloric price tag.

Mushroom–Blue Cheese Sliders

You'll Need:

- 2 tsp olive oil
- 1 clove garlic, minced
- 1½ cups sliced mushrooms
- Salt and black pepper to taste
- ½ lb ground sirloin
- 2 Tbsp steak sauce
- ¼ cup crumbled blue cheese
- 4 small soft rolls, about 2" in diameter (Martin's mini potato rolls are perfect for the job)

How to Make It:

- Heat a cast-iron skillet or sauté pan over medium heat. Add the oil and garlic and sauté for 60 seconds, until fragrant but not brown. Add the mushrooms and sauté for 2 to 3 minutes, until the mushrooms are nicely caramelized. Season with salt and pepper.

- Heat a grill pan or cast-iron skillet over medium heat. Season the sirloin with salt and pepper; form into 4 patties, being careful not to overwork the meat (which will create dense, chewy patties). Brush each patty with steak sauce. When the pan is hot, add the burgers and cook for 3 minutes on the first side, then flip. Add the blue cheese crumbles to the cooked side and continue grilling for another 2 to 3 minutes, until the patties are firm and the cheese has begun to melt.

- Remove the burgers. While the pan is still hot, toast the rolls. Brush them with a bit more steak sauce if you like, then top each with a burger and mushrooms.

Makes 4 appetizer servings or 2 meal servings / Cost per serving: $1.17

320 calories
18 g fat (7 g saturated)
400 mg sodium
(average of both)

Chipotle-Bacon Sliders

You'll Need:

- 2 Tbsp mayonnaise
- 1 Tbsp chipotle pepper
- ½ lb ground sirloin
- Salt and black pepper to taste
- ½ oz shredded sharp Cheddar cheese
- 4 small soft rolls, about 2" in diameter
- 4 strips cooked bacon
- Caramelized Onions (see page 305)

How to Make It:

- Mix the mayo and chipotle pepper. Prepare and cook the burgers as described to the left, omitting the steak sauce and subbing Cheddar for the blue cheese. Spread the rolls with a bit of the mayo mixture, then top with the burgers, bacon, and caramelized onions.

Makes 4 appetizer servings or 2 meal servings/ Cost per serving: $3.01

1,268 calories
79 g fat
75 g carbohydrates

Not That!

Ruby Tuesday Bacon Cheese Minis (4)
Price: $8.99

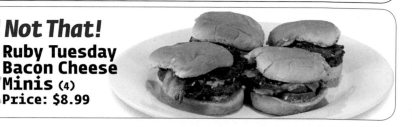

Save!
968 calories and $6.90! (on average)

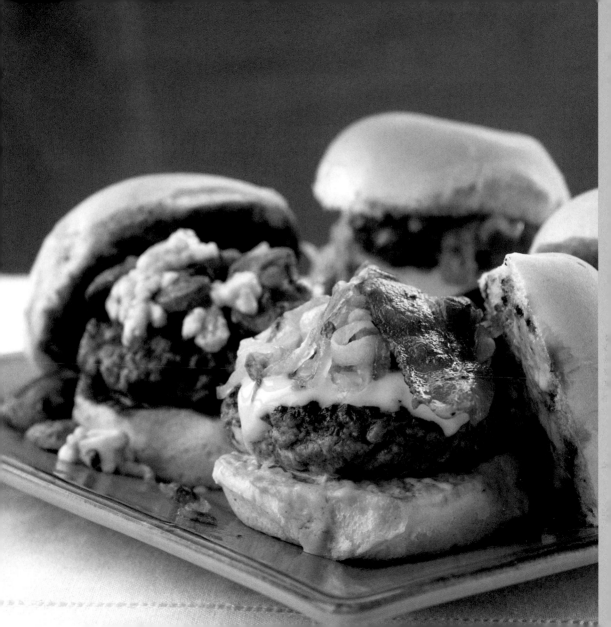

Crab Cakes with Mango-Avocado Salsa

In the skilled hands of a four-star chef or a seafaring Maryland man, the goal of a crab cake is simple: Use just enough ingredients to build flavor and bind the cakes, but never at the expense of the crab itself. The goal of the corporate cook is quite different: Make an inexpensive crab cake that will hold together under duress and leave them wanting more. That's why mayo and a deep fryer are invariably part of the process. Our cakes take the former route.

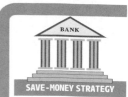

SAVE-MONEY STRATEGY

Crab—even canned crab—can be one of the most expensive ingredients in the supermarket, making crab cakes a fairly pricey endeavor. If you want to lighten the blow to the wallet, buy the regular (i.e., nonlump) canned stuff, which is considerably more affordable. Better yet, sub in a pound of fresh shrimp for the crab. Simply pulse the peeled and deveined shrimp a few times in the food processor, then follow the rest of the recipe. You'll save about 2 bucks a serving.

You'll Need:

- 1 can (16 oz) jumbo lump crab meat
- 2 Tbsp minced jalapeño
- 2 scallions, chopped
- ½ cup minced red bell pepper
- 1 egg, lightly beaten
- 2 tsp Dijon mustard

Juice of 1 lemon

- ¼ tsp Old Bay seasoning
- ½ tsp salt
- ¾ cup bread crumbs

Mango-Avocado Salsa (see page 174)

How to Make It:

- Preheat the oven to 425°F.
- Gently mix everything but ½ cup of the bread crumbs. Using your hands, loosely form the crab mixture into 8 patties.
- Spread the remaining bread crumbs on a plate and roll each crab cake over the crumbs to lightly and evenly coat. As the cakes are formed, place them on a nonstick baking sheet or in a baking dish coated with nonstick cooking spray. If the patties are misshaped, use the palm of your hand to press them down into an evenly shaped disk, the size of a small hockey puck.
- Bake until golden brown on the outside, 12 to 15 minutes. Serve with a scoop of Mango Salsa.

Makes 4 servings / Cost per serving: $3.38

Don't love mangoes? Improvise a healthy tartar by mixing equal parts mayo and plain yogurt with chopped pickles, capers, and fresh lemon juice.

240 calories
3.5 g fat
(0.5 g saturated)
800 mg sodium

1,037 calories

Not That!
California Pizza Kitchen Blue Crab Cakes
Price: $10.79

Save!
797 calories and $7.41!

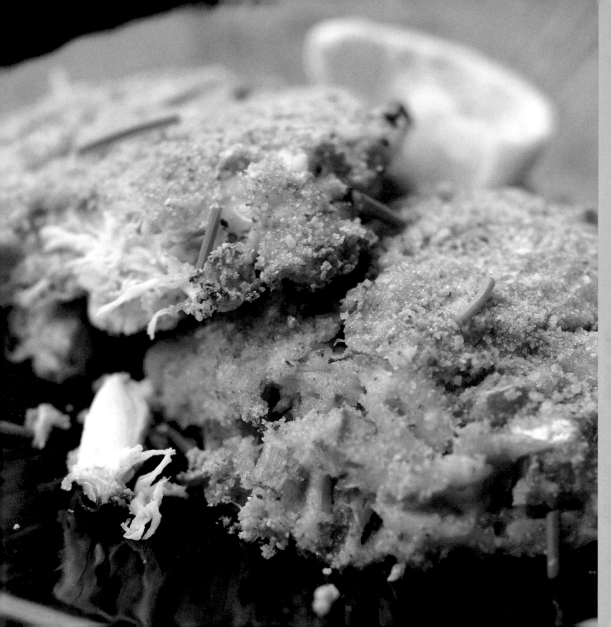

Nachos with Chicken & Black Beans

We've never found a nacho worth recommending in the restaurant world. The sad truth is that the tortilla chips are rendered a helpless vessel for thousands of calories of cheese, sour cream, and oily ground beef. And besides, who wants to dig through soggy nacho detritus in search of a chip crisp enough to bring from plate to mouth? This version ensures that every chip is evenly covered with protein-packed chicken and fiber-rich beans, plus enough salsa and lime-spiked sour cream to keep your mouth watering.

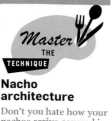

Master THE **TECHNIQUE**

Nacho architecture

Don't you hate how your nachos arrive covered in copious amounts of cheese and greasy add-ons, only to find the toppings all but disappear as you work through the layers? The secret to a great nacho is balance. Put too much on and that little chip grows soggy and overburdened. Add too little and they're not really nachos, are they? To hit the sweet spot, spread a single layer of chips (the bigger, the better) on a baking sheet. Start with beans, followed by cheese, meats, and vegetables. Save all cold toppings (guac, salsa, etc.) for after the nachos emerge from the oven.

You'll Need:

- 6 oz tortilla chips (round chips are preferable) •
- 1 can (16 oz) black beans, rinsed and drained
- 1½ cups shredded Monterey Jack cheese
- 1 cup cooked chicken, shredded
- ½ red onion, diced

Juice of 2 limes
- ½ cup light sour cream

Chopped cilantro

Salsa (either fresh, page 174, or your favorite bottled salsa)

Pickled Jalapeños (see page 304)

Want to boost fiber and lower the calorie content? Garden of Eatin' Black Bean are the best tortilla chips in America.

How to Make It:

- Preheat the oven to 425°F. Arrange the chips in a single layer on a large baking sheet. Spoon the beans evenly over the chips, then top with the cheese, chicken, and onion. Bake for 15 to 20 minutes, until the cheese is fully melted and bubbling. Remove.

- Combine the lime juice, sour cream, and cilantro. Spoon over the nachos. Top with the salsa and jalapeños.

Makes 6 appetizer servings / Cost per serving: $2.65

330 calories
12 g fat (6 g saturated)
500 mg sodium

2,020 calories
110 g fat
(41 g saturated)
2,980 mg sodium

Not That!
Baja Fresh Charbroiled Chicken Nachos
Price: $7.59

Save!
1,690 calories
and $4.94!

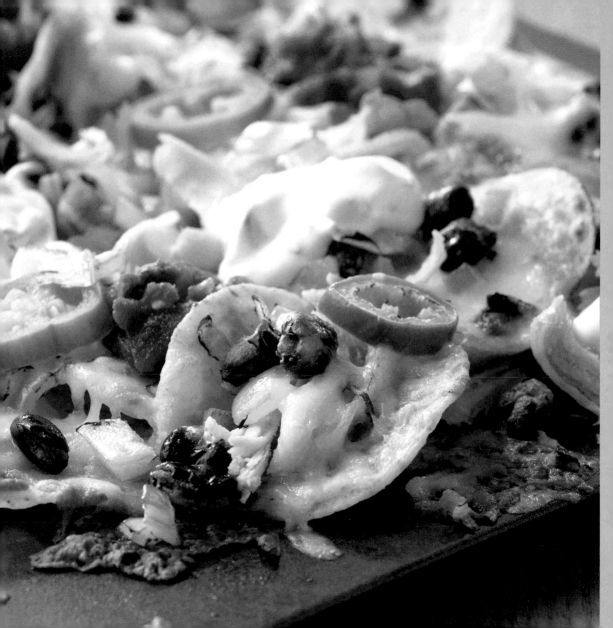

Tuna Satay Skewers

Appetizer sections are home to the densest caloric concentrations on America's menus. It's hard to find anything in the starters section that hasn't touched the deep fryer or isn't built entirely out of refined carbs and cheap fat. What you really want to start your meal with is a big dose of protein: Not only does it get your metabolism firing, protein also keeps your belly full, which helps ward off overeating later in the meal. Luckily, these grilled tuna skewers are nearly pure protein.

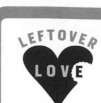

LEFTOVER LOVE

You'll Need:

½ Tbsp peanut or vegetable oil

1 Tbsp minced fresh ginger

1 clove garlic, minced

2 Tbsp peanut butter

1 cup light coconut milk

½ Tbsp low-sodium soy sauce

Juice of 1 lime

1 tsp sriracha or other hot sauce

1 lb ahi tuna, cut into 8 long pieces

Even easier than mincing ginger is shredding it on a cheese grater.

How to Make It:

• Soak 8 wooden skewers in cold water for at least 20 minutes.

• Heat the oil in a medium saucepan over medium heat. Cook the ginger and garlic until lightly toasted, about 1 minute. Add the peanut butter, coconut milk, and soy sauce. Simmer on low heat for 10 minutes. Add the lime juice and sriracha and remove from the heat.

• Heat a grill or stovetop grill pan until hot. Thread each piece of tuna onto a skewer and brush all over with the sauce. Cook for 2 minutes per side, until charred on the outside but still pink in the center. Serve the skewers with the remaining sauce.

Makes 4 servings / Cost per serving: $3.32

Find yourself with more peanut sauce than you need for the tuna? Perfect. It will keep in the fridge for up to 3 days and is perfect for quick stir-fries on busy weeknights. Heat a wok or sauté pan over high heat; sauté chicken, beef, or pork with broccoli, asparagus, bell peppers, and onions. When the produce and protein are almost fully cooked, dump in the peanut sauce, along with a splash of water or chicken broth to thin it out. Cook for 2 to 3 minutes more. Serve sprinkled with crushed peanuts and accompanied by lime wedges.

300 calories
8 g fat (2 g saturated)
270 mg sodium

1,750 calories
58 g saturated fat
1,300 mg sodium

Not That!

Cheesecake Factory Wasabi Crusted Ahi Tuna
Price: $21.95

Save!
1,450 calories and $18.63!

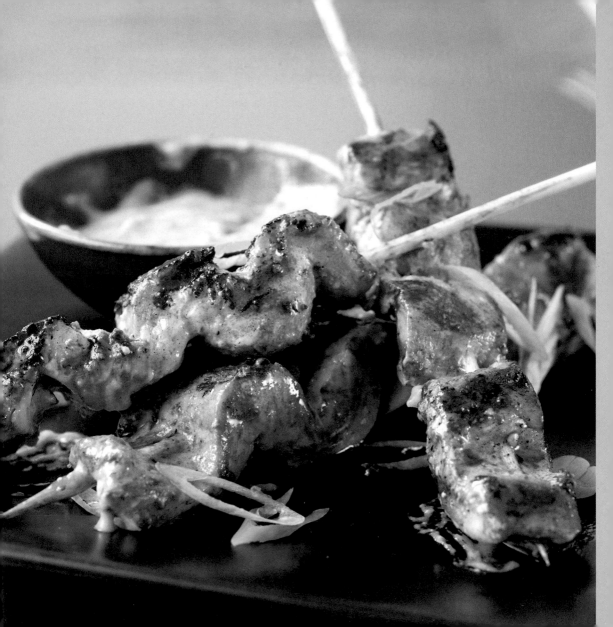

Cook This!
Bruschetta, 2 Ways

Bruschetta, the Italians' answer to chips and salsa, can make a perfectly healthy beginning to a meal. That's why it's especially shocking to see that restaurants like Carrabba's can turn a simple creation into a full-blown caloric calamity. Start your meal with something like this and you can forget about the rest of dinner (and breakfast the next morning).

You'll Need:

1 **baguette, cut on the diagonal into ½" slices**

TOMATO-BASIL

2 **large tomatoes, seeded and chopped**

2 **cloves garlic, minced**

½ **cup chopped fresh basil**

1 **Tbsp olive oil**

Salt and black pepper to taste

Italians don't love raw garlic, so instead they simply cut a clove in half and rub it across the toasted bread. Feel free to follow suit.

PEPPERONATA

½ **cup part-skim ricotta**

2 **cups Pepperonata (see page 305), warmed**

Make a big batch and save the leftovers to stuff into an omelet or scatter across sandwiches and pizza.

How to Make It:

- Preheat the oven to 450°F. Place the baguette slices on a baking sheet and bake until light brown (but still soft in the middle).

- While the bread bakes, mix the tomatoes, garlic, basil, and olive oil. Season to taste with salt and pepper.

- Remove the bread from the oven and arrange on a large serving plate or individual plates. Top half with the tomato mixture. Slather the other half with the ricotta, then top with a small scoop of the peppers.

Makes 4 appetizer servings / Cost per serving: $3.38

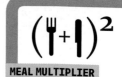

MEAL MULTIPLIER

These five flavor combinations also make beautiful bruschetta.

- Canned chickpeas sautéed with tomatoes and diced jalapeño
- Jarred tapenade (garlicky olive paste) and feta
- Sautéed Spinach (see page 295) and shaved Parmesan
- Canned white beans sautéed with jarred artichoke hearts
- Pan-Roasted Mushrooms (see page 295)

240 calories
7 g fat (2 g saturated)
410 mg sodium

1,119 calories

Not That!
Carrabba's Grilled Bruschette
Price: $7.50

Save!
879 calories and $4.12!

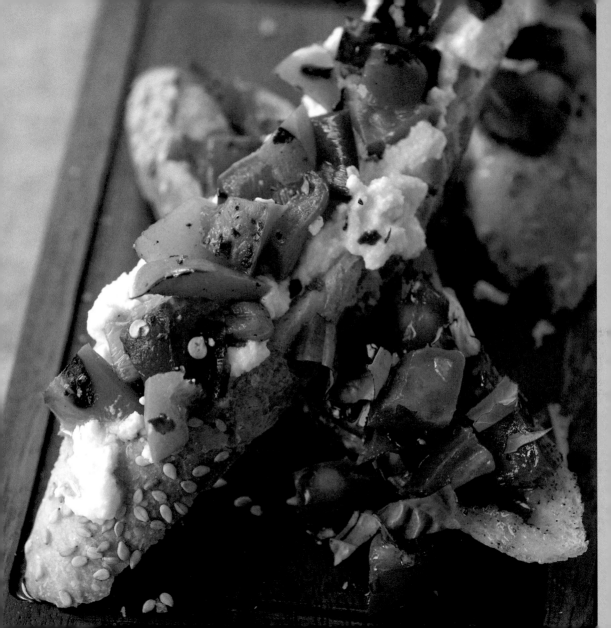

Chicken Fingers with Chipotle-Honey

Whether shaped like nuggets, stars, crowns, or fingers, deep-fried chicken bites do a major disservice to one of the planet's best sources of protein. Let the restaurant coat it in one of their special sauces and you could be downing nearly a full day's worth of calories on a food designed for children. In fact, Chili's popular Crispers pack in more calories than a dozen Fresco Beef Tacos from Taco Bell and more sodium than 24 small bags of Lay's potato chips. Make the switch to this oven-fried version once a week and you'll shed 25 pounds (and cut out 210,080 milligrams of sodium) in a year.

You'll Need:

- 1 lb boneless, skinless chicken tenders
- Salt and black pepper to taste
- 3 egg whites, lightly beaten
- 2 cups panko bread crumbs
- 2 Tbsp Dijon mustard
- 1 tsp chipotle pepper puree
- 1 Tbsp honey

How to Make It:

- Preheat the oven to 450°F. Season the chicken with salt and pepper. Place the egg whites in a shallow bowl. Place the crumbs on a plate and season those, too. Dip the chicken tenders into the egg, then toss in the crumbs, being sure to coat fully.

- Place the breaded chicken pieces on a baking sheet coated with nonstick cooking spray and bake for 10 to 12 minutes, until the crumbs have browned and the chicken is firm.

- Combine the mustard, chipotle, and honey in a large bowl. Toss the cooked chicken tenders in the mixture so they are all evenly coated with the spicy-sweet sauce.

Makes 4 servings / Cost per serving: $2.00

This dish is perfect for chicken finger-loving kids. Just be sure to cut the chiles from the sauce.

250 calories
1.5 g fat (0 g saturated)
350 mg sodium

SECRET WEAPON

Panko bread crumbs

Most oven-fried foods lack the satisfying crunch that comes with a long soak in bubbling fat. But trade in your blue canister of flavorless bread crumbs for this Japanese variety and you'll have the delicious crust of fried chicken without all the calories. Panko bread crumbs are coarse and flat, which provides an enduringly crunchy crust on any food they coat. Find a box in the international section of your supermarket or score them online at asianfoodgrocer.com.

Not That!

Chili's Crispy Honey-Chipotle Crispers
Price: $8.99

1,930 calories
108 g fat (17 g saturated)
4,390 mg sodium

Save!
1,680 calories and $6.99!

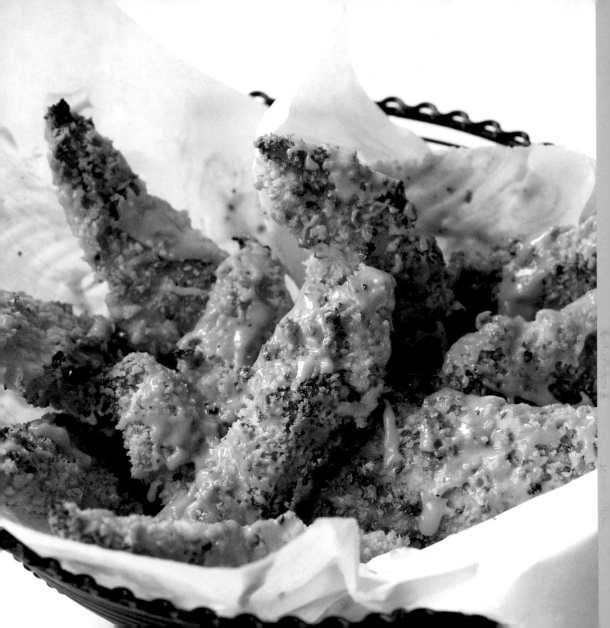

Melted Brie with Vegetables

To love the taste of melted cheese is to be an American. But the concept of breading sticks of cheese and dropping them into hot fat is an exercise in excess that we simply can't get behind. If cheese is the focus, surround it with a strong supporting cast. Brie is the unquestionable star here, but the sautéed vegetables add plenty of vital substance.

You'll Need:

- 1 wedge (6 oz) very cold brie (do not remove rind)
- ½ Tbsp olive oil
- 1 red onion, sliced
- 1 red bell pepper, sliced
- 1 ripe but firm pear, peeled and sliced •
- 1 medium zucchini, halved lengthwise and sliced
- ½ cup dry white wine
- Fresh thyme leaves (optional)
- Salt and black pepper to taste
- 12 slices baguette, toasted

How to Make It:

- Preheat the oven to 325°F. Place the brie wedge in the center of a large sheet of foil. Fold the foil over the brie, leaving some air space between the top of the wedge and the foil. Seal the edges to create a packet. Place the brie on a baking sheet and bake for 10 to 12 minutes, until very soft and oozing but not completely melted.

- Meanwhile, heat the oil in a large skillet or sauté pan over medium heat. Cook the onion and pepper until soft and lightly caramelized, about 5 minutes, then add the pear and zucchini and cook for another 3 minutes. Pour in the wine and add the thyme (if using); cook until most of the liquid has evaporated, 2 to 3 minutes. Season with salt and pepper.

- Transfer the vegetables to a large serving platter. Remove the hot, oozing brie from the packet and dump directly on top of the vegetables. Surround with the toasted baguette.

*Makes 6 appetizer servings /
Cost per serving: $2.94*

The pear may seem out of place with the slew of vegetables, but the sweetness is a perfect match.

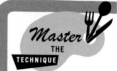

Master
THE
TECHNIQUE

Sautéeing vegetables

To get vegetables right every time take the following steps: First, cut everything to a similar size and shape. Next, stagger vegetables based on their cooking time, starting with firm veggies like peppers and carrots and ending with quick-cooking items like zucchini and peas. Finally, season at the right time. Salt early and vegetables give off liquid and create steam for a soft cook. If you're looking for caramelization, salt at the last second.

*310 calories
10 g fat (5 g saturated)
610 mg sodium*

970 calories

Not That!
IHOP Monster Mozza Sticks
Price: $4.99

Save!
*660 calories
and $2.05!*

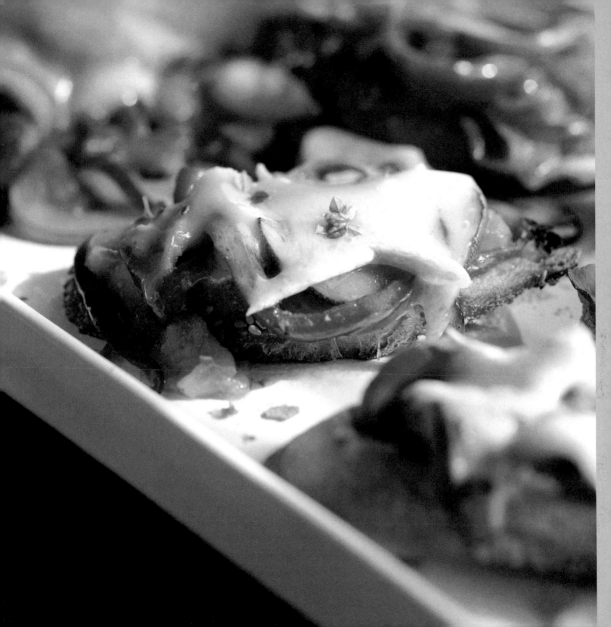

Chicken Pot Stickers

If you see these little Chinese dumplings on a menu, order them; even in their worst iteration (like the oily pan-fried version from T.G.I. Friday's), they trump 90 percent of the other items in the appetizer section. Luckily, making them at home is a 10-minute project and allows you to cut calories and boost nutrition by spiking the dish with mushrooms and snap peas. This works great as an appetizer for four, or you can cut the recipe down and make it a lean mean meal for one.

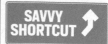

SAVVY SHORTCUT

Frozen pot stickers

You could go through the trouble of rolling out dough, making the filling, and pinching these little pockets of joy together by hand, but why bother when the frozen variety is perfectly delicious and usually quite healthy? Keep a bag or two on hand for quick weeknight dinners (either steamed or boiled, then pan-fried with fresh vegetables) or crowd-pleasing starters for your next dinner party. Our favorite version hails from Trader Joe's, but most markets carry a reliable rendition.

You'll Need:

- 24 **frozen pot stickers (chicken, pork, or vegetable)**
- 1 **Tbsp sesame or peanut oil**
- 4 **oz mushrooms (preferably shiitake), stems removed, sliced**
- 2 **cups sugar snap or snow peas, tough ends removed**
- 1 **Tbsp soy sauce**
- 1 **Tbsp rice wine vinegar**
- **Sriracha to taste**
- **Sesame seeds** (optional) •——
- **Sliced scallions** (optional)

How to Make It:

- Bring a large pot of water to a boil. Drop in the pot stickers and cook for a few minutes until tender but not gummy. Drain.

- Heat the oil a large nonstick skillet or sauté pan over medium heat. Add the mushrooms and cook for 2 to 3 minutes, until lightly browned. Add the cooked pot stickers to the pan and cook, undisturbed, until crispy and brown on the bottom, about 2 to 3 minutes per side. In the last minute of cooking, toss in the snap peas and warm through.

- Remove from the heat, stir in the soy sauce, vinegar, and sriracha. Divide among 4 bowls and garnish with sesame seeds and scallions (if using).

Makes 4 servings / Cost per serving: $3.92

Sesame seeds are a top source of magnesium, which help reduce stress and fight high blood pressure.

200 calories
9 g fat (2 g saturated)
520 mg sodium

830 calories

Not That!
T.G.I. Friday's Pot Stickers
Price: $7.49

Save!
630 calories and $3.57!

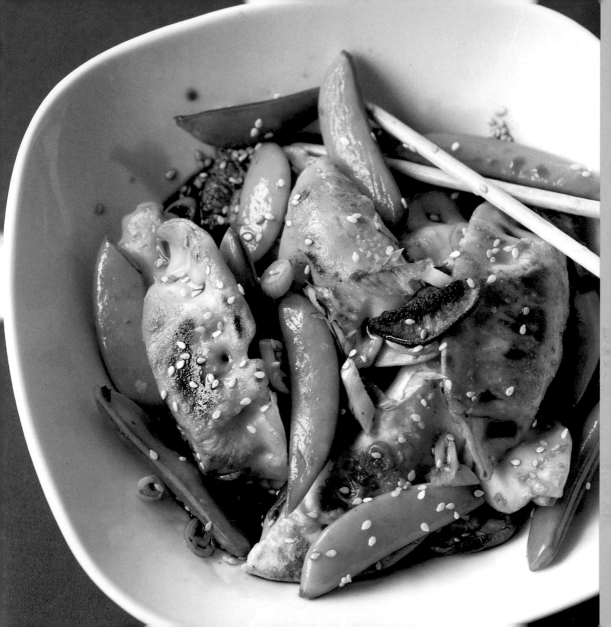

Mini Pizzas, 3 Ways

Personal pies are the bane of the pizza experience. Many pizza joints load individual pizzas with more than a day's worth of fat and sodium (and in the case of this Uno bomb, more than 2 days' worth of each). English muffins come with built-in portion control so no matter how lavishly you adorn them, you won't break the 400-calorie barrier.

Tomato Sauce

You'll Need:

1 can (14 oz) whole peeled tomatoes

½ tsp kosher salt

½ Tbsp olive oil

3–4 turns of a black-pepper mill

How to Make It:

- Combine the ingredients in a food processor or blender and pulse briefly until blended but still slightly chunky.

193 calories
8 g fat (4 g saturated)
563 mg sodium
(average of all)

Hawaiian

You'll Need:

¼ cup Tomato Sauce

2 English muffins, split

1 cup shredded mozzarella

2 slices deli ham, cut into strips

½ cup pineapple chunks

16 slices Pickled Jalapeños (see page 304)

How to Make It:

- Preheat the oven to 425°F. Spread the sauce among the 4 muffin halves, then top with cheese, ham, pineapple, and jalapeños. Place on a baking sheet and bake for 15 to 20 minutes, until the cheese is melted and bubbling and the bottoms of the English muffins are slightly crisp.

Pesto–Goat Cheese

You'll Need:

2 Tbsp basil pesto

2 English muffins, split

4 Tbsp goat cheese

2 Tbsp chopped green or kalamata olives

Red onion slices

4 bottled or canned artichoke hearts, quartered

How to Make It:

- Preheat the oven to 425°F. Divide the pesto among the 4 muffin halves, then top with the remaining ingredients. Place on a baking sheet and bake for 15 to 20 minutes, until the cheese is melted and the bottoms of the English muffins are slightly crisp.

Sausage and Pepper

You'll Need:

¼ cup Tomato Sauce

2 English muffins, split

1 cup shredded mozzarella

Cooked chicken sausage, sliced (Al Fresco and Bruce Aidell both make excellent products)

Pepperonata (see page 305) or ¼ cup roasted red peppers

Red pepper flakes

Fresh basil leaves

How to Make It:

- Preheat the oven to 425°F. Divide the sauce among the 4 muffin halves, then top with the cheese, sausage, and peppers; season with the pepper flakes. Place on a baking sheet and bake for 15 to 20 minutes, until the cheese is melted and bubbling and the bottoms of the English muffins are slightly crisp. Garnish with the basil.

Each recipe makes 4 appetizer servings / Average cost per serving: $1.87

2,310 calories
165 g fat (54 g saturated)
4,920 mg sodium

Not That!
Uno Chicago Classic Individual Deep Dish Pizza
Price: $10.50

Save!
2,117 calories and $8.63 (on average)

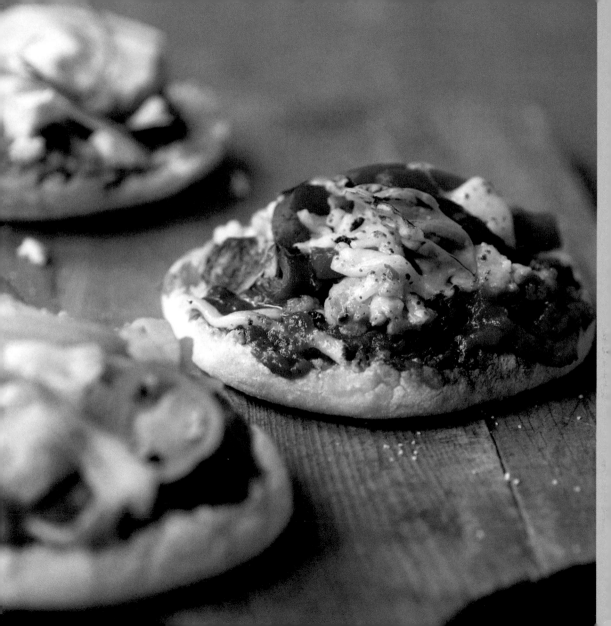

Spicy Potato Skins

In 1974, T.G.I. Friday's gave birth to the potato skin. That timeworn combination of potato, Cheddar, and bacon has since made its rounds across the menus of America, infiltrating nearly every pocket of this country with hypercaloric, frighteningly fatty facsimiles. We'll take this version—true to the original but with a few delicious twists—any day.

$$(\text{\Psi} + \text{\textbar})^2$$

MEAL MULTIPLIER

Truth be told, while these potato skins are a vast improvement on the kind offered by Friday's and their ilk, you could make some improvements by folding any of dozens of different vegetables and healthy flavor additions into the formula outlined here. Simply replace the bacon, Cheddar, and sour cream with the following:

- Steamed broccoli and Parmesan
- Sundried tomatoes, chopped olives, artichoke hearts, and pesto
- Caramelized onions and goat cheese
- Chicken, asparagus, and roasted red peppers

You'll Need:

- 4 small russet potatoes
- Olive oil
- Salt and black pepper to taste
- 1 cup 2% milk
- 2 Tbsp butter
- ½ cup shredded sharp Cheddar cheese, plus more for garnish
- 4 scallions, chopped, plus more for garnish
- ½ Tbsp minced chipotle pepper
- ¼ cup sour cream
- 6 strips bacon, cooked and crumbled
- Pickled Jalapeños (see page 304), optional

How to Make It:

- Preheat the oven to 400°F. Rub the potatoes with a bit of olive oil and lightly salt the skins. Bake for 35 to 40 minutes, until tender.

- Cut the potatoes in half and, when cool enough to handle, carefully scoop out the warm flesh into a bowl (leave a thin layer of potato intact around the skin to help prevent it from tearing). Add the milk, butter, cheese, and scallions and stir with a wooden spoon until smooth. Season with salt and pepper.

- Preheat the broiler. Carefully scoop the mashed potatoes into the hollowed-out potato halves. Top with a bit of extra cheese and place under the broiler until the tops are brown and crispy, 3 to 5 minutes.

- Mix the chipotle with the sour cream and place a dollop on top of each cooked potato. Finish each with a bit of crumbled bacon and jalapeños.

Makes 4 servings /
Cost per serving: $1.28

310 calories
11 g fat (5 g saturated)
490 mg sodium

1,310 calories

Not That!

T.G.I. Friday's Loaded Potato Skins (half order)
Price: $6.69

Save!
1,000 calories and $5.41!

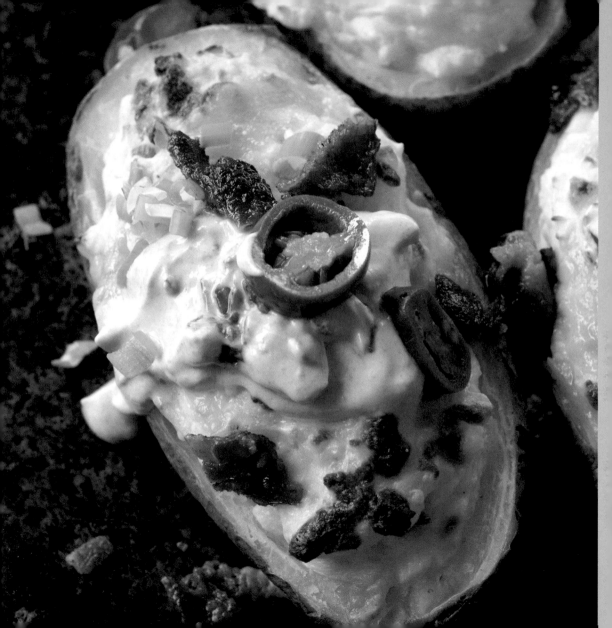

Chapter

5

Cook This, Not That!

Soups
&
Salads

When did "healthy" food get so bad for us?
And how do we rescue it?
You'll find the answers to both within.

Theoretically, having more choices is a good thing. But when ordering a coffee at Starbucks is like doing a mini dissertation in some vaguely Romantic language, and when picking out a jar of jelly at the supermarket requires an encyclopedic knowledge of every berry known to man, choices start to get overwhelming. Which is why, at the end of the day, when somebody asks, "Soup or salad?" most of us would rather bury our faces under the napkin than make even one more decision.

How Restaurants Turned Lettuce into a Junk Food

But your soups and your salads are critical. You know how the USDA wants you to get between five and nine servings of fruits and vegetables a day? And how, if you count the little red crispy things in the box of Franken Berry you ate that morning, maybe you got two? Well, think of the soup and the salad as your extra credit, your personal ace in the hole—the tiny little bit you do on the side that skyrockets your daily nutritional score from a C+ to an A-. A well-crafted soup or salad can give you three or four servings of vegetables and fruits, and presto, you go from failing the nutritional test to passing with flying colors. (And your best bet is to eat them first, before your big meal. When subjects in one study had a small bowl of chunky vegetable soup 15 minutes before their dinner, they ate a total of 20 percent fewer calories—even when you count the calories in the soup!)

But you're not always doing yourself a favor when said salad or soup comes from one of America's chain restaurants. At T.G.I. Friday's, for example, six out of seven salads on their menu come with 900 crunchy calories or more, including their almost pathological corruption of the entire salad concept, the Pecan Crusted Chicken Salad, with a whopping 1,360 calories. (You could have an all-you-can-eat buffet at Mr. McGregor's garden—and cook up a pot of Peter Rabbit stew on the side—and still not touch that calorie count.) So how you can cut down on calories, ring up your nutritional requirements, and not get bushwhacked by unexpected calories? This chapter of *Cook This, Not That!* is designed to give you personal power over your soups and salads, so the nutritional gods—and members of the opposite sex—will smile upon you.

Cook This!
The Dressing Matrix

Pop quiz: Most bottled salad dressing is a) overpriced, b) awash in excess sodium, c) polluted with dubious food additives, or d) all of the above? If we told you the answer was d, would you start making your own dressings at home? What if we also told you that you're never more than 60 seconds away from a perfectly balanced batch of dressing that could last for a week in your fridge? Would you be interested in that? Yeah, we thought so. Here's what you do:

Four Instant Salad Upgrades

Wind your way down the matrix and you're guaranteed to strike dressing gold. Consider these four inspiration for your own creations.

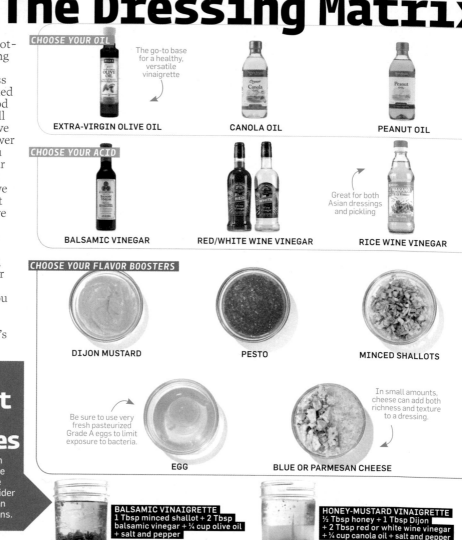

CHOOSE YOUR OIL

The go-to base for a healthy, versatile vinaigrette

EXTRA-VIRGIN OLIVE OIL

CANOLA OIL

PEANUT OIL

CHOOSE YOUR ACID

Great for both Asian dressings and pickling

BALSAMIC VINEGAR

RED/WHITE WINE VINEGAR

RICE WINE VINEGAR

CHOOSE YOUR FLAVOR BOOSTERS

DIJON MUSTARD

PESTO

MINCED SHALLOTS

Be sure to use very fresh pasteurized Grade A eggs to limit exposure to bacteria.

In small amounts, cheese can add both richness and texture to a dressing.

EGG

BLUE OR PARMESAN CHEESE

BALSAMIC VINAIGRETTE
1 Tbsp minced shallot + 2 Tbsp balsamic vinegar + ¼ cup olive oil + salt and pepper

HONEY-MUSTARD VINAIGRETTE
½ Tbsp honey + 1 Tbsp Dijon + 2 Tbsp red or white wine vinegar + ¾ cup canola oil + salt and pepper

The Rules of the Dressing

Step 1
Traditional vinaigrettes are made with 3 parts oil and 1 part vinegar or citrus. For a healthier (and livelier) dressing, start with a 2-to-1 ratio and adjust from there.

Step 2
Eggs and mustard are both emulsifiers, which means they help bind oil to vinegar smoothly and seamlessly. Add either and your dressing will be thicker, more uniform, and less acidic. If you don't like the idea of raw egg in your dressing, coddle the egg by cooking for about 60 seconds in boiling water.

Step 3
Vinaigrettes are normally made by slowly whisking the oil into the vinegar. The easier way to make one is to combine all the ingredients in a mason jar or other sealable glass jar and shake like crazy for 10 seconds. Simply pour what you need from the bottle, then store the rest sealed in the fridge for up to a week. Also great for sandwiches and any grilled food.

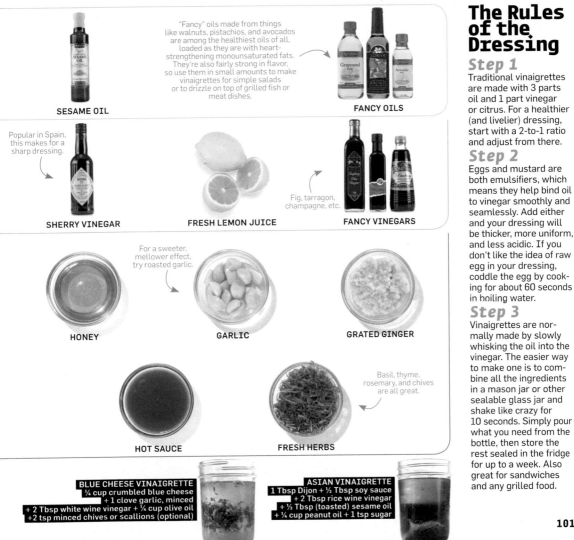

SESAME OIL

"Fancy" oils made from things like walnuts, pistachios, and avocados are among the healthiest oils of all, loaded as they are with heart-strengthening monounsaturated fats. They're also fairly strong in flavor, so use them in small amounts to make vinaigrettes for simple salads or to drizzle on top of grilled fish or meat dishes.

FANCY OILS

Popular in Spain, this makes for a sharp dressing.

SHERRY VINEGAR

FRESH LEMON JUICE

Fig, tarragon, champagne, etc.

FANCY VINEGARS

For a sweeter, mellower effect, try roasted garlic.

HONEY

GARLIC

GRATED GINGER

HOT SAUCE

FRESH HERBS

Basil, thyme, rosemary, and chives are all great.

BLUE CHEESE VINAIGRETTE
¼ cup crumbled blue cheese
+ 1 clove garlic, minced
+ 2 Tbsp white wine vinegar + ¼ cup olive oil
+ 2 tsp minced chives or scallions (optional)

ASIAN VINAIGRETTE
1 Tbsp Dijon + ½ Tbsp soy sauce
+ 2 Tbsp rice wine vinegar
+ ½ Tbsp (toasted) sesame oil
+ ¼ cup peanut oil + 1 tsp sugar

Grilled Caesar Salad

Caesar salad may be the most misleading food in America—it's the type of dish you order when you want to be good to your body, only to find out it's eating up half of your day's calories. This recipe transforms the high-calorie dressing into a lighter vinaigrette and adds substance, flavor, and nutrition in the form of sundried tomatoes and olives.

You'll Need:

DRESSING

2 Tbsp red wine vinegar

1 Tbsp mayonnaise

1 clove garlic, minced

2 anchovies (soak in milk for 10 minutes if you want to mellow the flavor)

1 tsp Worcestershire sauce

Juice of 1 lemon

6–8 turns of a black-pepper mill

½ cup olive oil

SALAD

4 hearts of romaine

2 English muffins, split

2 boneless, skinless chicken breasts (6–8 oz each)

Olive oil

Salt and black pepper to taste

¼ cup black or green olives, pitted and roughly chopped

¼ cup sundried tomatoes, chopped

¼ cup finely grated Parmesan

410 calories
29 g fat
(3.5 g saturated)
610 mg sodium

How to Make It:

- Preheat the grill. Combine all the dressing ingredients except the oil in a food processor and pulse to blend. With the motor running, slowly drizzle in the oil.

- Cut the romaine down the middle lengthwise, leaving the root end intact so the leaves hold together. Brush the romaine, English muffins, and chicken with olive oil and season with salt and pepper. When the grill is hot, add the chicken and grill for 4 to 5 minutes per side until firm and caramelized. Remove the chicken and allow to rest.

- Place the lettuce and English muffins on the grill. Cook the lettuce for 1 to 2 minutes, just enough to lightly char and wilt the leaves. Cook the English muffins until brown and crispy.

- Slice the chicken into thin strips. Cut the muffins into bite-size pieces. Arrange both, along with the olives and sundried tomatoes, over the individual lettuce halves. Drizzle with dressing and sprinkle with cheese.

Makes 4 servings /
Cost per serving: $3.76

Master THE TECHNIQUE

Grill outside the box

Seem strange to grill lettuce? How about potatoes? Or even peaches? Truth is, there are very few fresh foods that don't benefit from the char of a fiery grill. The concentrated heat teases out the natural sugars in food, which in turn creates caramelization (i.e., those nice grill marks) and extra layers of flavor. Test out the theory: Place a bunch of grapes directly over a low flame and turn a few times until soft (but still holding their shape). Toss with toasted almonds, feta, and baby spinach.

1,000 calories
64 g fat
(14.5 g saturated, 0.5 g trans)
2,380 mg sodium

Not That!

Quiznos Chicken Caesar Flatbread Salad (with bread)
Price: $5.89

Save!

590 calories and $2.13!

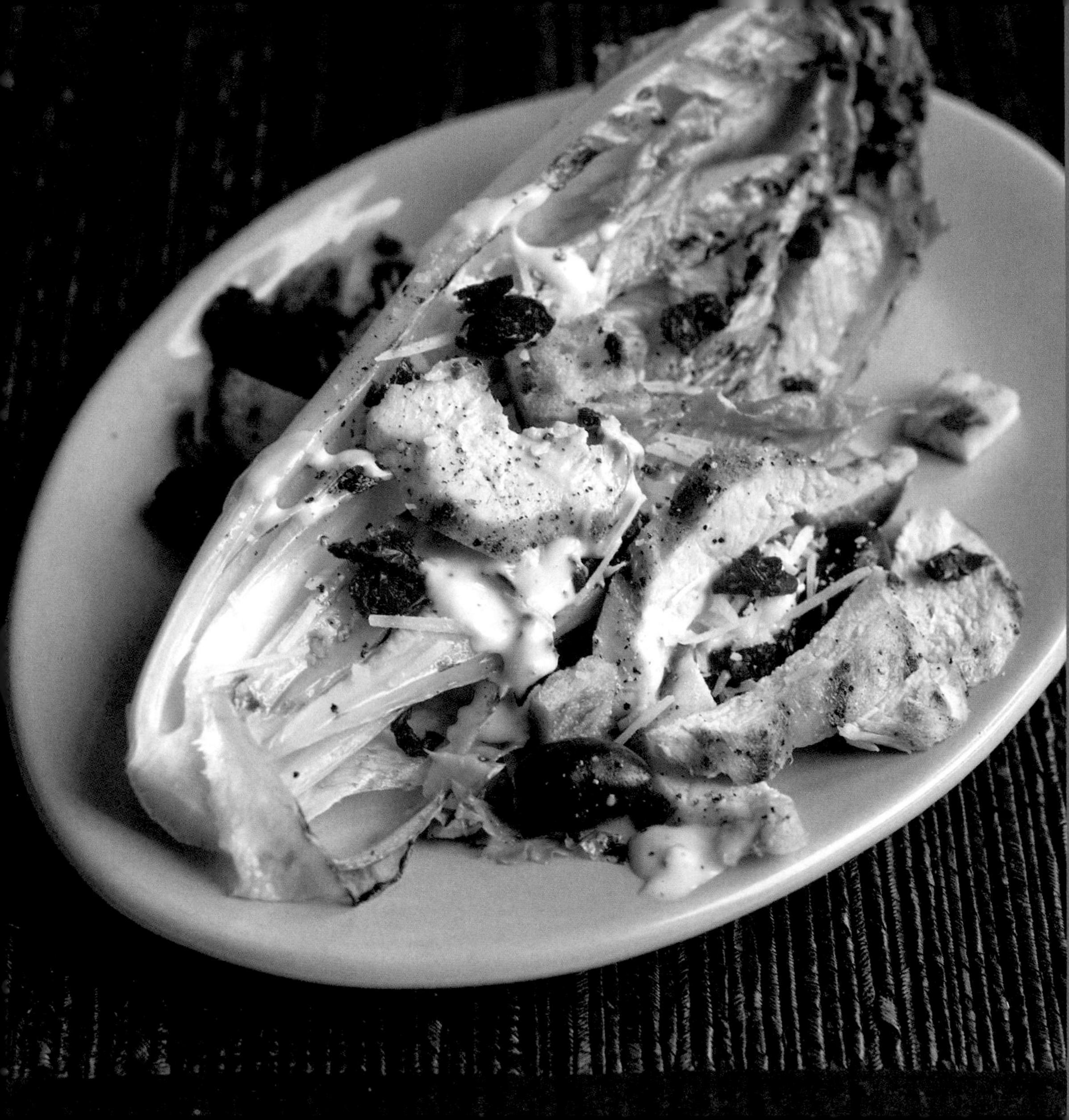

Warm Goat Cheese Salad

Can you believe that a salad with no meat and no cheese has more calories than a Wendy's Baconator and large fries? California Pizza Kitchen follows in the footsteps of nearly every other restaurant by serving their salads in troughs with buckets of dressing. If you want to drop 15 pounds this year, replace every restaurant salad you eat with a homemade version. Start with this one; the warm goat cheese crouton and sweet, crisp pear will make a salad believer out of anyone.

You'll Need:

- 1 log (4 oz) fresh goat cheese
- 1 cup bread crumbs
- 1 tsp dried thyme or Italian seasoning
- Salt and black pepper to taste
- 1 egg, lightly beaten
- ¼ cup walnuts
- 16 cups mixed greens or arugula (6-oz bag)
- Balsamic Vinaigrette (see page 100)
- 1 pear, peeled, cored, and sliced

How to Make It:

- Slice the goat cheese into four ½" disks (a piece of unflavored dental floss makes this job easy). If the cheese crumbles, use your hands to form it back into disks. Pour the bread crumbs onto a plate and toss with the thyme and a pinch each of salt and pepper.

- Dip the goat cheese into the egg, then into the crumb mixture and turn to coat evenly. Place the disks on a plate and into the freezer for 15 minutes to firm up.

- Preheat the oven to 450°F. Place the goat cheese on a baking sheet coated with nonstick cooking spray and bake for 10 minutes, until the cheese is soft and the crumbs are toasted. Remove. While the oven is still hot, toast the walnuts for 5 minutes.

- Toss the lettuce with the vinaigrette and pear. Divide among 4 cold plates. Top with the walnuts and goat cheese.

Makes 4 servings /
Cost per serving: $2.89

370 calories
22 g fat (6 g saturated)
660 mg sodium

1,372 calories

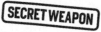

SECRET WEAPON

Fresh goat cheese

Break free from the reliance on Cheddar and mozzarella and discover some of the truly fantastic cheeses that too many serious eaters overlook. Fresh goat cheese has a tangy creaminess that makes it one of the most versatile in the dairy case, great for crumbling onto salads, spreading on sandwiches, or folding into warm pasta dishes. Our favorite goat cheeses are made by Cypress Grove Chevre and are available in supermarkets nationwide. An ounce has just 70 calories and 6 grams of fat, making it one of the healthiest cheeses you'll find.

Not That!

California Pizza Kitchen Field Greens Salad
Price: $10.29

Save!
1,002 calories and $7.40!

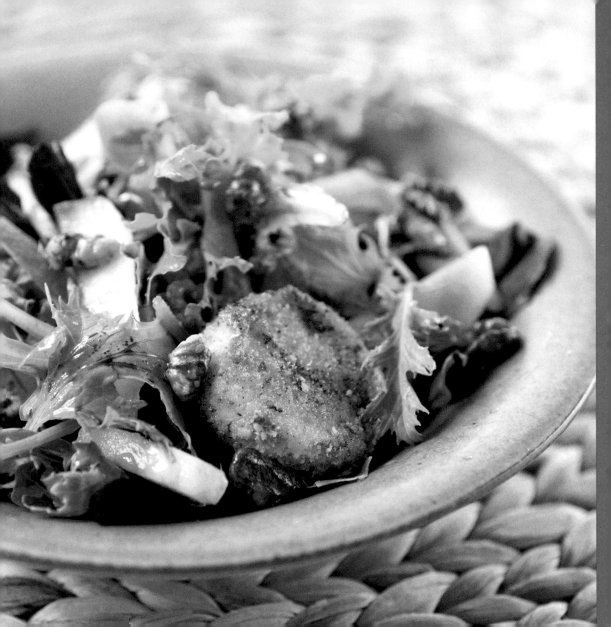

Spinach Salad with Warm Bacon Dressing

The word "spinach" creates a health halo for cooks and diners alike. People think that because the base of a salad is made with a superfood, the rest of the salad can be filled with whatever troubling toppings they like. That's how we end up with dozens of 1,000-calorie spinach salads at chain restaurants. This rendition smashes the halo to pieces.

You'll Need:

- 6 strips bacon, cut into small pieces
- ½ red onion, sliced
- 1 cup sliced mushrooms
- 8 oz shrimp, peeled and deveined
- Salt and black pepper to taste
- 2 Tbsp pine nuts
- 1 Tbsp Dijon mustard
- 3 Tbsp red wine vinegar
- Olive oil (optional)
- 1 bag (6 oz) baby spinach
- 2 hard-boiled eggs, sliced

How to Make It:

- Heat a large skillet or sauté pan over medium heat. Cook the bacon until crispy, 5 to 7 minutes. Use a slotted spoon to transfer to a paper towel on a plate and reserve.

- Add the onion and mushrooms to the hot pan and cook until the onions begin to brown, about 3 minutes. Season the shrimp with salt and pepper and add to the hot pan, along with the pine nuts. Cook until the shrimp are pink and firm, no more than 4 minutes (shrimp cook more quickly than nearly any other protein and no one likes overcooked shrimp). Stir the mustard and vinegar into the pan; season with salt and pepper. If the pan looks dry, add a splash of olive oil.

- Divide the spinach and eggs among 4 plates and top with the hot shrimp mixture and some of the liquid in the pan. Sprinkle with the bacon.

Makes 4 servings / Cost per serving: $4.48

Shrimp is one of nature's greatest sources of selenium, a micromineral that helps reduce joint inflammation and fight off cancer-causing free radicals.

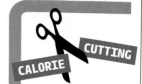

CALORIE CUTTING

So the idea of a warm bacon vinaigrette doesn't get you as excited as it gets us, huh? No worries. Replace the bacon in the recipe with a table-spoon of olive oil to begin with (for sautéing the vegetables, shrimp, and pine nuts) and another two on the back end, when you stir in the mustard and vinegar. You'll save about 75 calories per plate, plus you'll boost the meal with a solid dose of healthy mono-unsaturated fat.

220 calories
11 g fat (3 g saturated)
560 mg sodium

1,040 calories
11 g saturated
2,380 mg sodium

Not That!
Applebee's Grilled Shrimp 'N Spinach Salad
Price: $9.99

Save!
820 calories and $5.51!

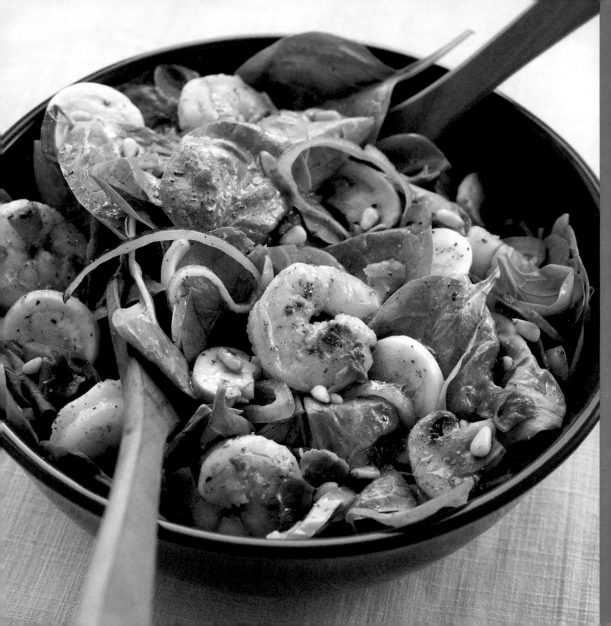

Caprese Tomato Towers

The classic tomato salad from Capri, Italy, is a study in simplicity: sweet, acidic tomatoes contrasted with creamy mozzarella slabs and the bright herbal bite of fresh basil. Why pay good money for such a simple pleasure you can make yourself only to let a restaurant screw it up with cheap parlor tricks? Make this one of your go-to summer salads.

You'll Need:

- 4 medium tomatoes (preferably different color heirloom tomatoes)
- 6 oz fresh mozzarella
- 16 large fresh basil leaves
- 1 Tbsp olive oil
- ½ tsp balsamic vinegar
- Salt and black pepper to taste

How to Make It:

- Slice the tomatoes into thick slices (each tomato should yield 4 or 5 slices). Slice the cheese into slightly thinner disks. There should be an equal number of tomato and cheese slices.
- Place a tomato in the center of small salad plate. Top with a mozzarella slice and a single basil leaf. Repeat until you've used up a quarter of the tomatoes, cheese, and basil (if you really want to nail this, salt and pepper each individual layer). If using different color tomatoes, alternate the slices throughout. Repeat with the rest of the tomatoes, cheese, and basil, making 4 towers in all. Drizzle each tower with a bit of olive oil and balsamic and season again with salt and pepper.

Makes 4 servings / Cost per serving: $3.20

Whether rare heirlooms or just a better beefsteak, tomatoes are best from farmers' markets. Seek out a local market and show up at the end of the day, when vendors are offering up great deals.

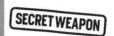

SECRET WEAPON

Heirloom tomatoes

This salad is probably not worth making in the winter, when lifeless tomatoes are flown in from below the equator. Come summer, though, when local tomatoes are abundant, there's nothing better to eat. Break out of the beefsteak box and explore the depth and variety of heirloom tomatoes now available. Each shape and color offers different levels of sweetness and acidity, and even just sliced and salted, make for an amazing salad.

170 calories
13 g fat (6 g saturated)
290 mg sodium

600 calories
36 g fat
(11 g saturated)
1,520 mg sodium

Not That!
Olive Garden Caprese Flatbread
Price: $6.35

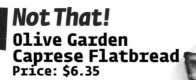

Save!
430 calories
and $3.15!

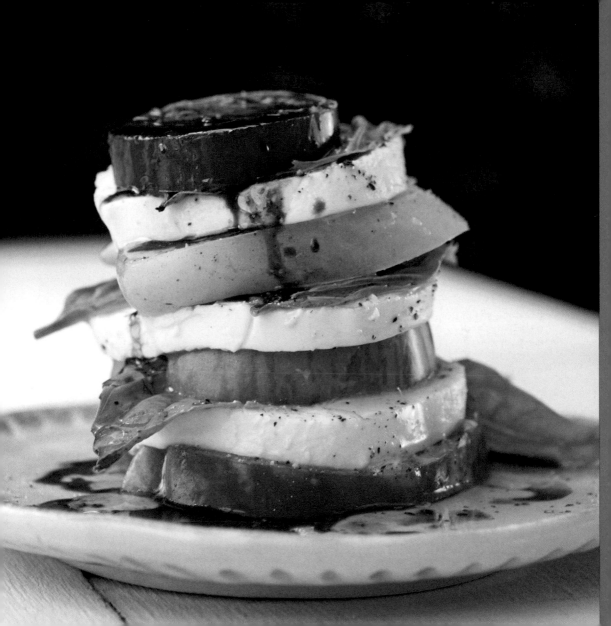

Grilled Chicken Salad

with Cranberries, Avocado, and Goat Cheese

There's no meal that's more necessary to make yourself than a salad. When put in the hands of a restaurant line cook, a harmless bowl of greens turns into an unmitigated mash-up of dressing deluges, cheese flurries, and crouton catastrophes. In fact, at CPK, the average entrée-size salad weighs in well above 1,000 calories! Make your salad in-house and you're guaranteed to cut that number in half.

You'll Need:

- 12 oz cooked chicken
- 12 cups arugula (1 prewashed bag)
- ¼ cup dried cranberries
- 1 avocado, pitted, peeled, and sliced
- ¼ cup crumbled goat cheese
- ¼ cup walnuts, roughly chopped
- ¼ cup Honey Mustard Vinaigrette (see page 100)
- Salt and black pepper to taste

How to Make It:

- Combine the chicken, arugula, cranberries, avocado, goat cheese, walnuts, vinaigrette, salt and pepper in a large bowl, using your hands or 2 forks to fully incorporate the dressing.

Makes 4 servings /
Cost per serving: $2.64

500 calories
24 g fat (3 g saturated)
660 mg sodium

Save!
1,144 calories
and $10.35!

1,644 calories

California Pizza Kitchen Waldorf Chicken Salad
Price: $12.99

STEP-BY-STEP

Pitting an avocado

No, you don't need to spend 45 minutes peeling the pebbly skin. Instead, follow these simple steps for all of your avocado needs.

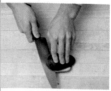

Step 1: *Work the blade carefully around the pit.*

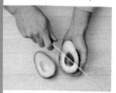

Step 2: *Thwack the pit with blade; twist and remove.*

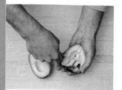

Step 3: *Slice or dice, then spoon out the soft flesh.*

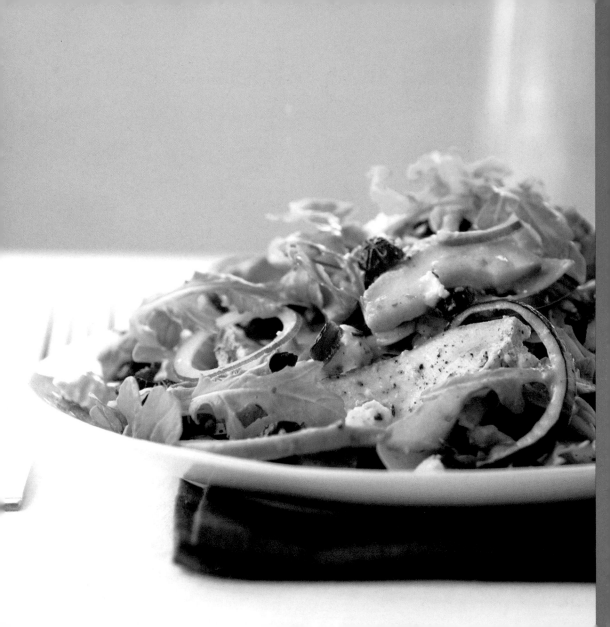

Tuna Niçoise

Tuna salad is a food industry euphemism for fish awash in a sea of mayo. But this French-inspired tuna salad may qualify as the healthiest meal in this (or any) cookbook. Tucked within the leaves are vitamin-dense green beans, lycopene-loaded cherry tomatoes, and omega-3-packed tuna, providing a perfect balance of protein, fiber, and healthy fat.

You'll Need:

4 eggs

Salt and black pepper to taste

1 lb red potatoes, quartered into ½" chunks

½ lb green beans, ends removed

2 tuna steaks (6 oz each)

16 cups baby mixed greens (8-oz bag)

¼ cup Honey-Mustard Vinaigrette (see page 100)

1 pint cherry tomatoes, sliced in half

¼ cup chopped black or green olives (kalamata and Niçoise are best)

How to Make It:

- Bring a large pot of water to a boil. Turn the heat to low until the water is just simmering and carefully lower in the eggs. Cook for 7 to 8 minutes (this should yield creamy, not chalky, yolks) and remove with a slotted spoon. Transfer to a bowl of cold water.

- Salt the same pot of water and add the potatoes. Cook for 15 to 20 minutes, until tender but not mushy. Right before the potatoes are done, toss in the green beans and cook for 3 to 5 minutes, until crisp-tender. (You can cook the green beans in their own pot, but why waste the water and the energy?) Drain both vegetables together.

- Heat a grill pan or cast-iron skillet over high heat. Season the tuna with salt and pepper. When the pan is very hot, add the tuna and cook for 2 minutes per side, until browned on the outside but still pink in the middle. Remove and let rest for a minute or two, then slice into thin strips.

- Peel the eggs and slice in half. Toss the greens with enough vinaigrette to just lightly cover. Divide among 4 chilled plates or bowls. In individual piles around the lettuce, arrange the potatoes, tomatoes, olives, green beans, and eggs. Top with slices of tuna and drizzle with extra vinaigrette, if you like.

Makes 4 servings /
Cost per serving: $5.14

350 calories
11 g fat (3 g saturated)
370 mg sodium

Not That!

Subway Tuna Salad with Ranch Dressing
Price: $5.44

610 calories
54 g fat
(8.5 g saturated, 0.5 g trans)
850 mg sodium

Save!

260 calories
and $0.30!

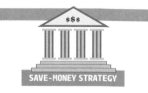

$$$

SAVE-MONEY STRATEGY

Fresh tuna is an amazing product that takes well to quick pan-searing and high-heat grilling. Trouble is, it can set you back up to $20 a pound. If you're looking to cut the cost of this dinner by about 60 percent (and speed things up a bit), ditch the fresh fish and reach for a high-quality can of tuna instead. If you can find canned or jarred tuna from Spain or Italy (Ortiz is a great brand), make it the new star of this dish. Regardless of the brand, figure half a can of tuna per salad.

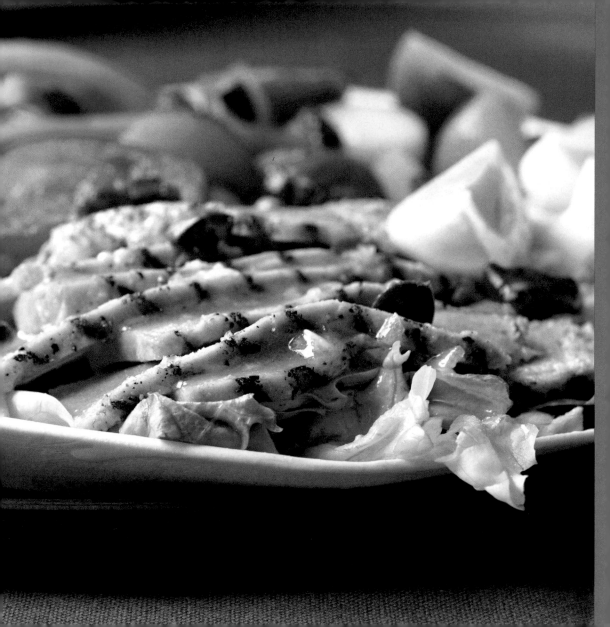

Cook This!
Chinese Chicken Salad

Chinese chicken salad is one of the world's ultimate fusion foods. It's an Eastern-inspired dish popularized by an Austrian chef (Wolfgang Puck) in Beverly Hills (at his restaurant Spago back in the 1980s). Whatever its disparate origins, it's undeniably one of the most popular—and ubiquitous—salads in America, sharing space on menus in four-star restaurants and Wendy's alike. Too bad most versions are nutritional disasters, bogged down by too much dressing and too many fried noodles. This lighter version is true to Wolfgang's original inspiration but with about a third of the calories.

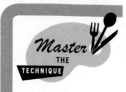

Master THE TECHNIQUE

Properly dressing salads

Most salads—both at home and in restaurants—end up overdressed, which compromises the flavor and the inherent nutritional value of the creation. For a properly dressed salad, the first step is to have perfectly dry lettuce leaves. Water on the lettuce repels the oil in the dressing, which means it won't cling to your salad. Invest in a salad spinner and use it religiously. Next, add the dressing a few tablespoons at a time immediately before serving (otherwise the lettuce begins to wilt) and use a pair of tongs to thoroughly distribute each new addition. Pluck a leaf from the bowl and taste; it should have a light sheen, not a heavy coat, of dressing and should still taste like lettuce.

You'll Need:

- 1 **head napa cabbage**
- ½ **head red cabbage**
- ½ **Tbsp sugar**
- 2 **cups chopped or shredded cooked chicken (freshly grilled or from a store-bought rotisserie chicken)**
- ⅓ **cup Asian Vinaigrette (see page 101)**
- 1 **cup fresh cilantro leaves**
- 1 **cup canned mandarin oranges, drained**
- ¼ **cup sliced almonds, toasted**

Salt and black pepper to taste

Make sure the mandarins are stored in water, not syrup. You don't want high-fructose corn syrup in your salad, do you?

How to Make It:

- Slice the cabbages in half lengthwise and remove the cores. Slice the cabbage into thin strips. Toss with the sugar in a large bowl.
- If the chicken is cold, toss with a few tablespoons of vinaigrette and heat in a microwave at 50% power. Add to the cabbage, along with the cilantro, mandarins, almonds, and the remaining vinaigrette. Toss to combine. Season with salt and pepper.

Makes 4 servings / Cost per serving: $3.30

380 calories
21 g fat (3.5 saturated)
23 g carbohydrates

1,430 calories
16 g saturated fat
93 g carbohydrates

Not That!
Applebee's Oriental Chicken Salad
Price: $9.49

Save!
1,050 calories and $6.19!

114

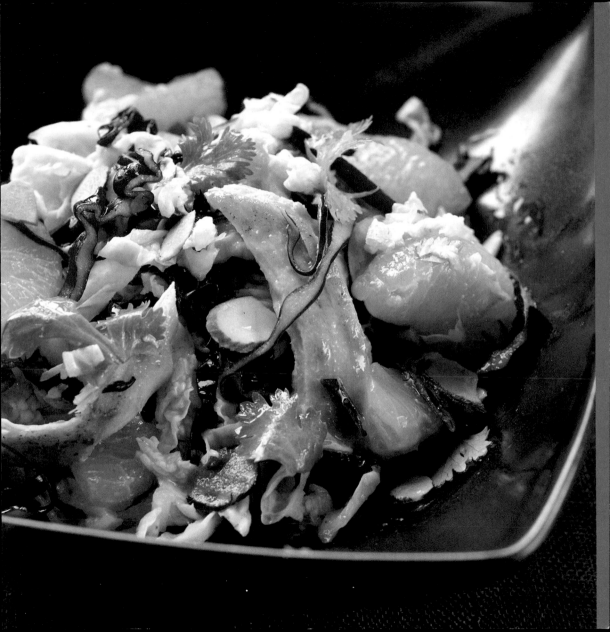

Cook This!
Butternut Squash Soup

We love tomato soup, but when it comes to vegetable soups, butternut is unbeatable. Beyond being super tasty, it's among the healthiest, packed with vitamin A, fiber, and omega-3s.

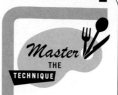

You'll Need:

1 **large butternut squash**

Olive oil

Pinch of grated nutmeg

Salt and black pepper to taste

2 **strips bacon**

1 **small onion, diced**

1 **Tbsp minced or grated fresh ginger**

1 **green apple, peeled, cored, and chopped**

4 **cups low-sodium chicken broth**

Chopped chives and light sour cream (optional)

How to Make It:

- Preheat the oven to 375°F. Slice the squash in half lengthwise and scoop out the seeds. Rub the halves with a touch of oil and season with nutmeg, salt, and pepper. Place on a baking sheet and roast until the flesh is very soft, about 35 to 40 minutes. Set aside to cool.

- Heat a large pot over medium heat. Add the bacon and cook until crispy, 5 to 7 minutes. Transfer to a plate and reserve. Add the onion and ginger to the hot pot and cook until the onion is translucent (but not browned), about 3 minutes. Add the apple and cook until soft, another 3 minutes or so.

- When the squash is cool enough to handle, scoop out the flesh and add it to a blender or large food processor. Add the contents of the pot and pour in enough broth to cover. (Be careful not to overfill; work in batches if necessary.) Process until very smooth and return to the pot. Stir in the remaining broth and bring to a simmer. Season with salt, pepper, and a touch more nutmeg. Garnish with crumbled bacon, chives, and sour cream (if using).

Makes 4 servings / Cost per serving: $1.89

The ginger gives this soup a subtle heat, but if you want to turn up the spice level, try a few shakes of cayenne or a tablespoon of chipotle pepper.

150 calories
3.5 g fat (1 g saturated)
490 mg sodium

370 calories
23 g fat
(12 g fat, 1 g trans)
740 mg sodium

Master THE TECHNIQUE

Spontaneous soups

Soups aren't rocket science; most don't even require recipes. Pureed soups (like this one) follow an especially predictable formula. Sauté 1 chopped onion and 2 minced garlic cloves until translucent, then add any of the following ingredients along with 4 cups chicken broth (the base of most soups); puree in a blender.

- 2 cans (14 oz) white beans; add 2 Tbsp chopped fresh rosemary after blending
- 1 can (28 oz) whole peeled tomatoes and ½ cup half-and-half; add 1 cup chopped fresh basil after blending
- 2 lb sautéed mushrooms and ½ cup half-and-half
- 2 cans (14 oz) black beans, juice of 2 limes, ¼ tsp each cumin and cayenne

Not That!
Panera Bread Creamy Tomato Soup with Croutons
Price: $5.00

Panera

Save!
220 calories
and $3.11!

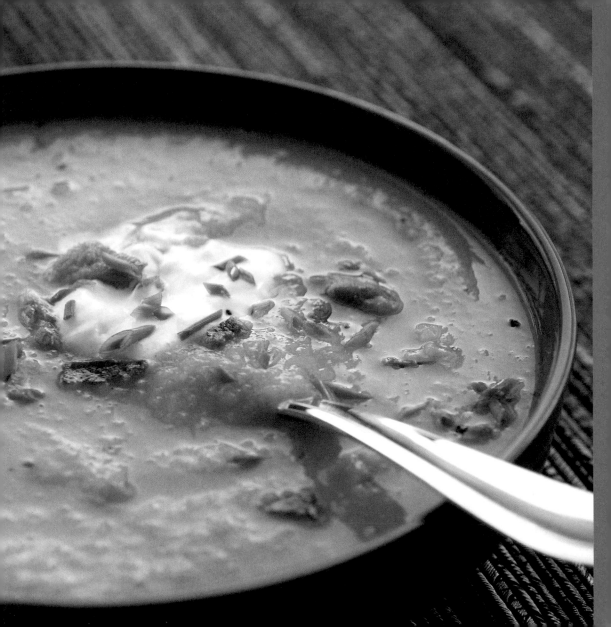

Tortilla Soup

Over the past 2 decades, tortilla soup has rivaled chicken soup as a comforting mainstay on major restaurant menus. Between the pulled chicken, the soothing tomato broth, and the pile of fixings, what's not to love? How about a bowl of soup with 86 percent of your day's sodium allotment? Unless you learn to enjoy it at home, that's what you're likely to get.

You'll Need:

- 1 Tbsp canola oil
- 1 onion, chopped
- 2 cloves garlic, chopped
- 1 can (14 oz) whole peeled tomatoes
- 1 Tbsp chipotle pepper
- 6 cups chicken broth
- ¾ lb boneless, skinless chicken breasts
- Salt and black pepper to taste
- 2 corn tortillas, cut into strips
- Juice of 2 limes
- Hot sauce (optional)
- ½ avocado, pitted, peeled, and cut into cubes
- Chopped onion, pickled jalapeños, sliced radishes, fresh cilantro (optional)

How to Make It:

- Heat the oil in a large pot over medium heat. Cook the onion and garlic until soft and translucent. Transfer to a blender and add the tomatoes (with juice) and chipotle; puree until smooth.

- Return to the pot and add the broth. Bring to a simmer. Season the chicken with salt and pepper. Drop the breasts into the liquid whole. Poach them in the soup until cooked all the way through, about 10 minutes. Remove and slice thin just before serving.

- Preheat the oven to 450°F. Lay the tortilla strips on a baking sheet and bake until lightly brown and crispy.

- Season the soup with the lime juice; adjust the seasoning with salt, pepper, and hot sauce (if using). Divide among 4 warm bowls. Top with the chicken, tortilla strips, avocado, and as many of the other garnishes as you'd like to use.

Makes 4 servings /
Cost per serving: $2.77

300 calories
11 g fat
(1.5 g saturated)
550 mg sodium

490 calories
25 g fat
(8 g saturated)
2,060 mg sodium

Upgrade

NUTRITIONAL

Homemade stock

None of the recipes call specifically for homemade stock, but if you have the time and some leftover chicken pieces, it's incomparably better than the sodium-soaked store-bought stuff. Place a pound or two of raw chicken pieces (or a leftover carcass from a roast or rotisserie chicken) in a pot with an onion, a few carrots, and a few stalks of celery. Cover with water and simmer for 90 minutes. Store in the fridge or freezer.

Not That!

On the Border Chicken Tortilla Soup (bowl)
Price: $4.99

Save!
190 calories
and $2.22!

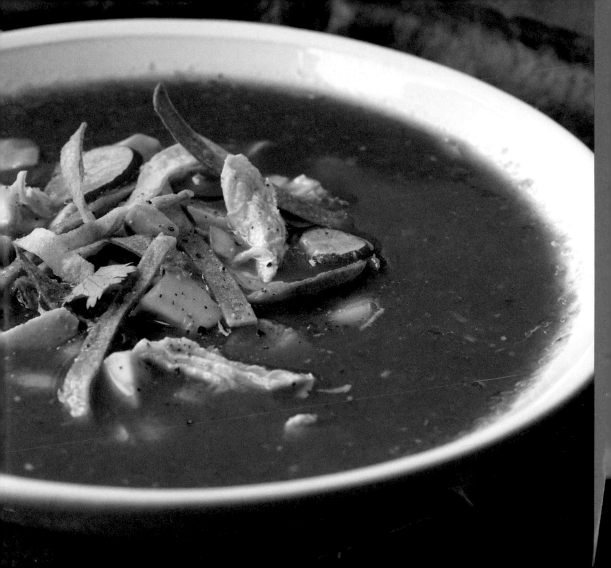

French Onion Soup

We're not going to lie: Good French onion soup takes time. But it takes almost no true effort, other than fighting back the tears as you chop your way through the five onions. And wouldn't you rather deal with a few errant tears than with a lackluster, overpriced bowl of soup that packs as much saturated fat as 20 strips of bacon and more sodium than nine bags of Lay's potato chips? Now that's a real reason to cry.

You'll Need:

- 1 Tbsp butter
- 5 medium onions (a mix of yellow and red is ideal), sliced
- ½ tsp salt
- 2 bay leaves
- 6 cups low-sodium beef broth •
- ½ cup dry red wine
- 4 or 5 sprigs fresh thyme (optional)
- Freshly cracked pepper
- 4 slices of baguette or sourdough bread
- ½ cup shredded Swiss cheese

How to Make It:

- Heat the butter in a large pot over low heat. Add the onions and salt. Cover the pot and cook the onions over low heat until very soft and caramelized, about 30 minutes. (Most of this is unsupervised. Check on the onions every 10 minutes or so and stir.)
- Add the bay leaves, broth, wine, and thyme (if using). Simmer on low heat for at least 15 minutes. Season with pepper. Discard the bay leaves.
- Preheat the broiler. Divide the soup among 4 oven-proof bowls. Top each with a slice of baguette and some cheese. Broil until the cheese is melted and bubbling, about 3 minutes.

Makes 4 servings / Cost per serving: $2.93

Chicken and vegetable broths are fine, too, but beef broth is best for bringing out the rich meatiness of the onions.

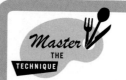

Master THE **TECHNIQUE**

Precision salting

Salt comes in dozens of shapes, sizes, and colors, but really it all comes down to three varieties: iodized salt (fine salt for use at the table), flaky sea salt (its crunchy texture is best used on cooked dishes like grilled steak and fish), and, most important, kosher salt. Chefs use kosher salt to season dishes as they're cooking because the coarse crystals allow them to season with precision. You should do the same, always using your hands (never a shaker!) to season.

230 calories
8 g fat (4 g saturated)
720 mg sodium

436 calories
32 g fat
(20 g saturated)
1,783 mg sodium

Not That!
Outback Steakhouse Onion Soup
Price: $3.95

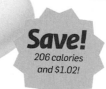

Save!
206 calories and $1.02!

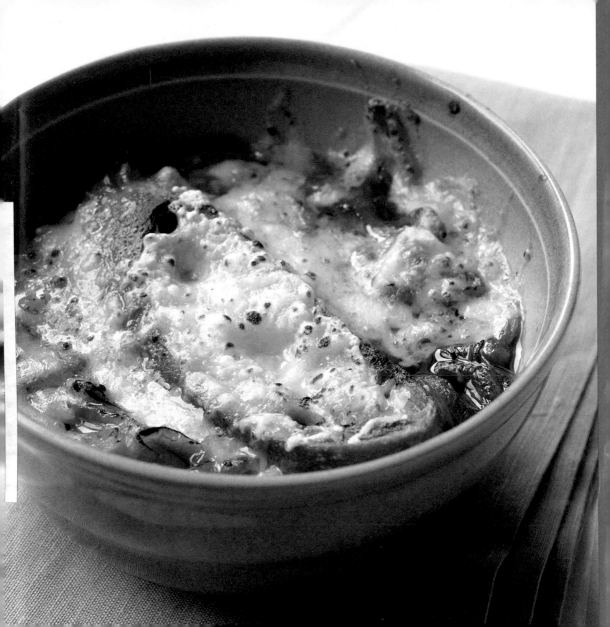

6

Cook This, Not That!

Sandwiches & Burgers

The food industry has hijacked our handheld heritage. Here's how you can take it back.

Two pieces of bread. That's the bedrock of every grinder, po'boy, hoagie, hero, hamburger, and sandwich on the planet. Food prep doesn't get more straightforward than that. With those virginal slices in hand you are the formidable Leonardo Da Vinci of your kitchen, free to build and create as far as your imagination—or gastrointestinal tract—will allow.

An exercise in excess

Now here's the caveat: With the power to create comes the power to inflate. For this there's no greater evidence than the greasy bread-boats being served at your local chain restaurant. Sure there are decent options out there, but more often than not the junk that comes stuffed between those two pieces of bread is enough to turn Mona Lisa into Homer Simpson. Want proof? Quiznos now serves more than a dozen sandwiches surpassing 1,000 calories apiece, and Arby's famous line of Market Fresh Sandwiches come enrobed in bread that has been injected with three types of sugar. Burgers are easier. Ruby Tuesday's average hamburger carries 72 grams of fat, and Cheesecake Factory sells at least three in excess of 1,700 calories. That's more of a Van Gogh approach to the culinary arts, but instead of slicing off an ear, these guys are trying to hijack your arteries.

That's why we've dedicated an entire chapter to the almighty sandwich. Our hope is that you'll hone your skills as crafter, learn to appreciate the versatility of the medium, and enjoy the satisfaction of tingling taste buds without falling into the same bad habits as the restaurant industry. To do just that, we show you the leanest cuts of meat, the best types of cheese, and the smartest toppings for you all your handheld creations. And we make one promise (that is, beyond the irrefutable fact that our burgers and deli concoctions are significantly easier on your waistline than those you'll find outside of the home): The sandwiches on these pages are as good or better than anything you will find on America's most popular menus.

So grab your palette of proteins and vegetables and get ready to start crafting. Consider these recipes your paint-by-numbers. The formulas are reliable, but if you feel the urge to stray, then by all means do it. Think your masterpiece needs an extra tinge of sweet? A soupçon of spice? You're the artist. Now get to work.

13 Instant Lunches

10-minute lunches to take on the go that will cut calories and save cash

1 Pack a stack of Triscuits, Swiss, and slices of smoked ham or turkey. It's like an adult Lunchables, only it's actually healthy.

2 Mix together a bit of mayo with grated horseradish. Spread on toasted rye or wheat bread, then top with roast beef, sharp Cheddar, sliced cucumbers, pickled onions, and arugula.

3 Place as many of the following items on a cutting board as you like: Ham, turkey, cucumber, bell pepper, tomato, olives, beans of any sort, scallions, blue cheese, and iceberg lettuce. Chop into tiny pieces. When you're ready to eat, dress the chopped salad with Honey Mustard (see page 100).

4 Chop two hard-boiled eggs and mix with diced pickles, a spoon of olive-oil mayonnaise, spicy mustard, and a pinch of cayenne. When you're ready to eat it, spoon the egg salad onto large romaine or Bibb lettuce leaves and eat like a burrito.

Want lunch for a whole work week for less than $15? Buy a rotisserie chicken at the supermarket. Remove the skin and shred every last bit of meat and do the following:

9 Monday Mix with barbecue sauce. Spread onto a large whole wheat or spinach tortilla and top with sautéed (or raw) onions and slices of avocado. Wrap tightly.

10 Tuesday Toss with chopped romaine, roasted red peppers, olives, artichoke hearts, and feta cheese. Bring one of your home-made dressings (page 100) to work and toss right before eating.

CHAPTER 6

5 *Mix a can of tuna with chopped pickles, minced onion, and equal parts Dijon and olive oil mayo. Stuff into a whole wheat pita.*

6 *Stuff a pita with black beans, guacamole, sliced tomato, crumbled feta cheese, and a handful of your favorite greens.*

8 Slice an avocado and remove the pit. Fill the round cavities with canned tuna and a squeeze of lemon, plus salt and pepper. Eat with Triscuits.

7 Mix equal parts of cooked brown rice and drained canned black beans. Top with leftover chicken or steak (or deli turkey), salsa, and guacamole. Eat with a small stack of tortilla chips.

11 Wednesday Bring a can of creamy tomato or wild mushroom soup to work. Heat. Stir in some of the shredded chicken. Wash it all down with a crisp apple.

12 Thursday Spread a thick layer of hummus onto an English muffin. Stack with arugula or mixed greens, roasted peppers, chicken, and a slice of smoked Gouda or provolone.

13 Friday Toss with cooked spaghetti, scallions, and red bell peppers. Dress with peanut butter mixed with soy sauce, lime, and hot sauce. Top with peanuts; eat hot or cold.

127

Grilled Chicken and Pineapple Sandwich

Not even the relatively healthy genre of grilled chicken sandwiches is a safe bet when you seek sustenance away from home. That's because places like Outback go long on the oil and the dressing, gobbling up (in this case) half of your day's saturated fat and sodium. Our sandwich is a spicy-sweet combination of teriyaki-glazed chicken, juicy grilled pineapple, and fiery jalapeños—a chicken sandwich to end all fatty chicken sandwiches.

You'll Need:

- **4 boneless, skinless chicken breasts (4–6 oz each)**
- **Teriyaki sauce**
- **4 slices Swiss cheese**
- **4 pineapple slices (½" thick)**
- **4 whole-wheat buns**
- **1 red onion, thinly sliced**
- **Pickled Jalapeños (see page 304)**

Whole-wheat buns are often made with a small percentage of whole grains and a surplus of sugar. Settle on a brand with 3 grams of fiber and fewer than 130 calories per bun. Nature's Own Whitewheat buns are the best in show.

How to Make It:

- Combine the chicken and enough teriyaki sauce to cover in a resealable plastic bag and marinate in the refrigerator for at least 30 minutes and up to 12 hours.

- Heat a grill until hot (you shouldn't be able to hold your hand above the grates for more than 5 seconds). Remove the chicken from the marinade and place on the grill; discard any remaining marinade. Cook for 4 to 5 minutes on the first side; flip and immediately add the cheese to each breast. Continue cooking until the cheese is melted and the chicken is lightly charred and firm to the touch. Remove and set aside.

- While the chicken rests, add the pineapple and the buns to the grill. Cook the buns until they're lightly toasted and the pineapple until it's soft and caramelized, about 2 minutes per side. Top each bun with chicken, red onion, jalapeño slices, and pineapple. If you like, drizzle the chicken with a bit more teriyaki sauce.

Makes 4 servings / Cost per serving: $2.64

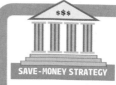

SAVE-MONEY STRATEGY

Cheaper chicken

Boneless, skinless chicken breasts may be America's most popular protein, but they're not exactly its cheapest. Want to cut the tab for this sandwich nearly in half? Switch to frozen. An in-house taste test at *Men's Health* found little to no discrepancy in flavor. The only real difference? Fresh chicken breast runs around $6 a pound, while a pound of frozen works out to be less than $4.

400 calories
11 g fat (6 g saturated)
640 mg sodium

696 calories
33 g fat (10 g saturated)
1,323 mg sodium

Not That!
Outback Grilled Chicken & Swiss Sandwich
Price: $7.95

Save!
296 calories
and $5.31!

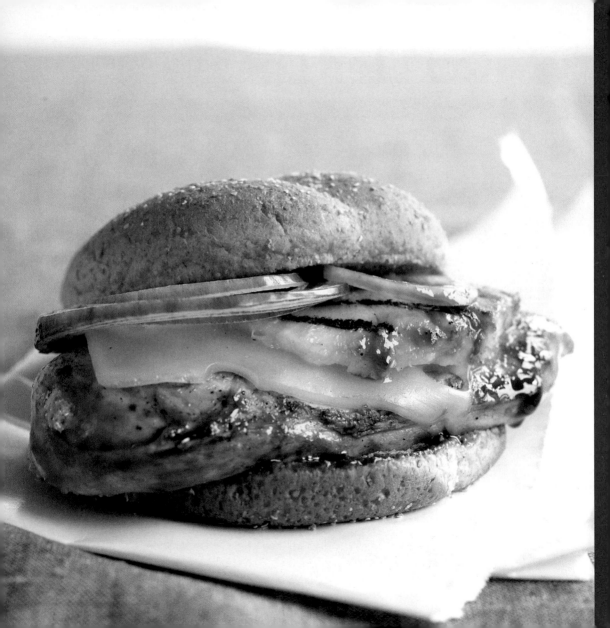

Grilled Cheese with Apples and Bacon

Funky versions of America's simplest sandwich have been popping up at national restaurants and quick-service chains more and more in recent years. Problem is, when restaurants start to get creative, it usually spells trouble for your waistline. Au Bon Pain's Prosciutto Mozzarella Sandwich is a perfect example of this "more is more" mantra, where a few thin slices of cured ham and a mozzarella blanket turn a lunchtime bite into a sandwich that packs as much saturated fat as 5 scoops of Breyers vanilla ice cream. We're all for innovating, but if you're going to do it, do it right. The curious combination of sweet apples, smoky bacon, and sharp cheese isn't just delicious, it contains less than half the calories of most other grilled cheese sandwiches out there.

$(\Psi+I)^2$

MEAL MULTIPLIER

We love a classic grilled cheese made with Kraft Singles as much as the next dude, but why limit yourself to that when so many other great combinations are waiting to be discovered? Here are a few worth trying.

- Gruyère or other Swiss cheese and caramelized onions (think French onion soup on bread)
- Blue cheese, arugula or frisée, and fresh figs
- Fresh mozzarella, tomato, and basil
- Pepper jack cheese, avocado slices, and salsa
- Brie, sliced ham, and sliced pear

You'll Need:

1 Tbsp butter

8 slices whole-grain bread (we love Martin's Whole Wheat)

1 Tbsp Dijon mustard

6 oz shredded sharp Cheddar cheese

1 Granny Smith apple, peeled, cored, and sliced

8 strips cooked bacon

How to Make It:

- Heat the butter in a large skillet or nonstick sauté pan over low heat. Slather 4 slices of bread with the mustard, then divide the cheese, apples, and bacon among them. Top with the other bread slices and add to the hot pan. The key to a great grilled cheese (i.e., crispy crust, fully melted cheese) is patience, so cook these sandwiches slowly until each side is deep brown and crunchy, about 10 to 12 minutes total.

Makes 4 servings /
Cost per serving: $1.55

330 calories
15 g fat
(6 g saturated)
790 mg sodium

810 calories
41 g fat
(16 g saturated)
2,290 mg sodium

Not That!

Au Bon Pain's Prosciutto Mozzarella Sandwich Price: $6.49

Save!
480 calories
and $4.94!

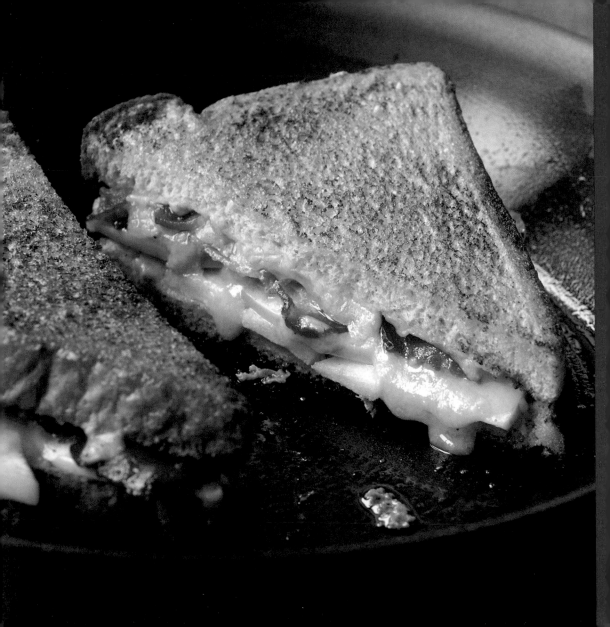

Shrimp Roll

Dead simple and insanely delicious, lobster rolls are one of America's greatest food inventions. Problem is, lobster meat is pricey (about $35 a pound as of this book's publication date), and restaurants too often drown out the fresh lobster flavor with an abundance of mayo and melted butter. We sub in ultra-lean shrimp—one of nature's best sources of immune-boosting, blood sugar-stabilizing zinc—for the lobster and go easy on the ingredients, letting the shrimp simply speak for themselves. The result: an amazing sandwich for half the calories and less than a quarter the price.

You'll Need:

- 1 lb cooked shrimp
- 2 stalks celery, diced
- ½ small red onion, minced
- 2 Tbsp minced chives
- 2 Tbsp mayonnaise
- Juice of 1 lemon
- 1 tsp hot sauce (we like sriracha)
- Salt to taste
- 4 hot dog buns (top-loading buns from Pepperidge Farm are best)

Top-loading buns are the traditional vessel of choice for lobster rolls across New England. If your supermarket doesn't carry them, any sturdy bun will do.

How to Make It:

- Mix the shrimp, celery, onion, chives, mayo, lemon juice, hot sauce, and salt together in a bowl, stirring to carefully incorporate.
- Heat a cast-iron skillet or sauté pan over medium heat. Add the hot dog buns and toast until the sides are nicely browned.
- Divide the shrimp mixture among the rolls. Garnish with chopped chives, if desired.

Makes 4 servings / Cost per serving: $2.96

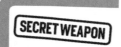

SECRET WEAPON

Sriracha

Our adoaration of this Asian-style hot sauce is well documented throughout this book. The reason is simple: Whereas most hot sauces bring fire, few actually add flavor, too. Sriracha—made from chiles, garlic, vinegar, salt, and sugar—brings a balanced attack of hot, salty, sour, and sweet to the table. But don't take our word for it: Try it on eggs, in stir-fries, or on sandwiches, like this one to the right.

300 calories
9 g fat (1.5 g saturated)
470 mg sodium

620 calories
26 g fat (4 g saturated)
1,240 mg sodium

Not That!
Uno Chicago Grill Lobster Sliders
Price: $14.04

Save!
320 calories
and $11.08!

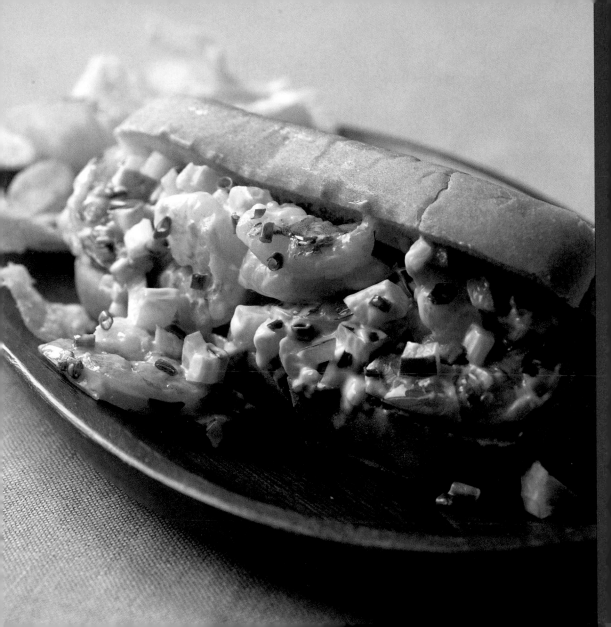

Grilled Lamb Gyros

One may be from Mexico and the other Greece, but burritos and gyros have everything in common. They're both handheld pockets stuffed with meat, vegetables, and sauces. Too bad most burritos pack twice as many calories as you'll find in this delicious gyro.

You'll Need:

- 2 lb butterflied leg of lamb
- 16 oz plain Greek-style yogurt
- 4 cloves garlic, minced
- 1½ tsp ground cumin
- 1 tsp salt
- 1 tsp freshly cracked pepper
- 6 whole-wheat pitas
- 2 beefsteak tomatoes, sliced
- 1 red onion, finely sliced
- Hummus (see recipe on page 304, or use store-bought)
- Hot sauce (we like sriracha)

How to Make It:

- Combine the lamb, yogurt, garlic, cumin, salt, and pepper in a container. Cover and marinate the meat for at least 2 hours or up to a full day.

- Heat a grill to medium. Remove the lamb from the marinade and wipe away most of the yogurt. Then place the meat on the grill. Cook 10 to 15 minutes a side, until the lamb is well charred on the outside and feels firm but yielding to the touch. For medium rare, a thermometer inserted into the thickest part of the lamb should read 125°F.

- Remove the lamb from the grill and let it rest for at least 10 minutes. In the meantime, warm the pitas on the grill for 30 seconds a side, or wrap them in foil and warm them for 5 to 7 minutes in a 350°F oven. Once the lamb has cooled slightly, slice it very thinly with a sharp knife and serve with the warm pitas, tomatoes, onion, hummus, and hot sauce.

Makes 6 servings / Cost per serving: $3.89

SECRET WEAPON

Greek-style yogurt

The Greeks know a thing or two about making yogurt—after all, they've been eating it for more than 4,000 years. The key to their yogurt supremacy comes from the fact that they strain off the watery whey, making a denser, creamier product with double the protein of American-style yogurts. Don't confine it to breakfast, though. Mixed with olive oil, minced garlic, fresh herbs, and lemon juice, Greek yogurt makes a killer marinade or sauce for grilled meats.

466 calories
12 g fat (3 g saturated)
833 mg sodium

970 calories
38 g fat (18 g saturated)
2,150 mg sodium

Not That!
Chipotle Steak Burrito
Price: $5.95

Save!
504 calories and $2.06!

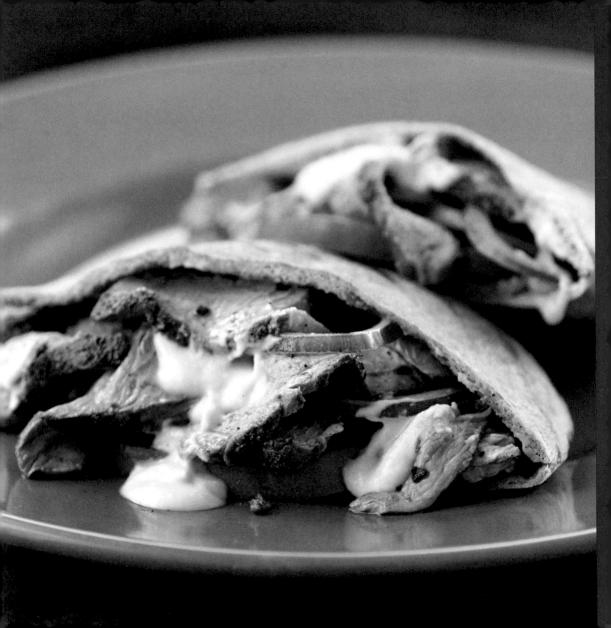

Chicken Panini with Pesto and Peppers

Paninis began their American invasion in the late '90s, taking over menus in big city Italian restaurants and corner cafés alike. Now they've spread nationwide, popping up on menus at places like Panera, Cosí, Au Bon Pain, and even Dunkin' Donuts. Problem is, these sandwiches usually suffer from a cheese and condiment overdose, racking up caloric totals akin to a half-pound hamburger. Keep it simple: A light, healthy spread like pesto, a low-calorie cheese like fresh mozz, and a layer of lean white meat chicken deliver all the flavor for a fraction of the calories.

You'll Need:

- 8 slices whole-grain sourdough bread
- 4 Tbsp homemade (see page 303) or prepared pesto
- 4 oz fresh mozzarella, thinly sliced
- ¾ lb cooked chicken
- ½ cup roasted red peppers

Olive oil

How to Make It:

- Heat a large cast-iron skillet or stovetop grill pan over medium heat. Spread 4 pieces of the bread with 1 tablespoon of the pesto each. Layer each piece with equal amounts of the mozzarella slices, chicken, and red peppers. Add a light film of olive oil to the pan; when hot, cook the sandwiches (2 at a time, if necessary) until the bread is crispy and the cheese is melted, 3 to 4 minutes each side. (For the best results, use a heavy pan to weigh down the sandwiches.)

Makes 4 servings / Cost per serving: $1.94

Fresh mozzarella is both tastier and lower in calories than regular mozz, but it's also more expensive. Any shredded part-skim mozzarella will work as a solid substitution.

$$$

SAVE-MONEY STRATEGY

Don't bother dropping $100 on a panini machine—they're one-trick ponies that take up precious kitchen storage space. (In fact, never buy any single-purpose kitchen equipment.) Instead, try using a George Foreman grill, which millions of Americans already keep on hand for indoor grilling. Simply slide the sandwich onto the preheated grates (sans butter or oil) and grill until crispy on the outside and melted on the inside. Don't have a Foreman? A hot skillet and something heavy to weigh down the sandwich work great in a pinch.

450 calories
15 g fat (6 g saturated)
820 mg sodium

980 calories
55 g fat (15 g saturated, 1 g trans)
2,340 mg sodium

Not That!
Panera Bread Chipotle Chicken on Artisan French Bread Price: $6.99

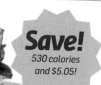

Save!
530 calories and $5.05!

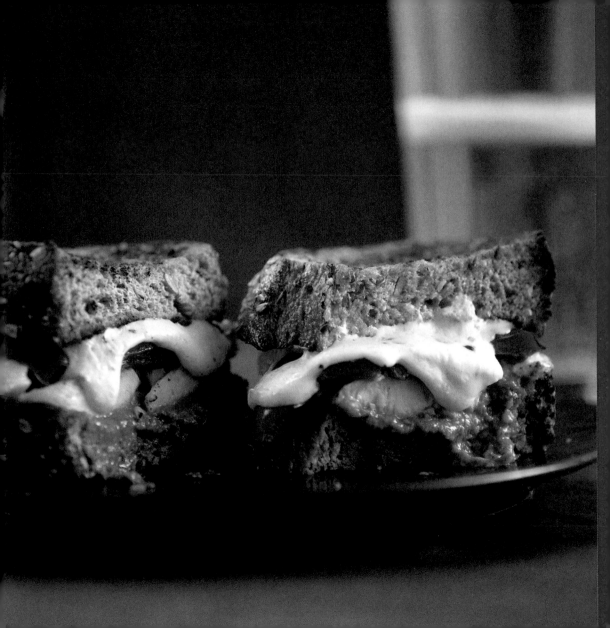

Cook This!
Patty Melt

This classic diner dish may be the most satisfying of all hamburger iterations: a thin, crusty patty crowned with a melting veil of cheese and plenty of sweet griddled onions, all held together between warm, crunchy slices of toasted rye. The bad news is you can't have this inspired creation, or any other restaurant-style burger, without a massive caloric investment. The good news is that our immensely satisfying 340-calorie version is never more than 15 minutes away in the comfort of your own kitchen.

You'll Need:

- 1 lb ground sirloin or ground turkey
- 1 tsp salt
- ½ tsp black pepper
- 1 Tbsp canola oil
- 1 large red onion, diced
- 4 slices Swiss cheese
- 8 slices rye bread, toasted

Both turkey and sirloin will produce perfectly lean, delicious results, so really, it's just a matter of personal preference.

Not only is Swiss traditional, but it also contains fewer calories and less sodium than Cheddar.

How to Make It:

- Season the meat with the salt and pepper and form into 4 large, thin patties. Heat the oil in a cast-iron skillet over medium heat. Add the patties and scatter the onion around the burgers. Stir the onion from time to time to keep it from burning.
- Cook the burgers for 3 to 4 minutes, then flip and immediately cover each with a slice of Swiss. Continue cooking until the burgers are cooked all the way through, about another 3 minutes. Remove, place on top of the toasted rye, cover with the sautéed onions, and top with other slice of rye.

Makes 4 servings / Cost per serving: $2.85

340 calories
12 g fat (5 g saturated)
640 mg sodium

Save!
690 calories
and $2.44!

1,030 calories
64 g fat
(19 g saturated)
1,250 mg sodium

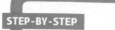

Not That!
Friendly's Patty Melt
Price: $5.29

STEP-BY-STEP

Diced onion

Fumble your way through an onion and you'll end up bathed in tears. Speed up your prep (and keep your eyes dry!) with these three simple steps.

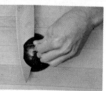

Step 1: *Slice off the top, leaving the root end intact.*

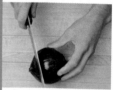

Step 2: *Make a series of horizontal and vertical cuts.*

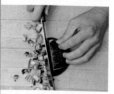

Step 3: *Chop across the onion in ¼-inch intervals.*

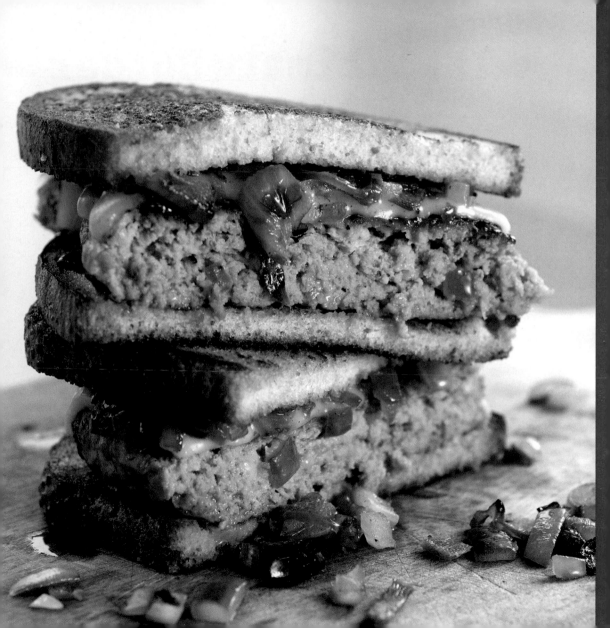

The Ultimate Burger

It is nearly impossible to find a burger at a sit-down restaurant with fewer than 1,000 calories. Blame the high-fat meat and heavy condiments. Here, we start with ground brisket, which is relatively lean but packed with perfect burger flavor. (The butcher at your local market should be happy to grind up a hunk for you.) We solve the condiment crisis by slowly caramelizing a red onion until it's sweet and moist. Combine that with the great beef and some peppery arugula for a first-class burger experience. If you must add cheese, a bit of crumbled blue goes well here.

Upgrade

You'll Need:

- 10 oz ground sirloin
- 10 oz ground brisket
- 1 tsp salt
- 1 tsp freshly cracked pepper
- 4 hamburger buns (preferably Martin's Potato Rolls), toasted
- 2 cups arugula
- ½ cup Caramelized Onions (see page 305)

Martin's Potato Rolls aren't just the perfect size (not too big or bready) for the burger—they also pack 3 grams of fiber apiece.

How to Make It:

- Heat a grill or stovetop grill pan until hot. Combine the sirloin, brisket, salt, and pepper in a bowl and gently mix. Form into 4 patties. Caution: Overworking the meat or packing your patties too tightly can make tough burgers.

- Cook the burgers for 2 to 3 minutes and flip. Cook on the other side for another 2 to 3 minutes, until nicely charred on the outside but still medium-rare to medium within. (The center of the patty should be firm but easily yielding—like a Nerf football.)

- After you remove the burgers, toast the buns briefly. Divide the arugula among the buns and top with the burgers and onions.

Makes 4 servings / Cost per serving: $2.98

NUTRITIONAL

Fresh ground beef

The prepackaged trays of ground hamburger meat at supermarkets may be convenient, but it's true mystery meat, usually made from a blend of beef scraps of dubious quality and age. Instead, pick out a fresh hunk of beef and ask the butcher to grind it for you on the spot; it's the single best way to instantly improve the quality of your hamburgers. When it comes to balancing flavor with an appropriate amount of fat, sirloin and brisket are the best picks in the meat case.

320 calories
12 g fat (6 g saturated)
710 mg sodium

890 calories
54 g fat
(20 g saturated)
2,040 mg sodium

Not That!
Carl's Jr
The Original
Six Dollar Burger
Price: $4.36

Save!
570 calories
and $1.38!

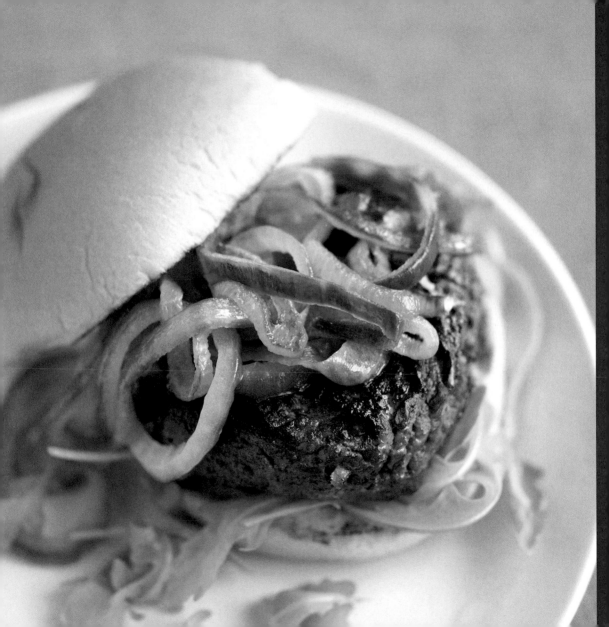

Cook This!
Green Chile Cheeseburger

As bad as fast-food burgers can be, they look like nutritional superstars when stacked next to sit-down restaurant burgers. The bulk of the burgers at Applebee's, Chili's, Ruby Tuesday, Outback, and T.G.I. Friday's weigh in at 1,000 calories or more—before the massive mound of French fries that invariably accompanies them. The key to keeping the calories down is finding a lean but tasty cut of beef (we love sirloin); using healthy, flavor-packed condiments (e.g., roasted chiles, not fried onion rings); and finding a small, fiber-rich bun to house the creation.

You'll Need:

- 1 lb ground sirloin or brisket
- Salt and black pepper to taste
- 1 can (4 oz) roasted green chiles, drained and chopped
- 4 slices Swiss cheese
- 4 potato buns (preferably Martin's Potato Rolls)
- 4 thick slices tomato
- 4 medium slices red onion

How to Make It:

- Heat a grill, stovetop grill pan, or cast-iron skillet. Season the beef with salt and pepper. Form 4 patties, being careful not to overwork the meat.
- When the pan is hot, add the burgers. Cook for 3 to 4 minutes on the first side (until nicely charred), then flip and immediately top each with a tablespoon of chiles and a slice of Swiss. For medium-rare burgers, continue cooking for another 3 to 4 minutes, until the patties are just firm. Remove the burgers and toast the buns on the hot grill or pan. Dress the bottom of the buns with the tomato and onion slices, then top each with a burger.

Makes 4 servings / Cost per serving: $2.62

Fresh chiles are even better. Grill poblano peppers until charred, then peel off the skin, remove the seeds, and slice.

$$\left(\text{\ding{}} + \text{\ding{}} \right)^2$$

MEAL MULTIPLIER

Burger-building
We wanted to fill this entire book with delicious burger recipes, but we decided to show some restraint. Here are some other great creations that didn't make the cut.

- Beef burgers with mozzarella, pesto, and roasted red peppers
- Beef burgers with pickled jalapeños, a slice of ham, and a fried egg
- Turkey burgers with pepper Jack cheese and fresh guacamole
- Salmon burgers with wasabi-spiked mayo

320 calories
11 g fat (4.5 g saturated)
420 mg sodium

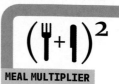

1,095 calories
68 g fat
1,508 mg sodium

Not That!
Red Robin Santa Fe Burger
Price: $9.79

Save!
775 calories and $7.17!

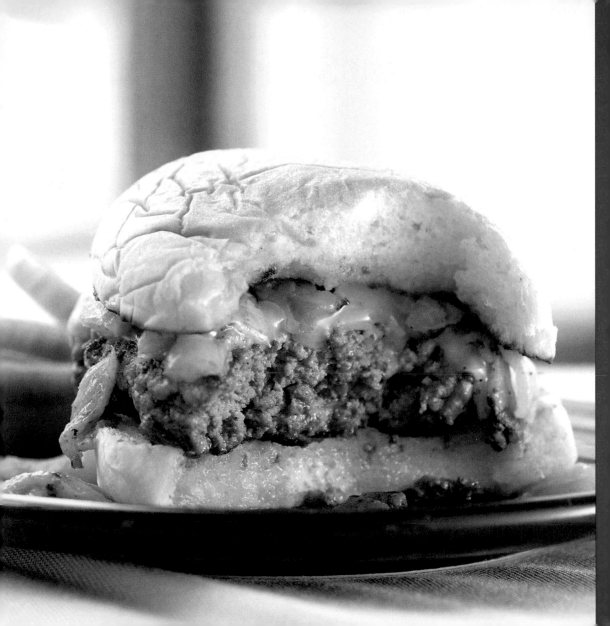

Turkey Sandwich with Guacamole and Bacon

As great as guacamole is with chips, it's even better slathered on a sandwich. Swapping in the avocado all-star for mayo not only shaves 70 to 100 calories from your sandwich but also replaces low-quality fats with healthy monounsaturated ones. Quiznos's creation fails because it doesn't rely solely on the guac but rather piles it on top of a slick of ranch dressing. Avoid this blunder by turning guacamole into your spread of choice for turkey, chicken, and grilled steak sandwiches.

You'll Need:

- 1 baguette
- 12 oz sliced turkey
- 4 slices Swiss cheese
- 1 large tomato, sliced
- ½ red onion, thinly sliced
- Pickled Jalapeños (see page 304)
- 4 strips bacon, cooked until crisp and patted dry
- ¼ cup Guacamole (see page 303) or store-bought guacamole

How to Make It:

- Preheat the broiler. Carefully slice the baguette in half horizontally and place on a large baking sheet. Layer the turkey and cheese on the bottom half of the bread.

- Place the sheet in the oven 6" below the broiler. Broil for 2 to 3 minutes, until the cheese has just melted and both halves of the bread are hot, but not too brown and crunchy.

- Remove from the oven and then layer the tomato, onion, jalapeños, and bacon on top of the turkey. Spread the top half of the baguette with the guacamole. Slice the baguette into 4 individual sandwiches and serve.

Makes 4 servings / Cost per serving: $3.54

Fresh jalapeños will work, too. Be aware that they're spicier when fresh, so slice them thinly.

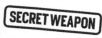

430 calories
13 g fat (4 g saturated)
1,070 mg sodium

810 calories
9.5 g saturated fat
2,700 mg sodium

Not That!
Quiznos Regular Turkey Bacon Guacamole Sub
Price: $5.39

Save!
380 calories
and $1.85!

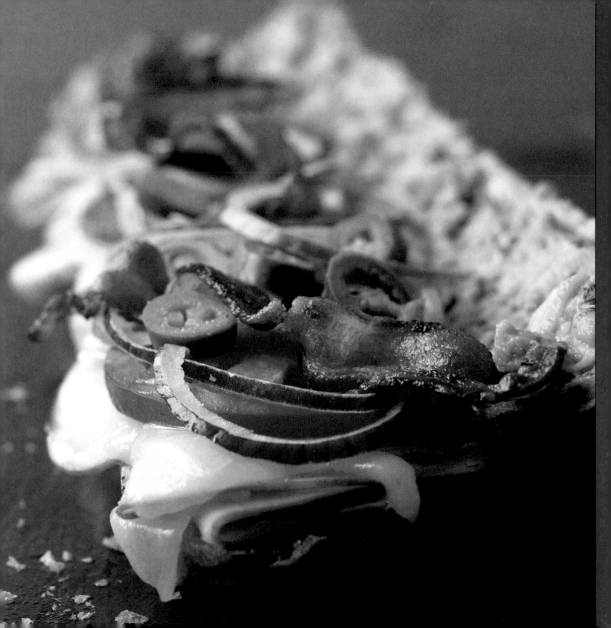

Chicken Salad Sandwich

with Curry and Raisins

Chicken and salad: two great foods on their own that make for a lousy dish when combined. That's because salad, when attached to chicken, is secret speak for mayo overload. In fact, chicken and tuna salad sandwiches are consistently the worst option you'll find on a deli menu, be it Subway or your neighborhood sandwich shop. We use a modest amount of olive-oil-based mayo, then punch up the flavor with plump golden raisins and the complex savory notes of curry powder. Make a big batch and bring it to work all week in sandwiches, stuffed in pitas, or crowning a bowl of mixed greens.

SECRET WEAPON

Curry powder

Curry powder is as ubiquitous throughout Indian cooking as it is diverse, with each cook preferring a different blend of spices such as coriander, cumin, fennel, and cardamom. One thing they nearly all have in common is that distinctive yellow tinge, which comes from turmeric, perhaps the world's healthiest spice. Studies have shown turmeric's vast antioxidant portfolio to be an effective defense against arthritis, prostate and colon cancers, and various other diseases. Get your dose by rubbing curry onto chicken and fish; mixing with yogurt, garlic, and ginger for a sauce or dip; or coating roasted nuts.

You'll Need:

- 3 Tbsp golden raisins
- 3 cups chopped cooked chicken
- 2 stalks celery, thinly sliced
- ½ onion, diced
- 1 carrot, shredded
- ½ tsp curry powder
- ¼ cup olive-oil mayonnaise
- Salt and black pepper to taste
- 4 large lettuce leaves (romaine, iceberg, or anything else)
- 8 slices whole-grain bread or English muffin halves, toasted
- 2 medium tomatoes, sliced

How to Make It:

- Cover the raisins with hot water and soak for at least 10 minutes (the warm water will help the raisins plump up); drain and place in a large bowl. Add the chicken, celery, onion, carrot, curry powder, and mayonnaise. Mix well and season with salt and pepper.
- Place the lettuce leaves on top of 4 bread slices, then top with tomatoes, chicken salad, and the remaining bread.

Makes 4 servings / Cost per serving: $2.66

From both a flavor and a nutritional standpoint, spices need to be replaced every 6 months to a year.

440 calories
15 g fat
(3 g saturated)
510 mg sodium

Not That!

Boston Market Classic Chicken Salad Sandwich
Price: $5.00

800 calories
41 g fat
(7 g saturated, 5 g trans)
1,900 mg sodium

Save!
360 calories
and $2.34!

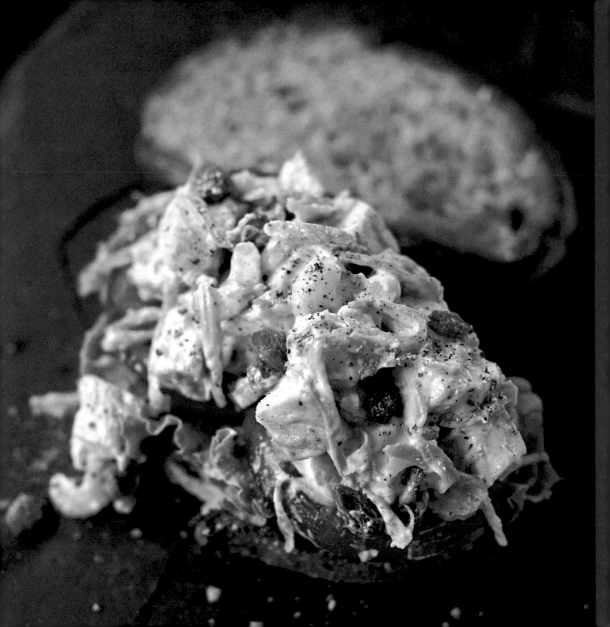

Cook This!

Blackened Fish Sandwich

The default fish sandwich in America is a slab of heavily processed mystery seafood, breaded and deep fried, bathed in a tartarlike sauce, and stuffed into an oversize squishy roll. You end up dropping anywhere between 600 and 800 calories and the better part of the day's sodium allotment for something that's supposed to be healthy. Our addictive fish sandwich replaces processed patties with fresh tilapia fillets, frying with blackening, and tartar sauce with creamy avocado and crunchy cabbage.

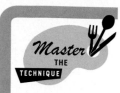

Master THE **TECHNIQUE**

You'll Need:

- 1 **cup plain Greek-style yogurt**
- 1 **tsp sriracha**
- **Juice of one lime**
- 1 **Tbsp canola oil**
- 4 **tilapia or catfish fillets (6 oz each)**
- 1 **Tbsp blackening seasoning**
- 4 **whole-wheat sesame seed buns**
- 1 **avocado, pitted, peeled, and sliced**
- 2 **cups shredded red cabbage**
- **Pickled Onions (see page 304)**

How to Make It:

- Combine the yogurt, sriracha, and lime juice. Set aside.
- Heat the oil in a large cast-iron skillet over high heat. Rub the fish fillets on both sides with plenty of blackening seasoning. When the oil in the pan is smoking, add the fish and cook, undisturbed, for 3 minutes, until a dark crust forms. Flip the fillets and cook for an additional 2 to 3 minutes, until the fish flakes with gentle pressure from your finger.
- While the fish is cooking, toast the buns (cut side up) under the broiler. Divide the avocado and cabbage among the buns. Top with the hot fish, yogurt sauce, and onions.

Makes 4 servings / Cost per serving: $3.68

Make sure it's American farmed tilapia; Asian tilapia is among the least environmentally friendly species of fish.

Blackening

Blackening is one of our favorite cooking techniques—not just because it's incredibly delicious, but also because the aggressive spice rub adds a potent layer of antioxidants to whatever it coats. Follow these three simple steps for fish, chicken, or pork.

- **Step 1:** Coat each piece of fish or meat on both sides with about ¾ tsp blackening seasoning.
- **Step 2:** Cook, undisturbed, in a very hot cast-iron skillet coated with canola oil until a dark crust develops.
- **Step 3:** Flip and repeat, until cooked all the way through.

460 calories
14 g fat
(2.5 g saturated)
620 mg sodium

640 calories
32 g fat
(5 g saturated, 0.5 g trans)
1,370 mg sodium

Not That!

Burger King Big Fish Sandwich
Price: $3.49

Save!

180 calories and 18 g fat!

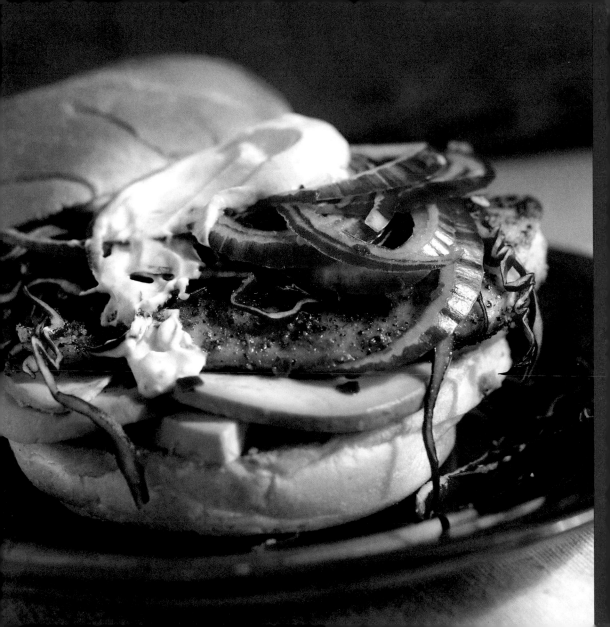

The Ultimate BLT

Is there any combination as rewarding and perfectly calibrated as a bacon, lettuce, and tomato sandwich? With the crispy, smoky bacon playing off the cool crunch of the lettuce and the acidic sweetness of ripe tomato, it's a top contender for Last Meal on Earth status. Bog down the BLT with bulky, sweetened bread and a sea of mayo, though, and the appeal vanishes—just as the caloric toll rises. Arby's self-proclaimed Ultimate BLT has nearly as many calories in the corn syrup–spiked bread (361) as you'll find in our entire sandwich. Plus ours is crowned with a soft, oozing fried egg—the only condiment you need.

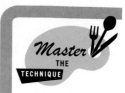

Master THE **TECHNIQUE**

Better bacon

Most people cook bacon in an over-crowded pan, which yields inconsistent results. Make life easier (and tastier) by using the oven instead. Lay bacon out in a baking dish at least 2" deep and bake in a 400°F oven for 10 to 12 minutes, until the meat just begins to brown and crisp around the edges (bacon, like other meat, will continue to cook after you remove it from the oven). Not only will the bacon be perfect every time, but the fat will also render out more thoroughly this way, meaning your bacon doesn't just taste better—it is better.

You'll Need:

- 1 egg
- 2 slices 7-grain or sourdough bread, lightly toasted
- Handful of arugula
- 3 thick slices tomato
- 4 strips bacon, cooked
- Salt and black pepper to taste

How to Make It:

- Heat a small nonstick skillet over medium heat. Coat with olive oil cooking spray and add the egg. Cook sunny side up until the white is set but the yolk is runny. Line the bottom half of the bread with the arugula, followed by the tomato slices and bacon. Set the cooked egg carefully on top and season with a pinch of salt and plenty of fresh cracked pepper. Top with the second slice of bread.

Makes 1 serving / Cost per serving: $1.98

There's been much debate over the perfect lettuce for a BLT. Some prefer the crunch of iceberg or romaine, others like leaves with a peppery bite, like watercress or arugula. It's your choice.

450 calories
20 g fat (6 g saturated)
840 mg sodium

880 calories
46 g fat (10 g saturated)
1,740 mg sodium

Not That!
Arby's Market Fresh Ultimate BLT
Price: $4.73

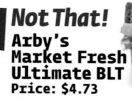

Save!
430 calories and $2.75!

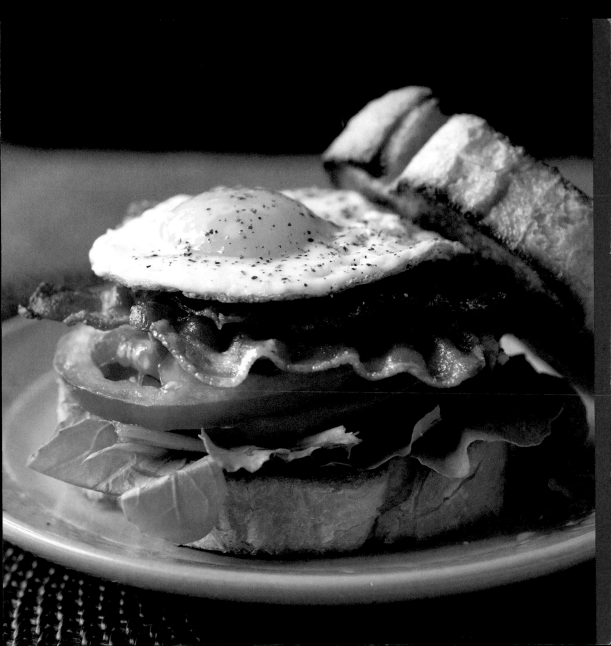

Meat Loaf Sandwich

Open-Face with Caramelized Onions

Meat loaf is like turkey: Half of the reason to make it is so that you can use the leftovers for sandwiches the next day. If you have leftover tomato chutney from the Turkey Meat Loaf recipe (see page 234), then pile it on.

You'll Need:

- 1 slice leftover meat loaf (½ inch thick)
- **Caramelized Onions** (see page 305)
- ¼ cup shredded smoked mozzarella •
- 1 slice sourdough bread, toasted
- Handful of arugula (optional)

How to Make it:

- Preheat the broiler. Top the meat loaf slice with the onions and cheese. Place underneath the broiler until the cheese is fully melted, about 2 minutes. Line the bread with the arugula (if using), then place the meat loaf on top.

Makes 1 serving / Cost per serving: $4.88

Smoked mozzarella is one of our favorite cheeses, but regular mozz, Swiss, or provolone all work excellently here.

$$(\text{\ding{202}}+\text{l})^2$$

MEAL MULTIPLIER

Open-face options

Open-face sandwiches have two great things going for them: (1) the missing slice of bread helps to mitigate the calories and carbs of the sandwich, and (2) the knife-and-fork treatment means you can be more aggressive with the sandwich construction. Here are a few of our favorite bold combinations:

- Roast chicken with black beans, salsa, and guacamole
- Grilled Steak with Red Wine Butter (see page 190)
- Guinness-Braised Short Ribs (see page 282)

510 calories
19 g fat (8 g saturated)
990 mg sodium

980 calories
46 g fat
(21 g saturated, 2 g trans)
2,350 mg sodium

Not That!

Boston Market Meatloaf Carver

Price: $6.29

Save!
470 calories and $1.41!

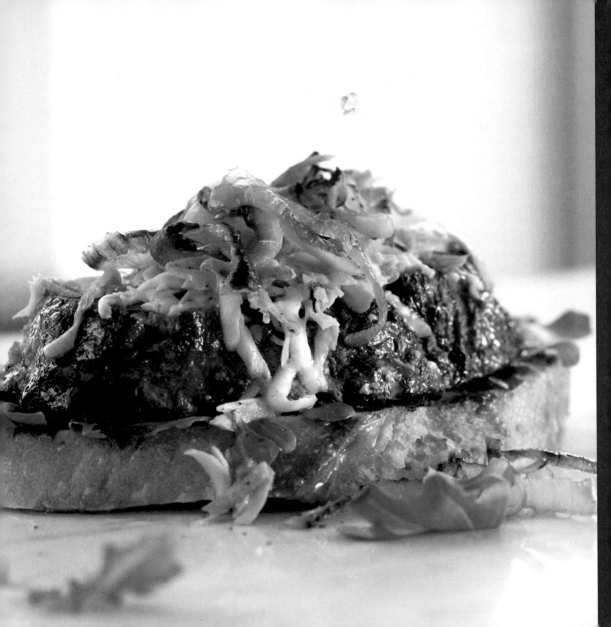

Pulled Pork Sandwich

Traditional North Carolina pulled pork is dressed with nothing more than a bit of spicy cider vinegar, used to accentuate the meat's flavor, not mask it. Unfortunately, when restaurants interpret this dish for a national audience, they use the same cheap trick unleashed on barbecued beef and racks of ribs: a bucket of sickeningly sweet sauce made from a slurry of sugar, corn syrup, and other insulin-spiking ingredients. The result: A single sandwich with as many calories as three Big Macs! We get back to the humble hog treatment and turn out a sandwich flush with flavor and light on calories.

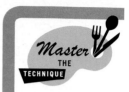

Master THE TECHNIQUE

Smoking pork

Not satisfied going the way of the Crock-Pot with your pork shoulder? Ed Mitchell, chef at The Pit in Raleigh, North Carolina, provides the details for an authentic, yet home-friendly smoked shoulder: Build a large charcoal fire on one side of the grill (called banking). Top the charcoal with a big handful of soaked hickory chips. On the other side, place a pan to catch meat drippings. Add the pork to the side with the pan, place the lid on top, and cook for 4 hours, refreshing the fire and the wood chips if the heat or the smoke dies down.

You'll Need:

- 1 **boneless pork shoulder (4–5 lb)**
- **Salt and black pepper to taste**
- ½ **Tbsp canola or vegetable oil**
- 1 **cup apple cider vinegar**
- 4 **cups low-sodium chicken broth**
- ½ **Tbsp liquid smoke**
- 4 **hamburger buns (preferably Martin's Potato Rolls)**
- **Coleslaw (see page 292)**

How to Make It:

- Heat a large skillet or sauté pan over medium-high heat. Cut the pork into 2 or 3 big pieces and season with salt and pepper. Add the oil to the pan and when hot, sear the pieces of pork until thoroughly browned on the outside. Remove the pork and place in a slow cooker.
- Add the vinegar to the hot pan and deglaze, scraping any bits of browned meat stuck to the bottom. Pour the vinegar over the pork, then add the broth and liquid smoke. Set the slow cooker to high and cook for 4 hours, until the pork falls apart with gentle pressure. Remove the pork from the liquid and shred. Toss with a bit more vinegar and serve on top of warm buns with coleslaw.

Makes 12 servings /
Cost per serving: $4.82

430 calories
18 g fat (5 g saturated)
540 mg sodium

1,590 calories

Not That!

Bob Evans Knife and Fork Pulled Pork Sandwich
Price: $6.84

Save!
1,160 calories and $2.02!

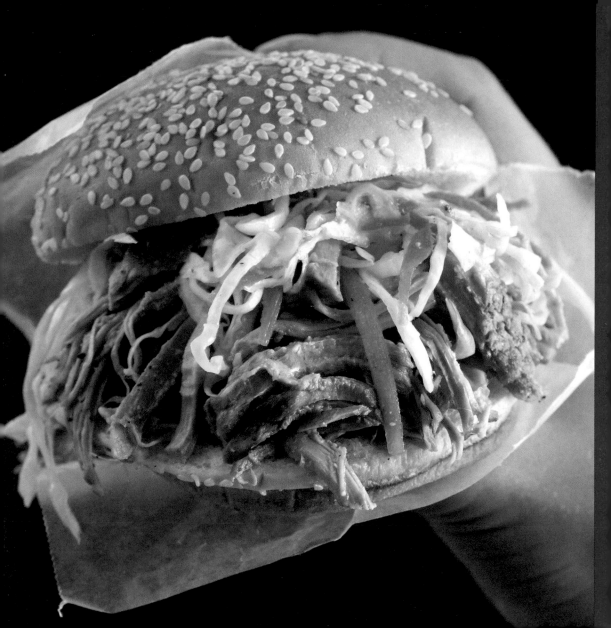

Cheesesteak Sandwich

The famous sandwich from Philly is a nutritionist's nightmare: mounds of greasy beef and fried onions; a massive, oil-soaked hoagie roll; and to top it all off, a viscous deluge of Cheez Whiz (that's right, traditional cheesesteaks are made with Whiz). But we want you to have your steak and eat it, too, so we came up with this version, which relies on a lean flank steak, a whole-wheat roll, and a yogurt-based blue cheese sauce. It's a bit fancier than the sandwich from the City of Brotherly Love, but to our tastes, it's also better.

You'll Need:

- 2 Tbsp plain Greek-style yogurt (we like Fage 2%)
- 2 Tbsp olive-oil mayonnaise
- ¼ cup crumbled blue cheese
- 16 oz skirt or flank steak
- Salt and black pepper to taste
- 2 cups arugula
- 2 tomatoes, sliced
- 4 whole-wheat sandwich rolls
- Caramelized Onions (see page 305)

Diffuse the caloric heft of mayo-based condiments by cutting the goop with 50 percent Greek yogurt.

How to Make It:

- Combine the yogurt, mayonnaise, and blue cheese. Set aside.
- Heat a grill, stovetop grill pan, or cast-iron skillet until hot. Season the steak with salt and pepper and cook for 3 to 4 minutes per side (for medium-rare), until the steak is firm but still gives with gentle pressure. Allow to rest for at least 5 minutes before slicing. Slice the steak into thin strips.
- Divide the arugula and tomatoes among the rolls. Top with the steak and caramelized onions and drizzle each sandwich with the blue cheese mayo.

Makes 4 servings / Cost per serving: $5.00

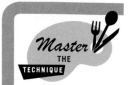

Master THE TECHNIQUE

Feel your way to perfect steak

Cut into a steak to see if it's done and you lose much of its precious juices. Instead, judge doneness by feel. Touch the center of the steak: Rare feels like a squishy dish sponge; medium is firm but yielding, like a Nerf football; and a well-done steak is hard yet springy, like a tennis ball. Regardless of feel, all meat needs to rest for 5 to 10 minutes, so the warm juices are reabsorbed by the meat, not your cutting board.

400 calories
14 g fat (4 g saturated)
730 mg sodium

1,070 calories
67 g fat
(16.5 g saturated, 1.5 g trans)
1,835 mg sodium

Not That!
Quiznos Regular Prime Rib Cheesesteak Sub
Price: $5.99

Save!
670 calories and $0.99!

156

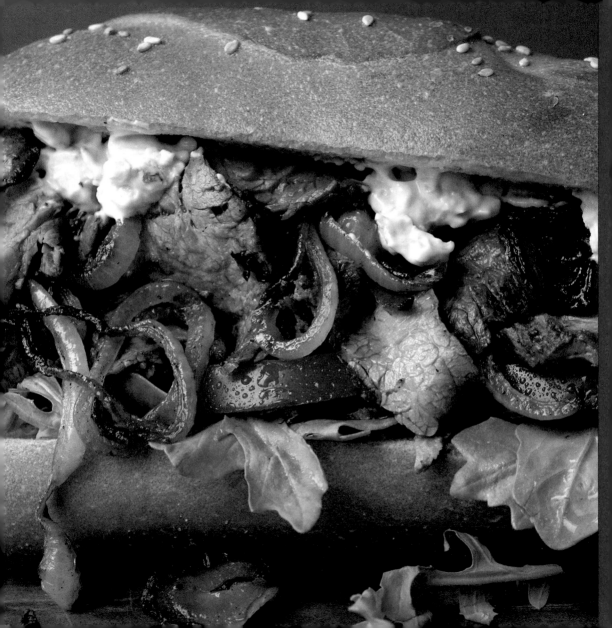

Mushroom Melts

Veggie burgers may seem like safe havens for nonmeat eaters and calorie counters alike. But the shocking truth we discovered after years of analyzing restaurant nutritional information is that vegetarian burgers offer little to no refuge from the onslaught of calories, fat, and sodium found in beef burgers. (Exhibit A: Ruby Tuesday's 952-calorie Veggie Burger.) We don't mess around with fake patties; instead, we go straight for a meaty portobello cap, rubbed in olive oil and balsamic and topped with a crown of melted mozz. Even if you're a beef buff, we think you'll like this meatless burger.

You'll Need:

- 2 Tbsp mayonnaise
- Juice of ½ lemon
- ¼ cup finely chopped roasted red peppers
- 1 clove garlic, minced
- 4 large portobello caps, stems removed
- 1 Tbsp olive oil
- 1 Tbsp balsamic vinegar
- 1 tsp dried Italian seasoning
- Salt and black pepper to taste
- ½ cup shredded mozzarella
- 4 slices red onion
- 4 potato rolls or whole-grain buns
- A few handfuls of mixed greens, arugula, or other lettuce

How to Make It:

- Heat a grill or grill pan. Combine the mayonnaise, lemon juice, red peppers, and garlic. (For a uniformly red mayo, puree in a food processor.)

- Rub the mushrooms with the olive oil, vinegar, Italian seasoning, and salt and pepper. Grill, top side down, for 2 to 3 minutes, flip, and immediately add the cheese. Cook for another 2 to 3 minutes, until the cheese is melted and the mushrooms are fully cooked. While the mushrooms are cooking, grill the onions until browned and toast the buns.

- Top each bun with greens, grilled onions, mushrooms, and the red pepper mayo.

Makes 4 servings /
Cost per serving: $3.17

370 calories
16 g fat (4 g saturated)
540 mg sodium

952 calories
53 g fat
95 g carbohydrates

Not That!
Ruby Tuesday Veggie Burger
Price: $8.69

Save!
582 calories
and $5.52!

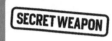
SECRET WEAPON

Flavored mayonnaise

Regular mayonnaise is boring; you just don't get a whole lot of flavor in exchange for your hefty calorie investment. By cutting the mayonnaise with ingredients like minced or roasted garlic, chipotle pepper puree, or roasted red peppers, you kill two birds with one stone: You up the flavor quotient while simultaneously lowering the caloric density of the mayo itself by bolstering it with healthier ingredients. Other great ingredients to flavor mayonnaise include balsamic vinegar, capers, fresh herbs, and wasabi powder. Just be sure to start with olive oil mayonnaise as your base; it's lower in calories and has a richer flavor.

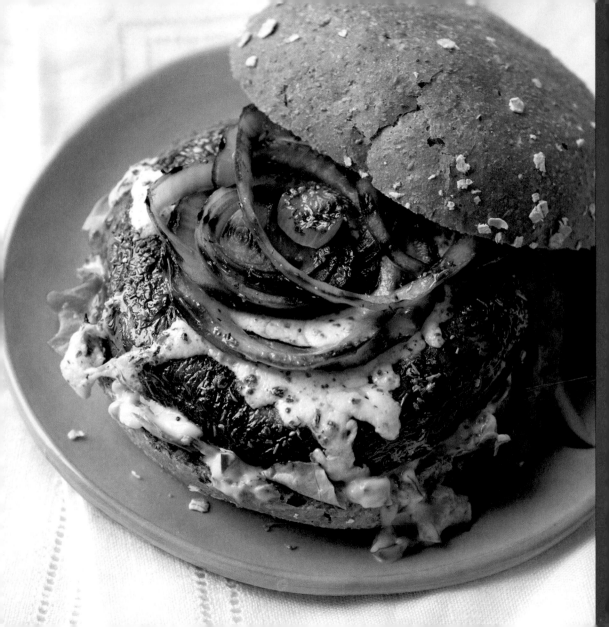

Cook This!
The Gobbler

If leftovers are the best thing about Thanksgiving, then this sandwich is the best thing about leftovers. But by all means, don't wait until Turkey Day to make this sandwich. With 900-calorie turkey sandwiches cluttering the menu boards of America's restaurants, you need as many cheap, delicious alternatives as you can get. Strewn with cranberry sauce, creamy avocado, and a bit of crispy bacon, this is the ultimate turkey sandwich. And if you want to shave an extra 100 calories, lose the bacon and make the sandwich on whole-grain bread; you'll still love the results.

You'll Need:

¼ cup whipped cream cheese

¼ cup whole-berry cranberry sauce

4 cups mixed greens or torn romaine

1 loaf focaccia or ciabatta, halved lengthwise and toasted

1 avocado, pitted, peeled, and thinly sliced

1 lb turkey (either sliced deli turkey or leftover chopped roasted turkey)

8 strips cooked bacon

How to Make It:

• Mix the cream cheese and cranberry until uniformly pink. Lay the lettuce across the bottom half of the bread. Top with the avocado, turkey, and bacon. Spread the cranberry cream cheese across the top part of the bread, top the sandwich, and cut into individual servings.

Makes 4 servings / Cost per serving: $3.86

As always, it's best if this is leftover from dinner, but if you buy it in the can, just be sure to skip the strange jello-like sauces.

If you do go for deli turkey, make it Hormel Natural Choice, the most promising of all packaged deli slices.

LEFTOVER LOVE

Want something to do with that extra Thanksgiving turkey that doesn't involve two slices of bread? Swap in turkey for some of our favorite chicken recipes to create these:

• Chicken Mole Enchiladas (see recipe on page 262)
• Thai Turkey Lettuce Wraps (see recipe on page 182)
• Grilled Caesar Salad (see recipe on page 102)
• Chicken Salad Sandwich (see recipe on page 146)
• Chicken Pot Pie (see recipe on page 226)

480 calories
16 g fat
(4.5 g saturated)
800 mg sodium

970 calories
54 g fat
(12 g saturated, 1 g trans)
1,970 mg sodium

Not That!
Panera Bread Sierra Turkey on Asiago Cheese Focaccia Price: $6.95

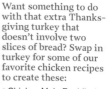

Save!
490 calories and $3.09!

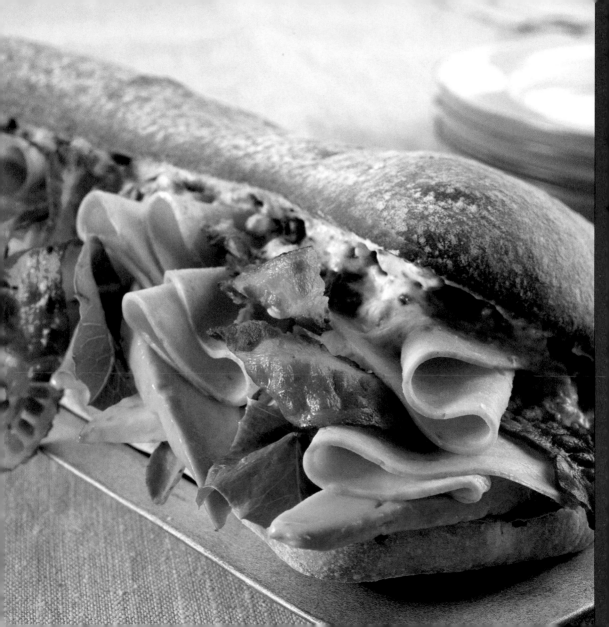

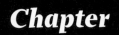

Chapter 7

Cook This, Not That!

Off the Grill

It's time to reclaim all that's good and great about America's favorite culinary pastime.

Ah, the Sunday barbecue—kids splashing in the pool, Mom mixing up some old-fashioned lemonade, Dad running around with a fire extinguisher, praying that the homeowners' insurance covers the decking. While everybody loves the idea of grilling, the reality is often less satisfying, and less flavorful, than we might dream—especially if Dad is a little overeager with the lighter fluid.

The Best Tool of All

Most of us grill one of four things: burgers, dogs, steaks, and chicken. And more often than not, the yield less resembles a gourmet dinner than it does a collection of hockey pucks. But in reality, the grill ought to be considered one of our most versatile weight loss tools. With a small array of skewers and racks, almost any meat or vegetable that can be boiled, broiled, fried, baked, or nuked can be cooked on the grill—and you'll reap untold weight loss benefits from giving a delicious diversity of foods their turn over the fire, especially the ones you don't normally eat. (Example: In a study published in the *European Journal of Clinical Nutrition*, subjects were fed equally caloric lunches consisting of either grilled fish or beef. Four hours later they ate dinner, and subjects were free to eat as much as they wanted. Those in the fish group needed 11 percent fewer calories to feel satisfied.)

That said, grilled food sometimes gets a bad rap, because many family grill-tenders have only two ways of cooking—raw or burnt. Well, from here on, that's a thing of the past. The information in this chapter is designed to introduce you to the many subtleties of grilled food, while quickly and efficiently making you master of the open flame. (And, hopefully, giving you enough great tastes and ideas to wean you off that bottle of sugary, calorie-laden commercial barbecue sauce.)

By becoming a baron of the barbecue, you'll easily overcome the "I'm too busy to cook" conundrum that keeps so many of us held hostage to the fry-cooks and grease purveyors at America's fast food restaurants. In about an hour on a Saturday afternoon, you can cook up an entire week's worth of entrées and side dishes, and simply call on your friend Mr. Tupperware to keep your meats and vegetables ready-to-eat in the fridge.

The Marinade Matrix

Marinades and spice rubs pack your food with flavor without the gut-busting calories of heavy sauces. They also break down tough muscle fibers and seal moisture into your food, turning even pedestrian cuts of meat into the type of succulent eats you pay serious cash for in a restaurant. With the help of Food Network chef Tyler Florence, we've created this easy-reference matrix for making the most of any meat.

Soak for your health: The polyphenols in marinade, drawn from a pool of herbs and spices, cut carcinogen deposits found in grilled foods by up to 88 percent, according to the Food Science Institute in Kansas.

Flavor Savers

The best marinades consist of three parts:

Acids

"Acid breaks down the muscle fibers and gives you a tender, moister piece of meat," says Florence. Expand your horizons with different vinegars: wine, sherry, or apple cider. Citrus juice, wine, and yogurt also do the trick.

Role players

These flavor builders add depth and character to a marinade. Olive oil, Dijon mustard, honey, fresh ginger, chipotle peppers, soy sauce, and others give your meat and fish an identity.

Accents

Fresh or dried herbs impart subtle notes, while assertive spices like cayenne and curry powder can shape an entire flavor profile. But beware of salt in your marinades. "Early salting creates osmosis, which pulls important moisture from your food," says Florence.

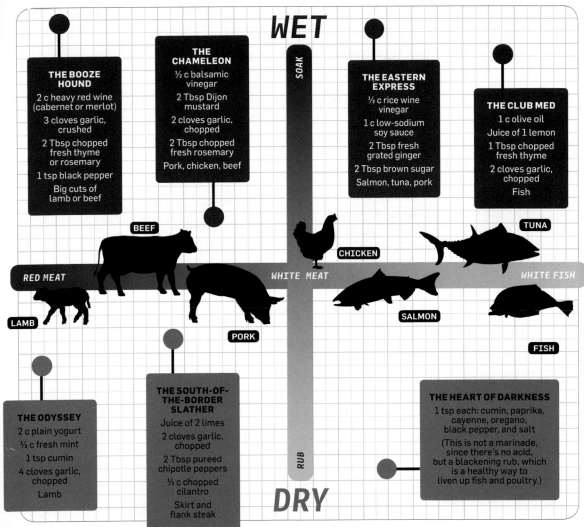

WET

SOAK

THE BOOZE HOUND

2 c heavy red wine (cabernet or merlot)

3 cloves garlic, crushed

2 Tbsp chopped fresh thyme or rosemary

1 tsp black pepper

Big cuts of lamb or beef

THE CHAMELEON

½ c balsamic vinegar

2 Tbsp Dijon mustard

2 cloves garlic, chopped

2 Tbsp chopped fresh rosemary

Pork, chicken, beef

THE EASTERN EXPRESS

½ c rice wine vinegar

1 c low-sodium soy sauce

2 Tbsp fresh grated ginger

2 Tbsp brown sugar

Salmon, tuna, pork

THE CLUB MED

1 c olive oil

Juice of 1 lemon

1 Tbsp chopped fresh thyme

2 cloves garlic, chopped

Fish

BEEF

CHICKEN

TUNA

RED MEAT

WHITE MEAT

WHITE FISH

LAMB

SALMON

PORK

FISH

THE ODYSSEY

2 c plain yogurt

½ c fresh mint

1 tsp cumin

4 cloves garlic, chopped

Lamb

THE SOUTH-OF-THE-BORDER SLATHER

Juice of 2 limes

2 cloves garlic, chopped

2 Tbsp pureed chipotle peppers

½ c chopped cilantro

Skirt and flank steak

RUB

THE HEART OF DARKNESS

1 tsp each: cumin, paprika, cayenne, oregano, black pepper, and salt

(This is not a marinade, since there's no acid, but a blackening rub, which is a healthy way to liven up fish and poultry.)

DRY

Cook This!
The Skewer Matrix

Whether you call them skewers or shish kebabs or dinner on a stick, there's hardly a better way to get your meat-and-vegetable fix than by grilling them in perfectly self-contained packages. The very nature of a skewer—lean meat, interspersed with a variety of fresh vegetables, and maybe brushed with a simple sauce—all but guarantees healthy eating. Best of all, they take but a few minutes to assemble and the potential for deliciousness is only limited by your imagination.

Four Super Skewers

To help get the party started, we've laid out the key players and a few of our favorite flavor combinations, but it's up to you to find the stick that suits you best.

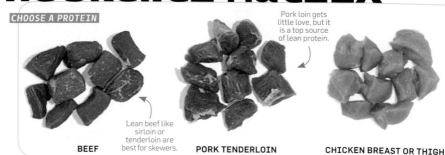

CHOOSE A PROTEIN

Pork loin gets little love, but it is a top source of lean protein.

Lean beef like sirloin or tenderloin are best for skewers.

BEEF

PORK TENDERLOIN

CHICKEN BREAST OR THIGH

CHOOSE PRODUCE

CHERRY TOMATOES

MUSHROOMS

CHOPPED ONIONS

CHOOSE A SAUCE

TERIYAKI

PESTO

BARBECUE SAUCE

TERIYAKI SALMON
salmon + mushrooms + pineapple + onion + teriyaki

PESTO CHICKEN
chicken + cherry tomatoes + zucchini + pesto

168

PEELED AND DEVEINED SHRIMP

SCALLOPS

SALMON

CHOPPED BELL PEPPERS

CHOPPED ZUCCHINI

Almost any firm fruit will do.

CUBED PINEAPPLE AND PEACHES

OLIVE TAPENADE

JERK SAUCE

OLIVE OIL, LEMON, AND HERBS

MEDITERRANEAN SCALLOP
scallops + zucchini + cherry tomatoes + onion + tapenade

JERK PORK
pork + onions + red bell pepper + peach + jerk sauce

Rules of the Skewer

Step 1

Soak wooden skewers in water for at least 20 minutes before loading them up. The moisture will prevent the wood from catching fire and scorching your dinner.

Step 2

The size of the produce on your skewer should be determined by the protein you're cooking them with. Shrimp and scallops cook quickly, so the produce should be cut smaller. Chicken and pork take time to cook, so pair with larger chunks of vegetables.

Step 3

When it comes to sauce, you can marinate the skewers before grilling—up to 2 hours for the meat, but no more than 30 minutes for the seafood. If not, brush the skewers before grilling and at least once during grilling. Marinate or no, it's always great to finish them with a light sheen of sauce before serving.

Step 4

You want a medium-hot grill—not so hot that it chars the outside before cooking the inside, but not so cool that the food doesn't fully caramelize.

14 Instant Outdoor Cla

Break out of your high-heat routines and add one of these bold grilled creations to your backyard repertoire.

1 Rub medallions of filet mignon (or any cut of beef) with equal parts ancho chile powder, ground coffee or espresso, and brown sugar, plus salt and fresh cracked pepper. Grill over medium-high heat to your desired doneness.

2 Season a chicken breast with salt and pepper, wrap in thin slices of prosciutto, and grill over low heat until the prosciutto is crisp and the chicken breast is firm. (Why not do the same with a fillet of halibut?)

3 Combine equal parts Dijon and honey, plus a chopped chiptole pepper. Spread half over the surface of a pork tenderloin or chicken breast. Grill until firm but still yielding and brush with the other half of the sauce before serving.

4 Mix curry powder with softened butter. Stuff under the skin of chicken breasts and thighs and grill until lightly charred and cooked all the way through.

5 Rub a tri-tip steak with salt, pepper, garlic salt, onion powder, and cayenne. Grill over medium heat until lightly charred on the outside and pink throughout, about 10 minutes per side.

6 Toss zucchini slices, eggplant planks, onion slices, and asparagus spears in olive oil, salt, and pepper. Grill until lightly charred, then remove to a cutting board and give them a rough chop. Toss with cooked bow-tie pasta, plus olive oil, the juice of a lemon, and grated Parmesan.

ssics

7 Shuck a dozen oysters. Top with softened butter mixed with lemon and Tabasco. Place the shells directly on the grill and cook until the butter begins to bubble, 3 to 5 minutes.

8 Place a hunk of haloumi cheese (found at Whole Foods or in Greek markets) directly on the grill. Cook until lightly charred on the outside, about 2 minutes a side. Top with olive oil and fresh herbs and serve with toasted bread.

9 Cut watermelon into ½"-thick squares. Rub with olive oil and grill until lightly caramelized. Toss with arugula, goat cheese, more olive oil, and balsamic vinegar.

10 *Mix plenty of olive oil with a few cloves of chopped garlic, red pepper flakes, salt and pepper. Marinate shrimp in half of the mixture for 20 minutes, then grill over high heat for 2 minutes a side, brushing with the remaining garlic oil.*

11 Roll a ball of pizza dough (store-bought or homemade) into 12" rounds. Cook on a well-oiled grill until the crust is firm enough to handle. Top with tomato sauce or pesto and your choice of cheese and toppings. Return to the coolest part of the grill, cover, and cook until the cheese begins to melt.

12 Toss chicken wings with soy, garlic, ginger, sriracha, and brown sugar and marinate for a few hours. Grill until charred and crispy.

13 Grill slices of pineapple until nicely caramelized. Top each with a scoop of vanilla ice cream and a drizzle of melted dark chocolate.

14 Rub chicken breasts with garlic, lime juice, and cumin. Grill until firm and serve sliced into warm tortillas with grilled onions and guacamole.

Beer Can Chicken

In the past decade, whole chickens mounted on beer cans have become a familiar sight at backyard barbecues the country over. And for good reason: The liquid creates steam that helps cook the chicken from the inside and keep it moist. Also, standing the chicken up vertically means the legs (which take the most time to cook) are exposed to the most intense heat, meaning the bird will cook evenly without drying out the breast. The result: one of the tastiest chickens imaginable with no heavy sauces or sides.

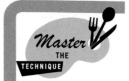

You'll Need:

1 **chicken** (3–4 lb)

24 oz Coca-Cola

¾ tsp salt

Freshly cracked pepper

1 can beer

Don't worry: You won't really be absorbing the calories from the Coke, since most of it is left behind in the brine. Don't have time to brine? Skip it. The chicken will still be obscenely good.

How to Make It:

- Combine the chicken and the Coke and soak overnight in the fridge (or for at least 2 hours).

- Heat a grill. If using charcoal, bank the hot coals to one side to create a cooler section for indirect cooking. If using a gas grill, leave one section of burners off and the others set on medium. Remove the chicken from the soda and dry all over. Rub with salt and pepper.

- Open up the beer can; drink half of it. Mount the chicken on top of the beer can, running the can through the chicken's cavity until it's firmly lodged and can stand up on its own. Place on the cooler side of the grill, cover, and cook until the a thermometer inserted into the thigh reads 160°F, about 1 to 1½ hours. You can baste the chicken with your favorite barbecue sauce in the last 20 minutes or so, but it's so moist, you don't really need it.

- Remove the chicken and allow to rest for 15 minutes before carving. Serve with baked beans and cole slaw.

Makes 4 servings / Cost per serving: $3.09

Brining meat

Lean meats like chicken, turkey, and pork tend to dry out easily, which is why they benefit immensely from a long soak in flavored liquid. A standard brine (and one that you can use here) is 6 cups water, 2 cups salt, and 2 cups sugar. Add any other flavor boosters (garlic, herbs, apple juice) and heat to dissolve the salt and sugar; cool before adding the meat. Store in the fridge for a few hours, or overnight.

410 calories
11 g fat
(2.5 g saturated)
730 mg sodium

1,000 calories

Not That!
T.G.I. Friday's Jack Daniels Chicken
Price: $14.89

Save!
590 calories
and $11.80!

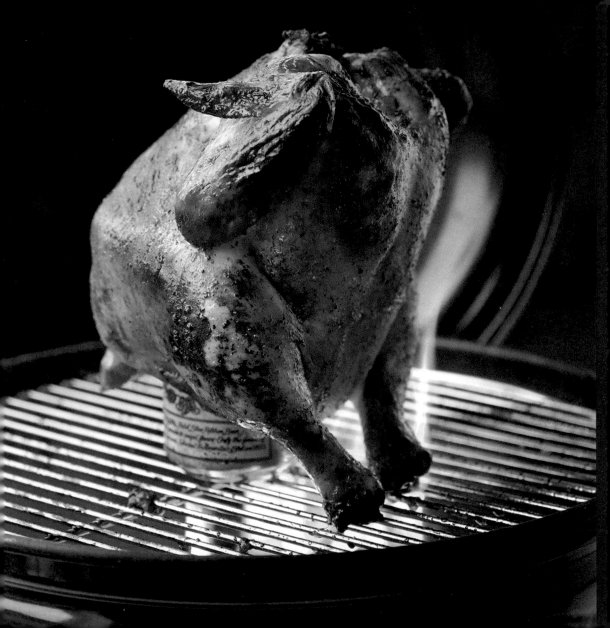

Cook This!
Grilled Fish Tacos

Who doesn't love fish tacos? South of the border, the fish is always battered and fried and served with an aggressive dousing of mayonnaise. We wanted to ditch the frying oil and mayo but maintain the flavor, so we subbed a spicy blackening seasoning and a nutrient-rich mango-avocado salsa, which cuts the heat and pairs perfectly with the fish. This salsa would make gardening gloves taste good.

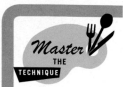

Master THE TECHNIQUE

Learn to salsa

Bottled salsas are fine in a pinch, but making fresh salsa is the type of effortless act that can instantly elevate your food and score you big points with anyone you cook for. All salsas follow a basic formula: 1 part aromatics + 2 parts flavor base. Begin with a finely chopped mix of onions, cilantro, and peppers (jalapeno, serrano, red bell). Add your flavor base: Tomatoes (roasted or raw) are favorites, but pineapple, mango, black beans, and corn can all play the role just as well. Finish with a bit of acid (lemon or lime juice, vinegar) and salt and pepper.

You'll Need:

- 1 mango, peeled, pitted, and cubed
- 1 avocado, pitted, peeled, and cubed
- ½ red onion, finely chopped
- Juice of 1 lime, plus wedges for garnish
- Chopped fresh cilantro
- Salt and black pepper
- Canola oil
- 2 large mahimahi fillets (1½ lb total)
- 1 Tbsp blackening spice (see page 167)
- 8 corn tortillas
- 2 cups finely shredded red cabbage

How to Make It:

- Mix the mango, avocado, onion, and the juice of 1 lime in a bowl. Season with cilantro, salt, and pepper.
- Heat a grill or stovetop grill pan until hot. Drizzle a light coating of oil over the fish and rub on the blackening spice. Cook the fish, undisturbed, for 4 minutes. Carefully flip with a spatula and cook for another 4 minutes. Remove.
- Warm the tortillas on the grill for 1 to 2 minutes or wrap in damp paper towels and microwave for 1 minute until warm and pliable.
- Break the fish into chunks and divide among the warm tortillas. Top with the cabbage and the mango salsa. Serve with the lime wedges.

Makes 4 servings / Cost per serving: $2.97

No ripe mangoes at the supermarket? Both pineapple and peaches would make perfect substitues.

380 calories
11 g fat (2 g saturated)
240 mg sodium

2,350 calories
152 g fat
(31 g saturated)
4,060 mg sodium

Not That!
On the Border Dos XX Fish Tacos
Price: $13.95

Save!
1,970 calories
and $10.98!

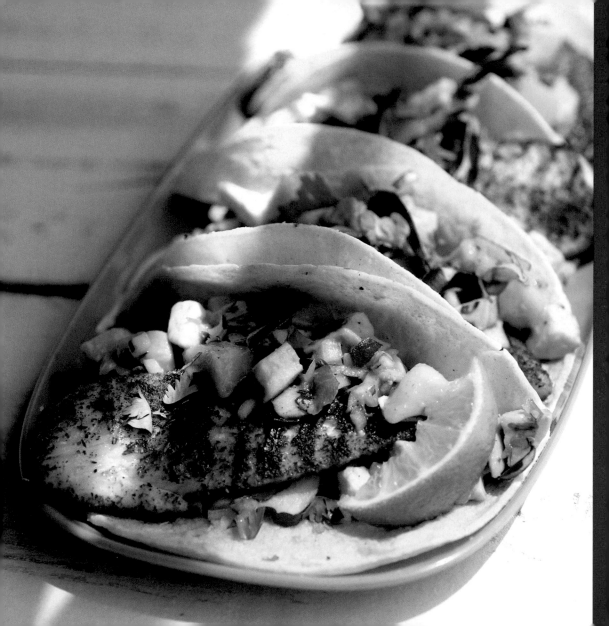

Grilled Pork & Peaches

Restaurant pork chops are usually Flintstonian in size and skirted with enough fat to keep a bear warm in the winter. The result (as witnessed here with the Romano's chop): 196 percent of your day's saturated fat, plus more sodium than you'd find in 36 cups of salted popcorn. Our dish takes its cue from classic pork chops and applesauce, using grilled fruit and blue cheese to punch up the flavor without skyrocketing the calorie count.

You'll Need:

- 4 **thick-cut (1"), bone-in pork chops (8 oz each)**
- Olive oil
- Salt and black pepper to taste
- 2 **firm peaches or nectarines, halved and pitted**
- 2 Tbsp **pine nuts, toasted**
- 1 **small red onion, thinly sliced**
- ½ cup **crumbled blue cheese**
- 1 Tbsp **balsamic vinegar**

How to Make It:

- Heat a grill to hot. Brush the pork with olive oil and season with salt and pepper. Grill for 4 to 5 minutes on each side. The outside should be charred (not burned), but the meat should be light pink in the middle.
- While the chops cook, brush the peach halves with oil and add them to the grill, cut side down. Grill for 5 minutes or until soft. Remove, slice, and toss with the pine nuts, onion, blue cheese, and vinegar; season with salt and pepper. Top each chop with half of the peach mixture and serve.

Makes 2 servings / Cost per serving: $7.71

Prepackaged pork chops are cut too thin, so they dry out easily. Have the butcher cut them thick and on the bone, which imparts moisture and flavor during cooking.

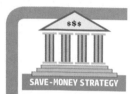

SAVE-MONEY STRATEGY

Savvy swaps

As much as we love the combination of funky blue cheese and sweet caramelized peaches, the ingredients aren't set in stone. Blue cheese pricey at your market? Try feta or goat cheese. Apricots or nectarines on sale today? Ditch the peaches for either. Price of pine nuts too high for your budget? Almonds, pecans, or walnuts all work beautifully. The point is, there's always room to adapt.

430 calories
24 g fat (8 g saturated)
530 mg sodium

1,380 calories
77 g fat (39 g saturated)
4,040 mg sodium

Not That!

Romano's Macaroni Grill Grilled Pork Chops
Price: $15.99

Save!
950 calories and $8.28!

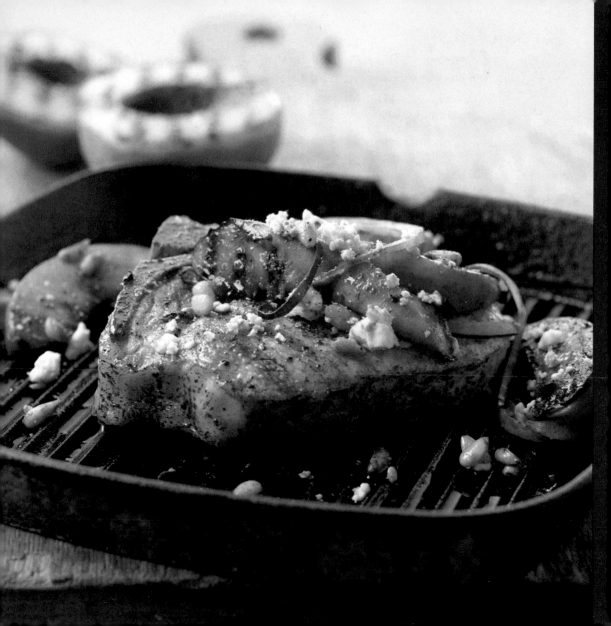

Cook This!
Grilled Salmon with Ginger-Soy Butter

Yes, even salmon can suffer at the hands of a restaurant chef who uses oil as a condiment and salt as a weapon. Whereas most of salmon's fat is of the heart-healthy monounsaturated variety, P.F. Chang's finds a way to cram nearly three-quarters of a day's worth of saturated fat into this otherwise super food.

You'll Need:

- 2 Tbsp unsalted butter, softened
- ½ Tbsp minced chives
- ½ Tbsp grated fresh ginger
- Juice of 1 lemon
- ½ Tbsp low-sodium soy sauce
- 4 salmon fillets (4–6 oz each)
- Salt and black pepper to taste
- 1 Tbsp olive oil

The best way to peel ginger? With a spoon. That's right; the edge of a spoon easily scrapes away ginger's thin skin without wasting any of the fragrant flesh inside.

How to Make It:

- Mix the butter, chives, ginger, lemon juice, and soy sauce. Set aside.

- Preheat a grill or grill pan. Season the salmon with salt and pepper and rub with the oil. Wipe the grill grates clean and rub with a paper towel dipped in oil. Add the salmon skin side down and cook for 4 to 5 minutes, until the skin is lightly charred and crisp.

- Flip the fish and cook for another 2 to 3 minutes on the flesh side, until the flesh flakes with gentle pressure from your finger but is still slightly translucent in the middle. (We believe salmon is best served medium, but if you want yours completely cooked, leave it on for another 2 to 3 minutes.)

- Serve the salmon with a generous spoonful of the flavored butter, which should begin to melt on contact.

Makes 4 servings / Cost per serving: $2.46

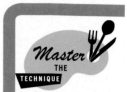

Master THE TECHNIQUE

Flavored butters

Spiking softened butter with assertive flavors is a great way to add an instant "sauce" to your dinner. And adding coins of compound butters (which keep for weeks in your fridge) to high-carb foods like baked potatoes can actually work to lower the glycemic impact of the dish, making a gentler ride for your blood sugar. Try any of these combinations on meat, fish, or vegetables.

- Crumbled blue cheese, chives, and black pepper
- Reduced balsamic vinegar and caramelized onions
- Minced sundried tomatoes and olives

390 calories
26 g fat (7 g saturated)
710 mg sodium

Not That!
P.F. Chang's Asian Grilled Salmon
Price: $17.95

734 calories
32 g fat
(14 g saturated)
1,306 mg sodium

Save!
344 calories
and $15.49!

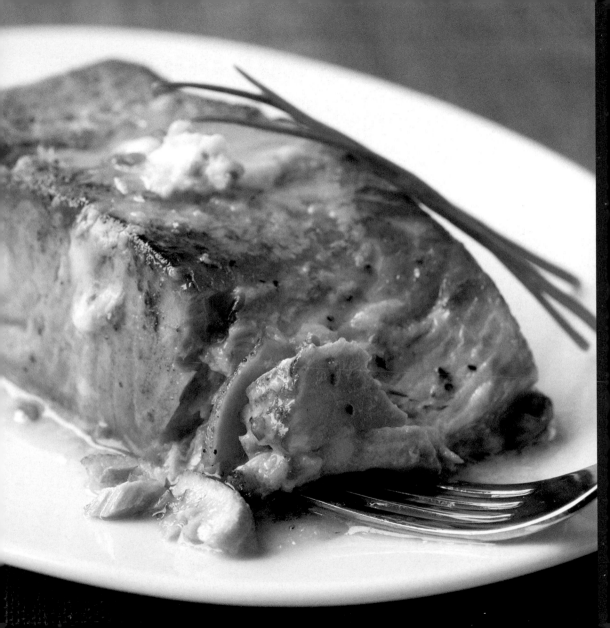

Mexican Hot Dogs

Hot dogs normally arouse the scorn of nutritionists and health-conscious eaters alike, but don't be so quick to dismiss the humble wiener. In the best circumstances, hot dogs are perfectly portioned, protein-packed vessels set to play host to a barrage of healthy, boldly flavored toppings. While finding that type of dog may be challenging at a restaurant, it's quick and effortless to create at home.

You'll Need:

- 4 hot dogs
- 4 scallions, bottoms trimmed
- 4 potato or whole-wheat hot dog rolls (we like Martin's)
- 4 Tbsp bottled salsa (preferably pico de gallo)
- Guacamole (see page 303)
- Pickled Jalapeños (see page 304)

How to Make It:

- Heat a grill or stovetop grill pan until hot. Add the hot dogs and scallions (work in batches, if necessary) and cook until lightly charred on all sides, about 10 minutes.

- Tuck the hot dogs into the rolls and top each with pico de gallo, guacamole, a grilled scallion, and jalapeños.

Makes 4 servings / Cost per serving: $2.06

If you're making these for a crowd, homemade salsa and guacamole are ideal, but if it's just you, go ahead and use a good store-bought product.

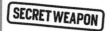

SECRET WEAPON

Applegate Farms Natural Big Apple Hot Dogs

Popular supermarket dogs like Ballpark and Nathan's can pack up to 200 calories and 10 grams of saturated fat—not exactly solid specimens to keep around the house. But this dog from Applegate Farms has just 100 calories and 3 grams of saturated fat, plus it's free of the chemical preservatives found in most franks. Just as important, the flavor is spot-on and the natural casing provides that perfect hot dog snap. Other favorite dog toppings include caramelized onions, sautéed mushrooms, chili sauce, and even the occasional fried egg.

330 calories
18 g fat
(6 g saturated)
900 mg sodium

570 calories
35 g fat
(15.5 g saturated)
1,216 mg sodium

Not That!

Five Guys Hot Dog with Onions and Relish
Price: $3.26

Save!

240 calories and $1.20!

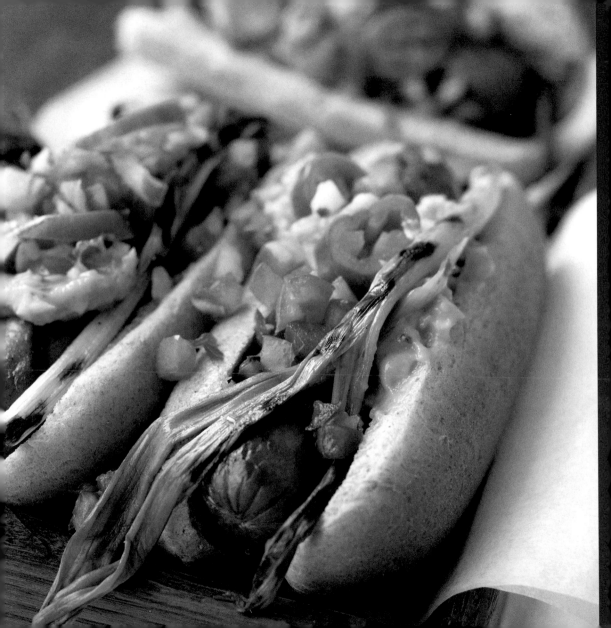

Thai Beef Lettuce Wraps

Asian cultures have known for hundreds (if not thousands) of years that wrapping things in lettuce makes an amazing snack or meal. Too bad the restaurant industry got their claws on the idea and fiddled with its simple brilliance. Now wraps at places like P.F. Chang's and Cheesecake Factory are overwrought affairs packing as many calories into an appetizer as you should have in an entire meal. Consider this Vietnamese-inspired version a blissful, healthy, flavor-packed return to the wrap's humble roots.

You'll Need:

- 12 oz flank, skirt, or sirloin steak
- Salt and black pepper to taste
- 1 Tbsp hot sauce (we like sriracha)
- 2 Tbsp fish sauce
- Juice of lime, plus wedges as garnish
- 1 jalapeño pepper, thinly sliced
- ½ red onion, thinly sliced
- ½ cup chopped fresh cilantro
- 1 carrot, grated
- 1 head Bibb lettuce, leaves separated

How to Make It:

- Heat the grill to hot or heat a grill pan over high heat for at least 5 minutes. Season the steak with salt and pepper and toss it onto the grill. Cook for about 4 minutes on each side, until it's firm but yielding to the touch. Let it rest for 5 minutes.

- Combine the hot sauce, fish sauce, and juice of 1 lime in a small saucepan over low heat.

- Slice the steak thinly (if it's flank or skirt steak, be sure to cut across the grain) and drizzle half of the warm sauce over it. Set out the jalapeño and onion slices, cilantro, carrot, and lettuce, along with the lime wedges and sauce. Use the leaves like tortillas to wrap up the steak slices with the other ingredients.

Makes 2 servings / Cost per serving: $4.86

$$\left(\Psi + \textbf{I} \right)^2$$

MEAL MULTIPLIER

Here are five other great culinary combinations that can be stuffed into lettuce leaves.

- Grilled mushrooms with goat cheese
- Curry chicken salad (see page 146)
- Grilled fish and guacamole (a lettuce fish taco!)
- Ground turkey sautéed with ginger, garlic, and soy sauce
- Carolina-style pulled pork (see page 154)

290 calories
8 g fat (3 g saturated)
1,020 mg sodium

Save!
683 calories and $7.09!

973 calories
10 g saturated fat
2,110 mg sodium

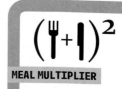

Not That!

The Cheesecake Factory Thai Lettuce Wraps
Price: $11.95

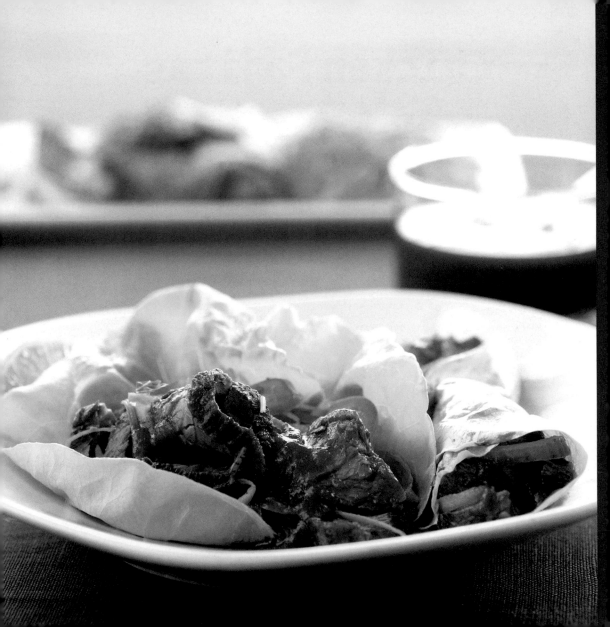

Chicken Fajitas

A skillet of sizzling chicken or beef strewn with fresh onions and peppers should be the base for a fantastic meal, but then why do Chili's, Chevys, Applebee's, and Baja Fresh all serve versions with more than 1,000 calories? Fattier cuts of meat, oversize tortillas, and hulking condiment trays are to blame. Thankfully, ours are boldly flavored, loaded with vegetables and protein, and healthy enough to eat twice a week.

You'll Need:

- ½ cup orange juice
- 2 Tbsp chopped chipotle pepper
- Juice of 1 lime
- 1 tsp ground cumin
- Salt and black pepper to taste
- 1 lb boneless, skinless chicken breasts
- 1 Tbsp canola oil
- 1 red bell pepper, sliced
- 1 green bell pepper, sliced
- 2 onions, sliced
- 8 small (6") flour tortillas, warmed
- Guacamole (see page 303)
- Salsa
- 1 cup shredded Jack or Cheddar cheese

How to Make It:

- Combine the orange juice, chipotle, lime juice, cumin, 1 teaspoon salt, and 1 teaspoon pepper in a sealable plastic bag. Add the chicken and marinate in the fridge for an hour.
- Preheat a grill or stovetop grill pan until hot. Remove the chicken from the marinade and discard what's left in the bag. Grill the chicken for 4 to 5 minutes per side, until lightly charred and cooked all the way through. Let rest for 5 minutes before slicing.
- While the chicken cooks, heat the oil in a large cast-iron skillet over high heat. Cook the bell peppers and onions until charred and caramelized on the outside, about 10 minutes. Season with salt and pepper.
- Slice the chicken into thin pieces. For a dramatic presentation, place the chicken on top of the hot peppers in the skillet and bring the skillet sizzling to the table. Serve with warm tortillas, guacamole, salsa, and cheese.

Makes 4 servings /
Cost per serving: $4.13

$(\dagger + \dagger)^2$

MEAL MULTIPLIER

Four other bases that make fantastic fajitas:

- Skirt steak or flank steak, swapping in for the chicken, soaked in the same marinade
- Medium shrimp, peeled and deveined, and soaked in the same marinade for 20 minutes or less
- Pork Chile Verde (see page 278), served with sautéed onions and peppers
- Portobello mushroom caps, seasoned with chili powder, grilled or sautéed

490 calories
19 g fat
(3.5 g saturated)
900 mg sodium

1,030 calories
56 g fat
(16 g saturated)
3,620 mg sodium

Not That!

Chili's Classic Combo Fajitas with 3 Tortillas and Condiments Price: $11.49

Save!
540 calories
and $7.36!

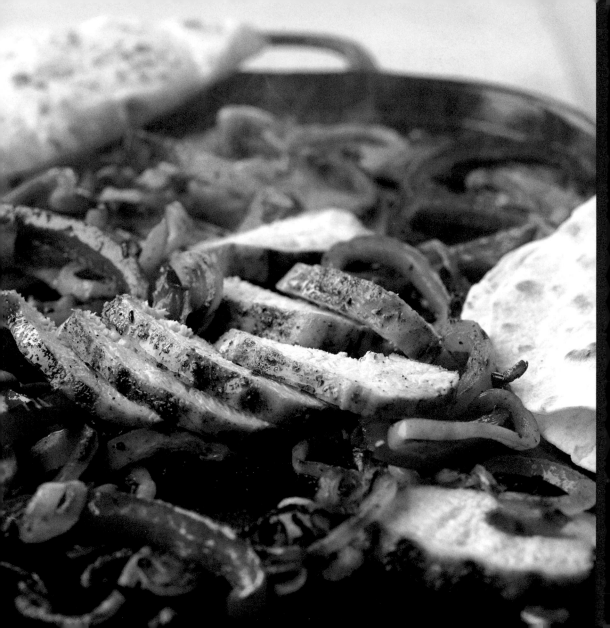

Grilled Flank Steak
with Chimichurri

Nobody knows steak like the Argentines. Theirs is a culture reared on steer; they eat 124 pounds of beef per person annually, nearly double what our cow-crazy citizenry consumes. Given the expertise, it's a shame that corporate chefs don't turn to them for inspiration when it comes to beefy matters. If they did, they'd find that chimichurri—a bright herbal sauce that plays the role of steak sauce in Argentina—is one of the most delicious (not to mention healthy) condiments on the planet. Serve it up with grilled scallions, pinto beans, and warm corn tortillas as a perfect replacement for fajitas.

You'll Need:

¼ cup red wine vinegar

3 tbsp water

4 cloves garlic, minced

Salt and coarsely ground black pepper

1 tsp red pepper flakes

¼ cup olive oil

1 cup finely chopped fresh flat-leaf parsley

1½ lb flank, skirt, or sirloin steak

2 bunches scallions

How to Make It:

• To make the chimichurri sauce, mix the vinegar, water, garlic, 1 teaspoon salt, 1 teaspoon black pepper, and pepper flakes. Whisk in the oil. When everything's blended, whisk in the parsley.

• Heat a grill or stovetop grill pan until hot. Season the steak with salt and pepper and place it on the hot grill. For medium-rare, cook it for 3 to 4 minutes on each side, or until an instant-read thermometer inserted into the thickest part reads 140°F. Trim the roots from the scallions and add the entire bunch to the grill just after you've flipped the steak. Cook the scallions until they're lightly charred, 4 to 5 minutes.

• Drizzle the steak with the chimichurri and serve with the grilled scallions.

Makes 4 servings /
Cost per serving: $4.71

Chimichurri has many interpretations. Fresh bay leaves and oregano often make it into the mix, as do red bell peppers and lime juice. Tweak and reinvent at will.

Save!
970 calories
and $7.29!

440 calories
31 g fat (7 g saturated)
570 mg sodium

1,410 calories

Not That!
Applebee's Sizzling Steak Fajitas
Price: $12.00

Upgrade

NUTRITIONAL

Most American cattle is raised on corn, which presents two major problems for the consumer (and even more for the cows). Not only does corn produce cows with more intramuscular marbling (i.e., fat), it also demands the use of antibiotics to keep the cows—which aren't naturally equipped to live on corn—from getting sick. In Argentina, most cows still live off of what they were born to eat: grass. The result is a leaner cut of beef free of antibiotics and rich in omega-3 fatty acids. You'll pay a bit more for grass-fed beef, but if you can afford the occasional splurge, consider it a down payment on a leaner, tastier life.

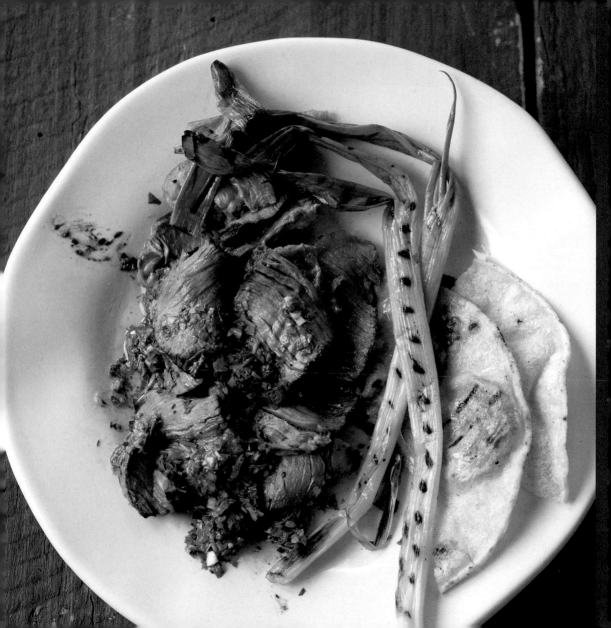

Cook This!
Grilled Mahimahi with Red Pepper Sauce

Menu descriptions can be so deceiving. "Red-chile seasoned fresh fillet of mahimahi grilled to perfection," as it reads on the On the Border menu, sounds like the healthiest dish ever devised by a chain restaurant. So how does it end up chewing through nearly half a day's calories? It's another unsolved restaurant mystery. As long as it's fresh, fish doesn't need much to make it delicious, and our simple, spicy African pepper sauce (called harissa) fits the bill. With just a few ingredients, it brings big flavor, plus heart-healthy fats and a monster dose of vitamin C, to any grilled protein it touches. If you don't feel like making it, try Mustapha's Moroccan Harissa (igourmet.com).

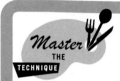

Crispy skin

Most people prefer their fish without skin, and we can't blame them: Who wants to eat chewy, flaccid fish skin? But skin does offer a number of excellent benefits. Not only does it contain a large percentage of fish's most virtuous nutrients (including omega-3s), but it also can protect the delicate fillet from drying out. Plus, if cooked properly, it provides a lovely crispy contrast to the soft flesh. Use paper towels to dry the skin thoroughly (wet skin won't crisp) and lightly oil it. Cook the fish skin side down for 75 percent of the time, until it's lightly charred and almost brittle, before turning to finish cooking briefly on the flesh side.

You'll Need:

- 1 jar (12 oz) roasted red peppers, drained
- ½ tsp cayenne pepper
- 1 clove garlic
- 2 Tbsp olive oil
- 1 tbsp sherry or red wine vinegar
- ½ tsp ground cumin
- Salt and black pepper to taste
- 4 mahimahi, sea bass, halibut, or snapper fillets (6 oz each)

How to Make It:

- To make the harissa, combine the red peppers, cayenne, garlic, olive oil, vinegar, and cumin in a blender and puree until smooth. Season with salt and pepper.
- Lightly oil a grill or stovetop grill pan and heat until medium-hot. Lightly season the flesh side of the fillets with salt and pepper and place them, skin side down, on the hot grill. Cook for 4 to 5 minutes, until the skins are lightly charred and crispy. Turn them over and cook another 2 to 3 minutes. When they're done, the fish should flake with gentle pressure from your fingertip.
- Serve immediately with a big scoop of harissa.

Makes 4 servings / Cost per serving: $5.64

Don't limit this sauce to fish alone. It's amazing on grilled steak, pork chops, roasted chicken, or tossed with grilled vegetables.

310 calories
15 g fat (2 g saturated)
480 mg sodium

970 calories
35 g fat (6 g saturated)
1,930 mg sodium

Not That!
On the Border Grilled Mahi Mahi
Price: $14.99

Save!
660 calories and $9.35!

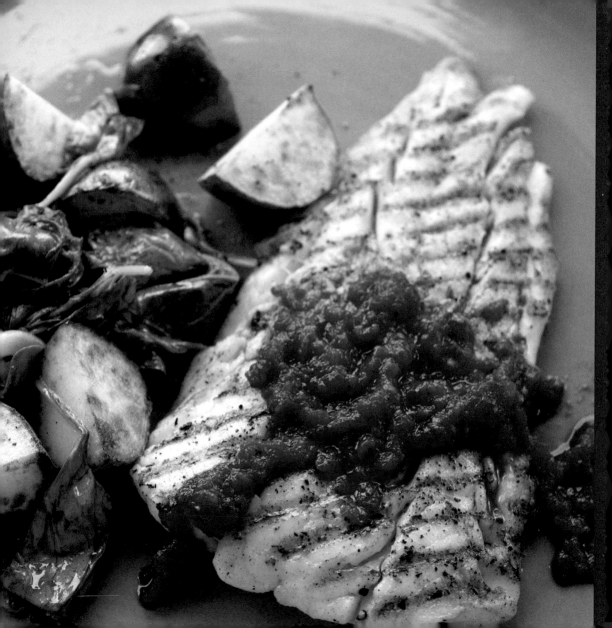

Cook This!
Grilled Steak with Red Wine Butter

Few meals satisfy like a good steak. And few things will ruin a good steak quicker than a heavy-handed sauce. That's why it's best to take your steaks simply grilled when eating out, lest you end up eating 2 days' worth of saturated fat. We'll give you steak and a slab of spiked butter for a quarter of the cost.

You'll Need:

- 1 cup dry red wine
- 1 shallot, minced
- 4 Tbsp butter, softened
- 1 tsp chopped fresh rosemary
- Black pepper to taste
- Salt to taste
- 4 steaks (flank, sirloin, skirt, or filet; 6 oz each)

How to Make It:

- Combine the wine and shallot in a small saucepan and simmer over medium heat until reduced to about 2 tablespoons (it will have a thick, syrupy consistency).

- Let the red wine syrup cool, then stir into the softened butter with the rosemary and a few cracks of black pepper. Once fully incorporated, spoon the butter onto a large piece of plastic wrap. Fold the wrap over the butter and twist the ends to create a log of red wine butter. Place in the fridge until ready to use.

- Preheat a grill, stovetop grill pan, or cast-iron skillet. Season the steaks with salt and pepper and cook until medium-rare (about 8 minutes total for skirt and flank and 10 to 12 minutes for the sirloin and filet). Remove the steaks and slice a coin of the butter over the top of each.

Makes 4 servings / Cost per serving: $3.72

Save!
515 calories and $11.23!

*380 calories
19 g fat
(10 g saturated)
470 mg sodium*

*895 calories
48 g fat
(25 g saturated)
2,905 mg sodium*

Not That!
Outback Steakhouse Roasted Filet Tenderloin with Port Wine Sauce Price: $14.95

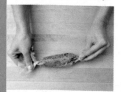

STEP-BY-STEP

Flavored butter

Having flavored butter on hand means you have sauce in a second. Combine the ideas on page 178 with the technique here for a potent flavor vehicle.

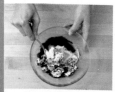

Step 1: *Mix softened butter with flavor add-ons.*

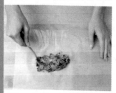

Step 2: *Place in the center of a piece of plastic wrap.*

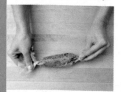

Step 3: *Twist the edges to form a uniform log.*

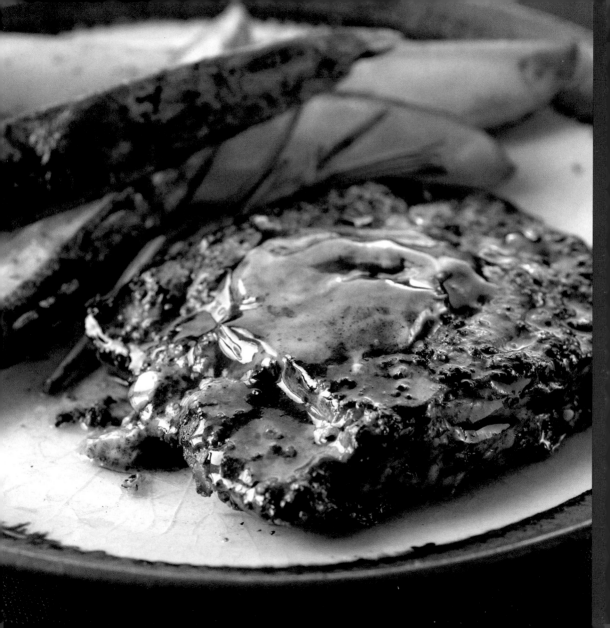

Dr Pepper Ribs

Order ribs at a restaurant and you could gain a pound of fat by the time the bill comes. Think we're kidding? The ribs at Outback, with more than 4 days' worth of saturated fat, are the Worst Food in America. And other restaurant ribs don't fare much better. We keep these ribs-sticking ribs lean by serving up half-slabs with a perfectly balanced sauce.

You'll Need:

- 2 **racks baby back ribs**
- 1 **bottle (2-liter) Dr Pepper**
- **Salt and black pepper**
- 1 **Tbsp chili powder**
- 1 **cup water**
- ½ **Tbsp canola or vegetable oil**
- ½ **onion, minced**
- 1 **clove garlic, minced**
- ½ **cup ketchup**
- 2 **Tbsp Worcestershire sauce**
- 2 **Tbsp apple cider vinegar**
- ⅛ **tsp cayenne pepper**

How to Make It:

- Place the ribs in a baking dish large enough to hold them comfortably. Pour in enough soda to cover, saving at least ½ cup for the barbecue sauce. Add ¼ cup salt and soak for at least 2 hours or overnight in the refrigerator.

- Preheat the oven to 350°F. Remove the ribs from the liquid and pat dry; discard the liquid. Sprinkle the ribs with the chili powder and return to the baking dish. Add the water and cover tightly with foil. Bake for 2 hours, until the meat is tender and nearly falling off the bone.

- While the ribs are in the oven, make the barbecue sauce. Heat the oil in a medium saucepan over medium heat. Sauté the onion and garlic until soft and fragrant, then add the ketchup, Worcestershire, vinegar, cayenne, and the reserved ½ cup soda. Simmer for 15 to 20 minutes, until the sauce thickens.

- Heat a grill until hot. Brush the ribs with barbecue sauce and grill for 10 to 15 minutes, rib side down, on a cooler part of the grates. Flip over and cook on the other side until lightly charred and smoky. Remove from the grill, brush with more sauce, and serve.

Makes 4 servings /
Cost per serving: $5.17

400 calories
15 g fat (4 g saturated)
1,140 mg sodium

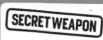

Dr Pepper

No, Dr Pepper isn't healthy—not even close, which is why you should rarely drink the stuff. But in moderation, it makes an amazing flavor booster. By soaking the ribs in a bath of Dr Pepper, you end up with tender meat in-fused with a touch of sweetness and salt, but you leave all the cal-ories behind. Yes, the soda does come into play in the sauce, but it takes the place of maple syrup or brown sugar, adding a measure of sweetness, along with a variety of complex flavor.

Not That!

Outback Steakhouse Baby Back Ribs Full Rack
Price: $12.95

3,021 calories
242 g fat
(90 g saturated)
4,678 mg sodium

Save!

2,621 calories
and $7.78!

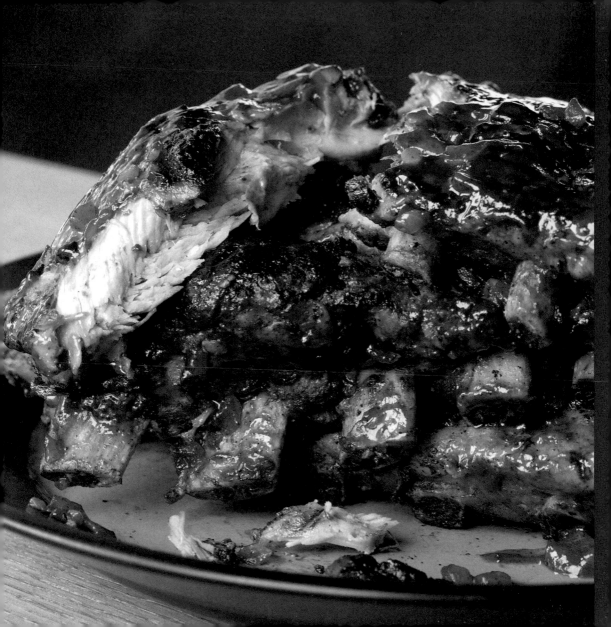

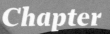

8

Cook This, Not That!

Pasta

In the age of the 3,000-calorie pasta plate, you need a little help to get your healthy noodle fix.

There's no greater comfort food than a heaping plate of noodles basking in a warm Jacuzzi of sauce. Ever since the first Italian grandmother comforted her brood with a bowl of spaghetti, pasta has been the go-to dish for any crisis. It's a high-energy carb fix and just about the easiest, fastest thing you can whip up—indeed, knowing how to boil water and toss in some hard linguine has turned many an inept bachelor into a first-class kitchen Casanova, even if the sauce came out of jar.

But the easiest way to cook up seduction has become the easiest way to lose out on said seduction, when the pasta comes from your favorite chain restaurant. Today's restaurant portion of spaghetti and meatballs has ballooned from a modest 500 calories just 20 years ago into a full-blown inflationary crisis, with the average serving now carrying 1,025 calories—and there's no sign of this bubble bursting any time soon. That's bad news if all you really want is a romantic night on the town.

Solving the Pasta Problem

Pasta has gotten a reputation as a food that fattens—Hollywood legend has it that Martin Scorsese got Robert De Niro out of fighting shape and into his late-life Jake LaMotta lard by fattening him up on pasta for the second half of *Raging Bull.* But that reputation isn't fair, because pasta is one of the original health foods. Even regular spaghetti is made from some whole grains, and you can boost the weight loss benefits of your next at-home dish even more by opting for whole-grain pasta: Switching to whole wheat noodles can triple the fiber load in your pasta, not to mention add a nutritional cache of B vitamins, manganese, and tryptophan. Not surprisingly, a Tufts University study found that eating more whole grains was associated with improved readings on nearly every significant health indicator, including BMI, blood pressure, LDL cholesterol, fasting blood glucose, and fasting insulin levels.

And the sauce ought to be an added boost as well. You probably already know that tomatoes are a great source of lycopene, an antioxidant that's been shown to be a powerful cancer fighter and can help protect skin from sun damage. But turn the humble tomato into a marinara sauce and

its protective powers really bloom: Turns out the now-famous antioxidant proliferates in a hot pan. That means as the tomatoes are simmered into marinara, lycopene concentrations multiply by a factor of about seven, making that sweet red sauce the most lycopene-rich food you'll ever eat.

So what's happened to restaurant pasta? It's simple: Portion sizes have grown exponentially, and sauces have become more sophisticated—fettuccine Bolognese (basically, marinara with meat in it) isn't as sexy to order as, say, "fettuccine Alfredo." But uttering those two words to a waiter at your local Olive Garden is like putting your tailor on notice that he's going to have to let out your pants. It more than doubles the number of calories in the sauce. And the math on that one is simple: bigger portions plus fattier sauces? Alfredo, we knew it was you! You broke our hearts!

Pasta made at home is incredibly cheap to buy, easy to cook, and packed with healthy ingredients. Pasta at a restaurant is cheap to buy (for the restaurant, at least), easy to eat lots of, and packed with more calories than you might ever imagine. It's time to start using your noodle and avenge the good name of Italian grandmothers everywhere.

The Pasta Matrix

Italians have pasta creation in their blood. Give a clueless young dude from Rome a box of noodles and a bottle of olive oil and watch him work wonders. But there's no reason all of us without the pasta gene can't do the same, especially once grasping a few techniques, tricks, and flavor combinations. Learn to cook pasta properly, sauce it skillfully, and portion it appropriately, and you can enjoy delicious 20-minute meals healthy enough to eat any night of the week.

Four Standby Pastas

In the time it takes you to boil water and cook noodles, you can whip up a sauce loaded with lean protein, fresh vegetables, and antioxidant-dense flavor boosters. Here are four favorites.

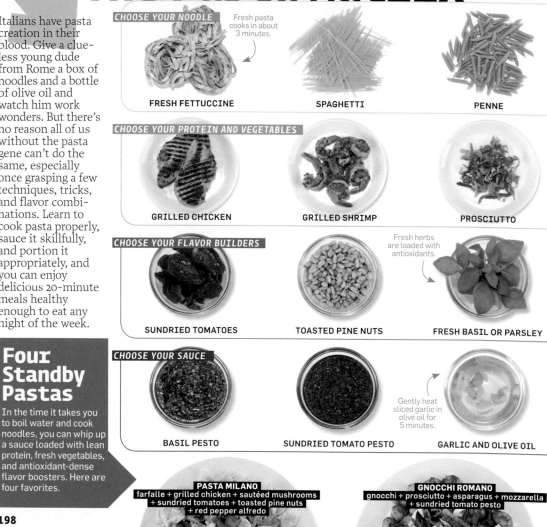

CHOOSE YOUR NOODLE

Fresh pasta cooks in about 3 minutes.

FRESH FETTUCCINE   SPAGHETTI   PENNE

CHOOSE YOUR PROTEIN AND VEGETABLES

GRILLED CHICKEN   GRILLED SHRIMP   PROSCIUTTO

CHOOSE YOUR FLAVOR BUILDERS

Fresh herbs are loaded with antioxidants.

SUNDRIED TOMATOES   TOASTED PINE NUTS   FRESH BASIL OR PARSLEY

CHOOSE YOUR SAUCE

Gently heat sliced garlic in olive oil for 5 minutes.

BASIL PESTO   SUNDRIED TOMATO PESTO   GARLIC AND OLIVE OIL

PASTA MILANO
farfalle + grilled chicken + sautéed mushrooms + sundried tomatoes + toasted pine nuts + red pepper alfredo

GNOCCHI ROMANO
gnocchi + prosciutto + asparagus + mozzarella + sundried tomato pesto

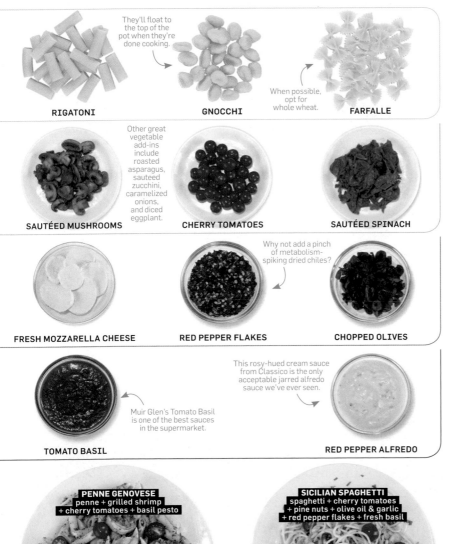

They'll float to the top of the pot when they're done cooking.

RIGATONI

GNOCCHI

When possible, opt for whole wheat.

FARFALLE

Other great vegetable add-ins include roasted asparagus, sautéed zucchini, caramelized onions, and diced eggplant.

SAUTÉED MUSHROOMS

CHERRY TOMATOES

SAUTÉED SPINACH

Why not add a pinch of metabolism-spiking dried chiles?

FRESH MOZZARELLA CHEESE

RED PEPPER FLAKES

CHOPPED OLIVES

This rosy-hued cream sauce from Classico is the only acceptable jarred alfredo sauce we've ever seen.

Muir Glen's Tomato Basil is one of the best sauces in the supermarket.

TOMATO BASIL

RED PEPPER ALFREDO

PENNE GENOVESE
penne + grilled shrimp
+ cherry tomatoes + basil pesto

SICILIAN SPAGHETTI
spaghetti + cherry tomatoes
+ pine nuts + olive oil & garlic
+ red pepper flakes + fresh basil

The Rules of Pasta

Step 1
In Italy, it's all about the noodle, but if you want to fill your belly without filling out your waistline, you should tilt the ratio to heavily favor the sauce and toppings.

Step 2
That said, cooking the noodles properly is still the most important step in making good pasta. Forget package instructions. Instead, spear noodles periodically to taste for doneness. Al dente ultimately means your pasta has the barest bite in the center.

Step 3
Before draining your pasta, dip a coffee mug into the pot and scoop up the cooking water. If the noodles look dry, add a few splashes of this magical stuff. The starchy water not only moistens the dish, but it helps the sauce cling to the noodles.

Step 4
Always toss the pasta with the sauce in the pan. Combining the two on the stovetop and cooking for 30 seconds ensures even distribution and allows sauce and noodle to meld.

199

Cook This!
Spaghetti & Meatballs

Traditional meatballs are made with a mixture of beef, pork, and veal. Turkey, lean and tender, replaces the latter two in these meatballs, saving you major calories. And if anything, go heavy on the meatballs and light on the pasta.

You'll Need:

- 2 slices bread, soaked in milk for 5 minutes
- 12 oz ground turkey breast
- 12 oz 85% lean ground beef
- 1 egg
- ½ cup chopped parsley, plus more for garnish
- 2 Tbsp grated Parmesan, plus more for garnish
- ¾ tsp salt
- ½ tsp pepper
- 1 onion, minced
- 3 cloves garlic, minced
- 2 Tbsp olive oil
- 1 can (28 oz) whole peeled tomatoes (we love Muir Glen)
- 1 lb DeCecco Whole Wheat Spaghetti

How to Make It:

- Remove the bread from the milk, squeeze out most of the liquid, and tear into tiny pieces. Mix the turkey, beef, egg, parsley, Parmesan, salt, pepper, half of the onion, and half of the garlic. Form into golf ball–size balls.

- Heat half of the olive oil in a large nonstick skillet or sauté pan and cook the meatballs over medium heat until well browned. Set aside.

- Heat the remaining tablespoon of olive oil in a saucepan and cook the remaining onion and garlic over medium heat until translucent. Add the tomatoes and bring to a simmer. Add the meatballs and cook for 15 to 20 minutes.

- Cook the pasta according to the package instructions until al dente. Divide it among 6 plates or bowls, top with meatballs and sauce, and garnish with parsley and Parmesan.

Makes 6 servings / Cost per serving: $2.48

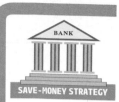

SAVE-MONEY STRATEGY

Think fresh tomatoes are the key to a great pasta sauce? Think again. Not only are they up to three times as expensive as canned tomatoes, they also require more prep work and produce inconsistent results (especially during winter, when tomatoes are shipped in from the southern hemisphere). Canned tomatoes are picked at the height of tomato season and canned on the spot. Whole peeled tomatoes are your best bet, since they're minimally processed and retain the most intense tomato flavor.

510 calories
12.5 g fat
(5 g saturated)
740 mg sodium

1,110 calories
50 g fat
(20 g saturated)
2,180 mg sodium

Not That!
Olive Garden Spaghetti & Meatballs
Price: $9.25

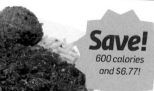

Save!
600 calories and $6.77!

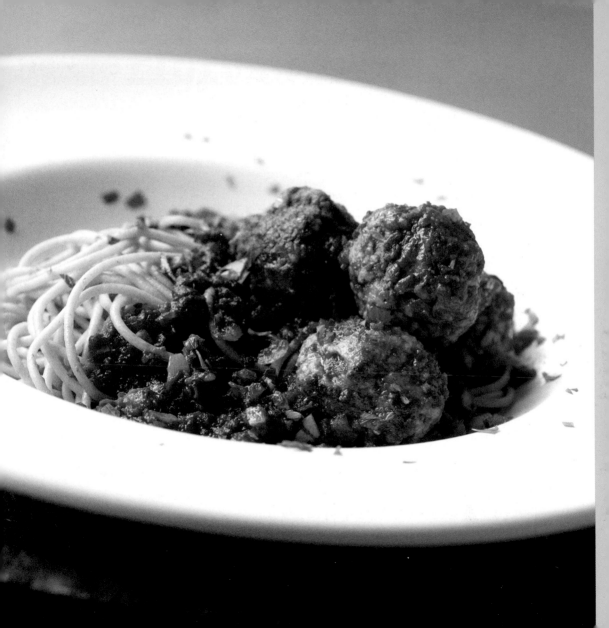

Cook This!

3-Cheese Ravioli with Cherry Tomatoes

"Four cheese" anything in the food world doesn't just mean four different types of cheese; it usually signifies quadruple the quantity, too. Here you get the depth and nuance of creamy ricotta, smoky mozzarella, and salty, sharp Parmesan, plus a sauce that would make anything (chicken, fish, shoe leather) taste great, for just 510 calories.

You'll Need:

- 1 cup part-skim ricotta
- ½ cup shredded smoked mozzarella (if you can't find smoked, regular mozzarella will do)
- 2 Tbsp grated Parmesan, plus more for garnish
- 48 wonton wrappers
- 2 egg whites, lightly beaten
- 2 Tbsp olive oil
- 2 pints cherry tomatoes (a combination of red and yellow works especially well)
- 2 cloves garlic, thinly sliced
- 1 cup fresh basil leaves, torn, plus more for garnish

Salt and black pepper to taste

How to Make It:

- Bring a large pot of water to a boil over high heat. Mix the three cheeses together. Working on a clean, floured surface, lay down a single wonton wrapper and place a spoonful of the cheese mixture in the center, being careful not to overstuff. Paint the edges of the wrappers with egg whites, then top with another wonton wrapper. Press firmly around the edges to secure the filling inside the ravioli. Repeat to create 24 ravioli.

- Heat the oil in a large skillet or sauté pan over medium heat. Cook the tomatoes and garlic for 5 to 7 minutes until the tomatoes are lightly colored on the outside and about to burst. Use a fork to lightly crush a few tomatoes to give this a more saucelike quality. Add the basil and remove from the heat.

- Salt the boiling water and turn down the heat to medium so that it's gently boiling. Carefully drop in the ravioli and cook for 3 minutes, then drain. Divide the ravioli among 4 warm plates or bowls, then top each with the tomatoes. Top with grated or shaved Parmesan and more fresh basil.

Makes 4 servings /
Cost per serving: $3.68

510 calories
16 g fat (6 g saturated)
790 mg sodium

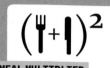

$$(\math{\Psi} + \math{I})^2$$

MEAL MULTIPLIER

Once you've mastered the art of ravioli-making, the possibilities for stuffing and saucing are endless. Here are some other excellent combinations.

- Ricotta cheese filling with Bolognese sauce (see page 216)
- Shredded chicken and roasted red peppers filling with pesto
- Fresh goat cheese filling with fresh tomato sauce
- Peas pureed with mint filling with butter and grated Parmesan

1,060 calories

Not That!

California Pizza Kitchen Four Cheese Ravioli with Sautéed Mushrooms
Price: $12.79

Save!
550 calories
and $9.11!

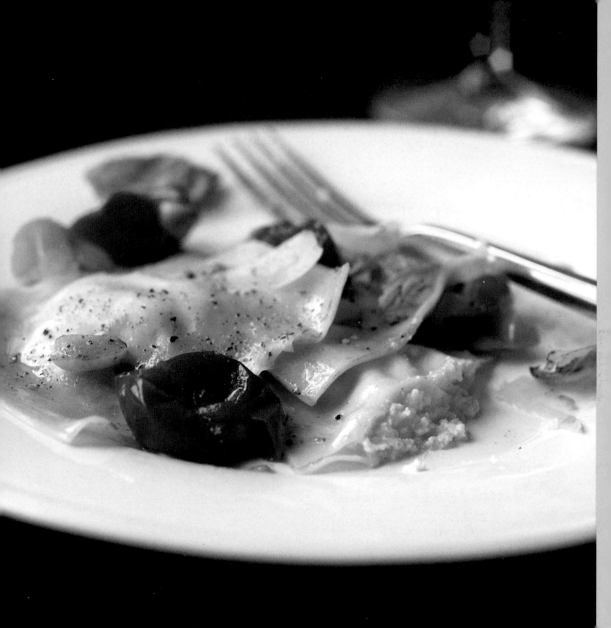

Cook This!
Linguine with Clams

The inimitable combination of briny bivalve and slick noodle is one of our favorites, but problem is, most versions are so short on clams you need flippers and a scuba tank to find them. Our bowl is more clam than pasta—a tastier and healthier ratio.

You'll Need:

- 4 strips bacon, cut into thin strips
- 1 red onion, diced
- 2 cloves garlic, minced
- Generous pinch of red pepper flakes
- 32 littleneck clams, scrubbed clean
- 1 cup dry white wine
- 12 oz whole wheat linguine
- ¼ cup fresh chopped parsley leaves

How to Make It:

- Heat a large skillet or sauté pan over medium heat and add the bacon. Cook until the fat renders and the bacon is well browned, about 5 minutes. Remove the bacon and reserve; pour out all but a thin film of the fat.

- Return the pan to the heat and add the onion, garlic, and pepper flakes. Cook, stirring occasionally, until the onion is translucent, about 3 minutes. Add the clams and wine and continue to cook over medium heat until most of the wine has evaporated and the clams have all opened—this should take about 10 minutes. (If the clams aren't opening, top the pan with a lid until they do. Discard any that never open.)

- Cook the pasta according to the package instructions until tender yet still al dente. Drain the pasta, reserving a cup or so of the cooking water, and add the cooked linguine directly to the pan with the clams. Stir in the parsley and cook for 30 seconds, adding a bit of pasta water if the noodles look dry. Divide the clams and pasta among 4 warm bowls and serve immediately.

Makes 4 servings / Cost per serving: $5.27

Curly parsley may be reserved as a lifeless garnish for steaks, but flat-leaf parsley (also called Italian parsley) is a great and versatile herb, perfect to garnish pastas, soups, and soft scrambled eggs.

470 calories
6 g fat (1 g saturated)
590 mg sodium

1,340 calories

Not That!
Carrabba's Linguine with Clams
Price: $16.51

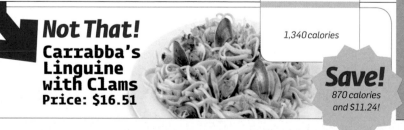

Save!
870 calories and $11.24!

STEP-BY-STEP

Mincing garlic

Bottled garlic lacks the character and the nutrients of the fresh stuff, since you lose most of its essential oils. Mince your own in 30 seconds or less.

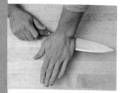

Step 1: *Press the heel of your knife to flatten the clove.*

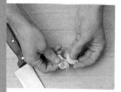

Step 2: *Peel off the papery skin.*

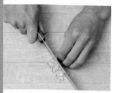

Step 3: *Cut in thin planks, then mince the planks.*

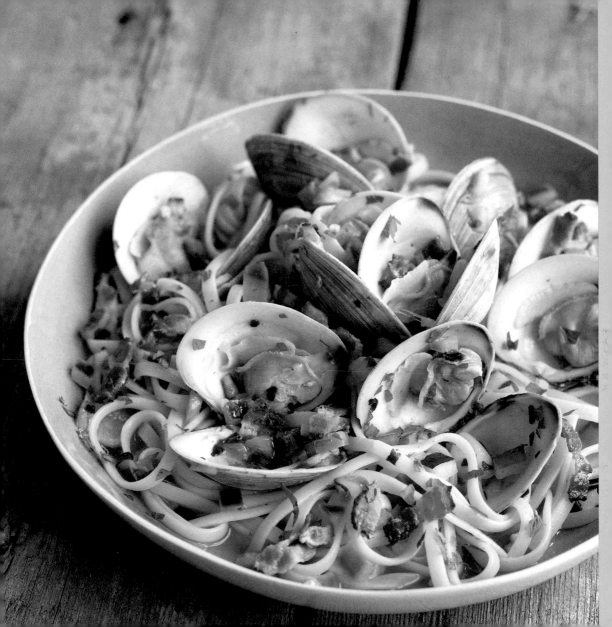

Hearty Lasagna

In the wrong hands, lasagna turns into a soupy, oily, hypercaloric mess. The wrong slice can easily hijack two-thirds of your day's precious calories. We'd rather save those for wine and dessert, so we improve matters considerably by trading the flurry of mozzarella and deluge of fatty ground beef for a low-fat ricotta sauce and lean chicken sausage.

You'll Need:

- 1 container (15 oz) part-skim ricotta
- ½ bunch fresh basil, chopped
- 2 links precooked chicken sausage, diced (we love Al Fresco Sundried Tomato and Basil)
- ⅓ cup 2% milk
- 2 garlic cloves, minced
- ½ tsp red pepper flakes
- ⅛ tsp salt
- 2¼ cups Muir Glen Tomato Basil Pasta Sauce
- 8 no-boil lasagna noodles •——

These brilliant noodles save you the time and trouble of boiling water and cooking noodles before the actual baking. Barilla makes a great version.

- ¼ cup grated Parmesan

How to Make It:

- Preheat the oven to 425°F. Mix the ricotta, basil, sausage, milk, garlic, pepper flakes, and salt.

- Spread ½ cup of the tomato sauce on the bottom of an 8" × 8" baking dish. Lay 2 noodles over the sauce; cover with one-fourth of the ricotta mixture and another ½ cup of the tomato sauce. Repeat with noodles, cheese mixture, and sauce twice more. Top with a last layer of pasta, the remaining ricotta mixture and sauce, and Parmesan.

- Cover with foil and bake for 20 minutes. Remove the foil and bake for another 15 minutes, until the top is golden. (Note: This recipe is good for a big crowd and very easy to double up on.)

Makes 4 servings / Cost per serving: $3.50

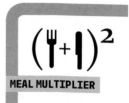

$(\text{\textservings} + \text{\textservings})^2$

MEAL MULTIPLIER

No-boil noodles put lasagna in reach even on busy weeknights. Take advantage with any of these alternative versions.

- Replace the ricotta with béchamel (see page 214) and the tomato sauce with Bolognese (see page 216)
- Trade the chicken sausage for sautéed spinach, mushrooms, and roasted red peppers
- Trade the sausage for shrimp and the tomato sauce for pesto

430 calories
13 g fat
(4.5 g saturated)
810 mg sodium

1,360 calories

Not That!
Carrabba's Lasagne
Price: $13.00

Save!
930 calories and $9.50!

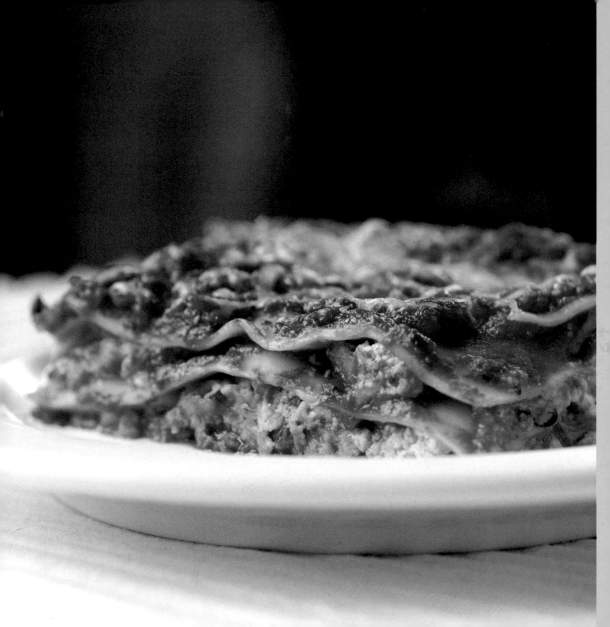

Butternut Ravioli with Sage Brown Butter

It's a sad state of affairs when a meat-free pasta can swallow up 95 percent of your day's saturated fat, but we've come to expect that from chain restaurants. This butternut ravioli is everything a vegetarian dish should be: healthy, exciting, and supertasty.

You'll Need:

- 1 can (16 oz) butternut squash or pumpkin puree
- ½ Tbsp balsamic vinegar
- Pinch of ground nutmeg
- 2 Tbsp grated Parmesan, plus more for garnish
- Salt and black pepper to taste
- 48 wonton wrappers
- 2 egg whites, lightly beaten
- 4 Tbsp butter
- 16 fresh sage leaves, plus more for garnish

How to Make It:

- Bring a large pot of water to a boil over high heat. Mix the squash, vinegar, nutmeg, and Parmesan; season with salt and pepper.

- Working on a clean floured surface, lay down a single wonton wrapper and place a small spoonful of the squash mixture in the center, being careful not to overstuff. Paint the edges of the wrapper with the egg whites, then top with another wonton wrapper. Press firmly around the edges with your fingers to secure the filling inside the ravioli. Repeat with the remaining wrappers to create 24 ravioli.

- Salt the boiling water and turn down the heat to medium so that it's gently boiling. Carefully drop in the ravioli and cook for 3 minutes, then drain.

- In the meantime, heat a large skillet or sauté pan over medium heat and add the butter and sage. Cook until the butter is lightly brown and begins to give off a nutty aroma. (Do this carefully, as you don't want the butter to burn.) Add the cooked ravioli to the pan, tossing gently to make sure they don't break. Divide among 4 warm plates and garnish with Parmesan and sage.

Makes 4 servings / Cost per serving: $3.08

450 calories
14 g fat (8 g saturated)
620 mg sodium

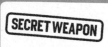

SECRET WEAPON

Wonton wrappers

Do you have the time on a busy weeknight to make fresh pasta by hand? We doubt it. Found in the refrigerated section of most supermarkets, wonton wrappers are a perfect, inexpensive substitute for fresh pasta, enveloping your filling of choice in thin sheets of flour, egg, and water. The secret to successful ravioli is threefold: **(1)** Don't overstuff the wrapper—a little less than a tablespoon of filling should do. **(2)** Seal the wrapper firmly, using egg wash as an adhesive around the perimeter. **(3)** Dust the assembled ravioli—and your work surface—with flour to keep the surface of the wrappers from sticking.

790 calories
44 g fat
(19 g saturated fat)
990 mg sodium

Not That!

Romano's Macaroni Grill Mushroom Ravioli
Price: $11.49

Save!

340 calories
and $8.41!

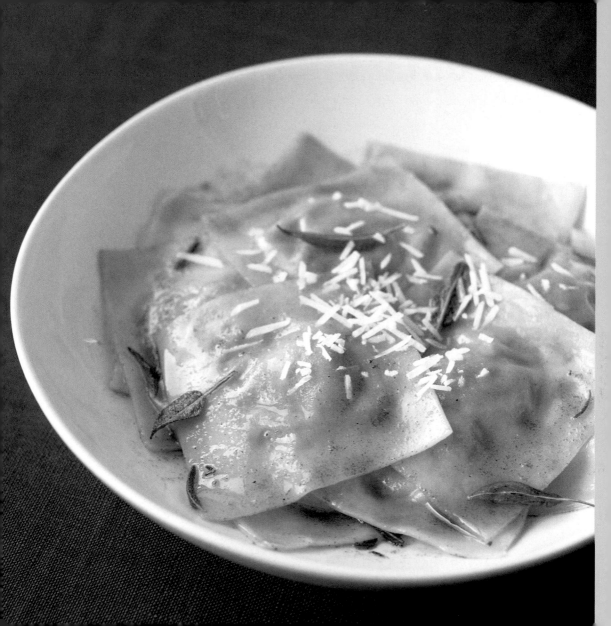

Pesto Gnocchi with Green Beans and Tomatoes

Depending on where you order, pesto can be a crapshoot. Individually, its components—olive oil, basil, garlic, pine nuts—are loaded with antioxidants and healthy fats, but if the balance is askew, then your nutritional intake will be too. Mess with the simplicity of pesto by adding things like cream and you can kiss your chances of healthy eating good-bye. When you make pasta with pesto, figure 2 tablespoons per plate—and throw in some healthy extras like tomatoes and green beans to bring substance and balance to the bowl.

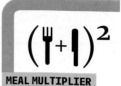

$$(\text{\textnumero}+\text{\textbardbl})^2$$

MEAL MULTIPLIER

Though it may pain some Italians to admit it, the pesto possibilities don't start and stop with basil, pine nuts, and Parmesan. Pesto can be made from dozens of different ingredients and used not just to top pasta but also to spike vinaigrettes, sauce grilled chicken, or spread on sandwiches. Combine any of the following with olive oil in a food processor.

- Sundried tomatoes, walnuts, and Parmesan
- Jalapeño, almonds, and red onions
- Cilantro, garlic, and pumpkin seeds

You'll Need:

- 1 Tbsp olive oil
- 1 lb green beans
- 1 pint cherry tomatoes
- Salt
- 1 package (16 oz) potato gnocchi
- ½ cup pesto
- 1 cup bite-size cubes of fresh mozzarella
- Freshly grated Parmesan

How to Make It:

- Set a large pot of water over high heat. Heat a large skillet or sauté pan over medium heat. Add the olive oil and green beans to the skillet and cook for 3 minutes, then toss in the tomatoes and continue to cook until the green beans are tender (but still crisp) and the tomatoes are browned on the outside. Remove from the heat.

- Salt the water after it reaches a boil. Drop the gnocchi in and cook until they float to the surface (4 to 5 minutes). Drain and add the gnocchi to the pan with the green beans and tomatoes. Stir in the pesto and mozzarella. Divide among 4 warm plates or bowls and top with a bit of grated Parmesan.

Makes 4 servings / Cost per serving: $2.26

Gnocchi are usually made from three parts potato and one part flour. They're available in the pasta aisle of most supermarkets.

490 calories
22 g fat (7 g saturated)
830 mg sodium

1,347 calories
49 g saturated
1,915 mg sodium

Not That!
California Pizza Kitchen Pesto Cream Penne
Price: $10.29

Save!
857 calories and $8.03!

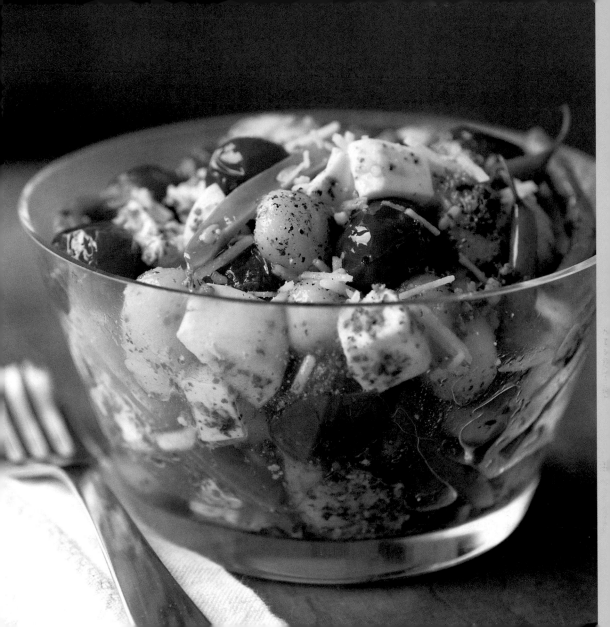

Shrimp Fra Diavolo

Curiously enough, seafood-based pasta is usually the worst type of pasta on the menu. (Look no further than Cheesecake Factory's 2,819-calorie Bistro Shrimp Pasta for proof.) Restaurants feel the use of a lean protein like shrimp entitles them to the use of egregious quantities of butter, cream, and cheese, all but drowning out any chance of actually tasting the seafood in question. Instead, we turn to a Little Italy favorite: spicy Shrimp Fra Diavolo, made from little more than crushed tomatoes, white wine, and a pinch of red pepper flakes.

You'll Need:

¾ lb shrimp, peeled and deveined

Salt and black pepper to taste

½ Tbsp olive oil

2 tsp red pepper flakes

1 small onion, chopped

2 cloves garlic, minced

¼ tsp dried oregano or thyme

1 can (28 oz) crushed tomatoes

1 cup dry white wine

8 oz spaghetti

2 Tbsp chopped flat-leaf parsley

How to Make It:

- Season the shrimp with salt and pepper. Heat the oil in a large skillet or sauté pan over medium heat. Add the shrimp and cook for 1 to 2 minutes, until just firm. Remove to a plate.

- Add the pepper flakes, onion, garlic, and oregano to the pan; cook until the onions are soft. Add the tomatoes and wine and simmer for 10 to 15 minutes.

- Meanwhile, cook the spaghetti according to the package instructions. Drain and return to the pot.

- Season the sauce with salt and pepper. Fold the cooked shrimp into the sauce. Pour the pasta and toss. Serve garnished with the parsley.

Makes 4 servings/Cost per serving: $3.16

470 calories
8 g fat (1 g saturated)
1,075 mg sodium

900 calories
40 g fat (17 g saturated)
3,490 mg sodium

Not That!

Olive Garden Grilled Shrimp Caprese
Price: $11.95

Save!
430 calories
and $8.79!

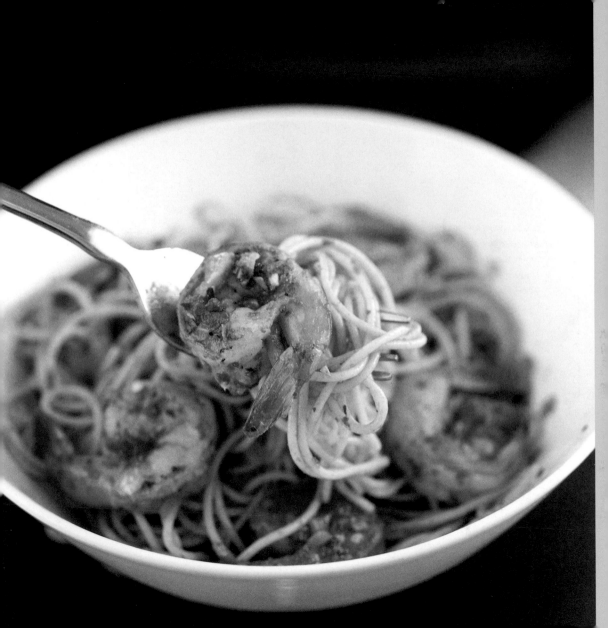

Loaded Alfredo with Chicken and Vegetables

Here's how restaurants make Alfredo: cream, butter, and cheese. We ditched the cream and made a basic béchamel sauce with flour, milk, butter, and Parmesan. We solved the other major shortcoming of pasta Alfredo (that is, a dearth of any true nutrition) by adding chicken, broccoli, mushrooms, and, for good measure, sundried tomatoes.

You'll Need:

- 2 Tbsp unsalted butter
- 3 Tbsp flour
- 3 cups 2% milk
- 2 cloves garlic, chopped
- 2 Tbsp grated Parmesan

Salt and black pepper to taste

- ½ Tbsp olive oil
- 2 cups bite-size broccoli florets
- 8 oz cremini mushrooms, sliced
- ¼ cup chopped sundried tomatoes
- 8 oz cooked chicken breast, thinly sliced (store-bought rotisserie chicken works well)
- 12 oz whole-wheat fettuccine (we like Ronzoni Healthy Harvest)

How to Make It:

- To make the béchamel, melt the butter in a saucepan over medium-low heat. Whisk in the flour. Cook for 1 minute. Slowly whisk in the milk to prevent any lumps from forming. Add the garlic and simmer, whisking often, for 10 to 15 minutes, or until nicely thickened. Stir in the Parmesan and season with salt and pepper. Keep warm.

- Heat the oil in a large skillet or sauté pan over medium-high heat. Add the broccoli and cook for 3 to 4 minutes. Add the mushrooms and tomatoes. Cook for 5 minutes, or until the vegetables have lightly caramelized. Stir in the chicken. Season with salt and pepper.

- Meanwhile, cook the pasta according to the package instructions. Drain, reserving 1 cup of the cooking water. Return the pasta to the pot, add the sauce and the chicken mixture, and toss to coat. If the sauce is too thick, add some of the pasta water to thin it. Serve immediately.

Makes 4 servings /
Cost per serving: $3.63

540 calories
14 g fat
(6 g saturated)
520 mg sodium

SECRET WEAPON

Parmigiano-Reggiano

That powdered stuff you've been shaking out of the green can all these years? That's not Parmesan. Parmigiano-Reggiano, as dictated by the Italian government, comes only from cows from northern Italy and is aged a minimum of 12 months. The result is one of the world's finest cheeses, at turns salty, nutty, and sweet. Look for the dotted stamp on the cheese rind, a sure sign of authenticity. It's pricey, but an $8 hunk will hold you over for months.

Not That!
Olive Garden Fettuccine Alfredo
Price: $12.00

1,220 calories
75 g fat
(47 g saturated)
1,350 mg sodium

Save!
680 calories
and $8.37!

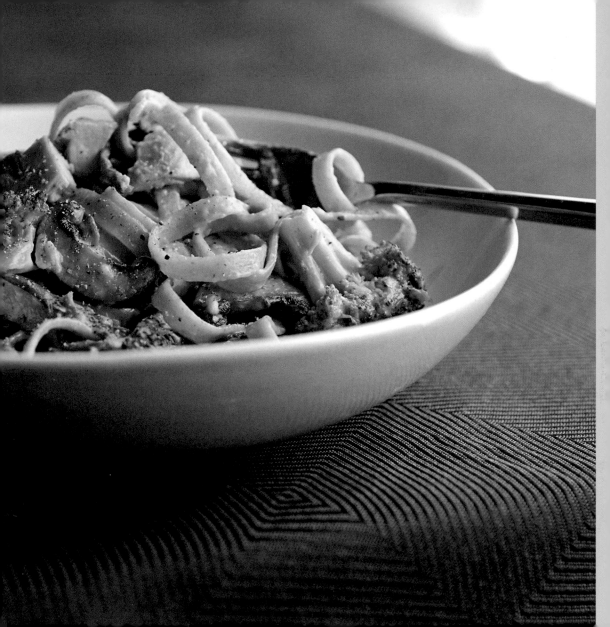

Pasta Bolognese

Call it meat sauce, call it ragù, call it whatever you want, but there's no denying that a well-made pasta sauce is one of life's finest pleasures. The Italians traditionally make Bolognese with pork, veal, and beef—a rich combination that makes for a delicious but calorie-laden bowl. This Bolognese follows the same technique used for an authentic, velvety sauce but subs in turkey for veal and lean sirloin for fattier beef. You can serve this over dried spaghetti or fettuccine, but fresh pasta really is best.

You'll Need:

- ½ Tbsp olive oil
- 3 cloves garlic, minced
- 1 medium carrot, diced
- 2 stalks celery, finely chopped
- 1 medium yellow onion, diced
- 6 oz ground turkey
- 6 oz ground pork
- 6 oz ground sirloin
- 1 can (28 oz) diced tomatoes
- 2 Tbsp tomato paste
- 1 cup reduced-sodium chicken or beef broth
- 1 cup milk
- 2 bay leaves
- Salt and black pepper to taste
- 1 package fresh or 1 lb dried fettuccine
- Parmesan, grated

How to Make It:

- Heat the oil in a large skillet over medium heat. Add the garlic, carrot, celery, and onion and sauté until the vegetables are cooked through, about 5 minutes. Add the turkey, pork, and ground sirloin and stir with a wooden spoon until the meat is no longer pink.
- Drain any accumulated fat from the bottom of the pan and add the tomatoes, tomato paste, broth, milk, and bay leaves. Turn the heat down and simmer for at least 30 minutes (and up to 2 hours), until the sauce has thickened. Season to taste with salt and pepper and keep warm.
- Cook the pasta in a large pot of salted boiling water according to the package instructions. Drain the pasta and toss with hot sauce. Serve sprinkled with Parmesan.

Makes 6 servings /
Cost per serving: $2.47

590 calories
14 g fat (5 g saturated)
840 mg sodium

780 calories
12 g fat
(3.5 g saturated)
1,650 mg sodium

Not That!
Fazoli's Spaghetti Bolognese
Price: $4.99

Save!
190 calories
and $2.52!

LEFTOVER LOVE

This sauce keeps (and freezes) perfectly, so go ahead and double the recipe. But don't limit yourself to serving it over spaghetti or fettuccine. Rich Bolognese is great served over soft polenta or used to dress 3-Cheese Ravioli (see page 202), and it is a critical component in a rich, lusty, authentic Italian lasagna (see page 206).

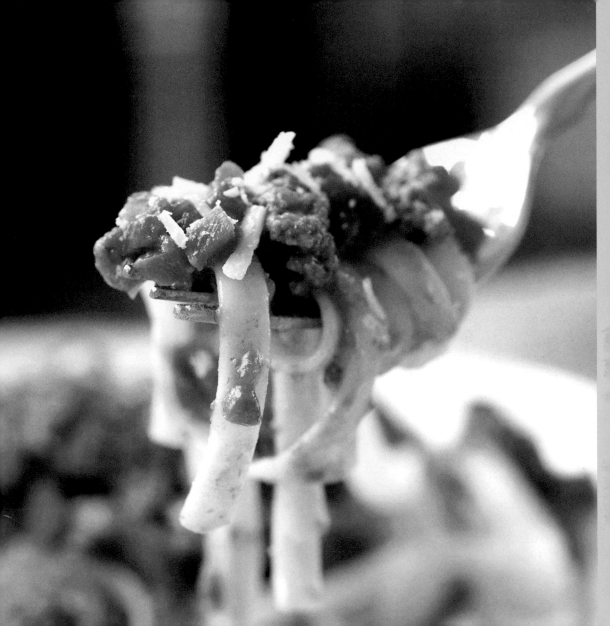

Chapter

9

Cook This, *Not That!*

American Classics

In a land where more is more, it takes finesse to turn your favorite foods into healthy eats.

Sometimes food is more than just something that comes in a box, which you buy through the window of your car. Sometimes food is a rallying point around which an entire nation defines its ideals and identity. During World War I, for example, Americans stopped eating sauerkraut, because it was redolent of the hated Germans—instead, we consumed the same recipe, but called it "Liberty cabbage." And when France said "no bien" to the American invasion of Iraq, our legislators responded by banning French fries from the congressional cafeteria, serving instead "Freedom fries." (Although "grilled rack of lobbyist" would have done the country more good.)

Not-So-Comforting Food

Americans define themselves through food. Describe someone as "a meat-and-potatoes kind of guy," and people instantly recognize him as "American as apple pie." And the American classics described in this chapter will instantly trigger memories of happier days—or at least, of *Happy Days,* because every one of these recipes could have come out of Mrs. Cunningham's kitchen.

That said, over the years classic American fare has been hijacked by "improvements" that have loaded it with caloric bells and whistles and supersize portions, turning former dietary muscle cars into minivans. And that's not just bad for you—it's bad for America.

Really! Consider this: In one study, Canadian researchers fed subjects two separate dinners, one with fast-digesting breads and potatoes and another with slow-digesting lentils and whole grains. Predictably, blood sugar levels spiked higher in the first group than the second. What's shocking though, is that the next morning at breakfast, despite both groups eating the same bowl of cereal, the blood sugar levels of those in the bread-and-potatoes group spiked higher once again! That means that when you eat a poor dinner, you're more likely to be tired, irritable, and impulsive at lunchtime. (Maybe they need to open some healthier restaurants on Wall Street?)

So if you want to spark a patriotic fervor and a personal economic recovery, watch what you eat. And the best way to take charge of that is to eat at home, if for no other reason than that you control portion size. When researchers in Pennsylvania varied the oversize portions of macaroni and cheese that they fed to the subjects of their study, they found that the more they put down on the plates, the more the subjects put away. With servings over a pound, subjects ate about 67 percent of the mac. When the portions bulged to more than 2 pounds, they ate nearly a quarter-pound more, which amounted to an extra 676 calories on their meal.

Here are some classic American meals, stripped of the fancy upgrades and turbo charged with all the fat-busting nutrition you could want.

The Law of Leftovers

Limp, lifeless, and soggy, leftovers invoke a near-universal sense of dread and disappointment in hungry eaters everywhere. *Not that again!* Truth is, many foods actually taste better the next day, after the flavors in a given dish have had a chance to spend some valuable time hanging out together. But reheat leftovers using the wrong method and you'll sacrifice moisture, texture, and any shot at having a satisfying second helping. Follow these four rules to breathe delicious life back into last night's dinner.

Make it fast! You might think that since leftovers are already cooked, slow reheating would be ideal. In reality, slow reheating allows food to stay in the "danger zone" of between 40 and 140 degrees for too long. Best to blast food with high heat—325°F at the very lowest—for a short time to take it from cool to hot quickly.

Stock it. Safety aside, taste and texture are hugely important factors to consider when reheating leftovers. And sadly, the reheating process too often leaves foods dry and unpalatable. Our favorite secret weapon is low-sodium chicken stock. Splash a bit on top of whatever you're reheating—pastas, meats, even vegetables—and the moisture will be reabsorbed by the food, bringing life and flavor back to the dish.

Dress it up. As often as possible, add a layer of fresh flavor to leftovers after they've been heated. Pasta and soups benefit from a sprinkle of fresh parsley or basil, plus a drizzle of olive oil. Stir-fries could use some chopped scallion, toasted peanuts, and a spritz of lime. Meat and fish scream out for some fresh lemon juice and a sprinkling of flaky sea salt.

(Don't!) Just heat it. Though convenient, the microwave reheats food unevenly and has an uncanny ability to make crisp foods soggy and moist foods dry. Take the time to reheat your food correctly and you'll be rewarded. Here's how to handle it.

• *Pizza:* Microwaving cold pizza is only good if you like soggy, greasy slices. Instead, place one or two slices in a cast-iron pan set over low heat. Warm until the bottoms have crisped up slightly and the cheese has remelted. (Doing a large pie and want to

Freezer Burned!

There's nothing more disappointing than reaching into the freezer and discovering food that looks like it survived the Ice Age. The good news is, freezer burn doesn't mean your food is unsafe—it just won't taste as good. If you can trim away the burned portions, the rest of your food should be good as new. In the future, prevent freezer burn by double-wrapping food in freezer-specific bags, and squeeze out as much air as possible before storing.

save time? Place on a cookie sheet and cook in a fully preheated 500-degree oven for 4 to 5 minutes.)

• *Steak, roasted chicken, and pork chops:* Leave the meat out on the counter for 20 minutes before cooking. Preheat an oven to 350°F. Heat a thin film of oil in a cast-iron skillet over medium heat. When hot, add the meat and cook until a nice crust has been reestablished on one side of the meat—2 to 3 minutes. Flip and place the whole skillet in the oven for 5 to 7 minutes, depending on the thickness of the leftovers.

• *Chili, soup, and braises:* The meat and vegetables in soups, stews, and braises absorb liquid as the leftovers sit, so to achieve the proper consistency, heat them slowly in a large sauce pan with up to a cup of low-sodium chicken stock (or vegetable stock or water). Stir constantly to ensure even heating.

• *Pasta and Asian noodle dishes:* Noodles act like sponges, soaking up moisture as they lie in wait with their saucy collaborators. (Which is why, if you have leftover noodles and sauce, try to store them separately.) Heat a nonstick skillet with a bit of olive oil. Add the pasta, along with a ¼ cup of low-sodium chicken stock or water per serving. Cook until the noodles are hot and the sauce is bubbling, about 3 to 4 minutes. Garnish with fresh chopped herbs (basil or parsley) and grated cheese.

• *Burgers and chicken sandwiches:* Preheat the oven to 350°F. Place the patties and chicken on a baking sheet and heat in the oven for 5 to 6 minutes, until the outside is hot to the touch. Toast a fresh bun and apply a new round of produce and condiments.

Good Timing

It's easy to let leftovers sit in the fridge for days (weeks?) on end, but for your safety it's important to eat or toss them before they go bad. Remember, if it looks, smells, or tastes weird, it's probably a good sign you need to throw it out. Can't tell? This chart breaks it all down.

Source: USDA Guidelines

Dish	Refrigerator Storage	Freezer Storage
Uncooked sausage	1–2 days	1–2 months
Cooked meat	3–4 days	2–6 months
Pizza	3–4 days	1–2 months
Lunch meat (once opened)	3–5 days	1–2 months
Deli salads with mayo	3–5 days	Do not freeze
Casseroles	3–5 days	2–3 months
Hot dogs	1–2 weeks	1–2 months
Frozen dinners and entrees	Do not refrigerate	3–4 months
Frozen fruits and vegetables	Do not refrigerate	Up to 2 years

Cook This!
The Crock-Pot Matrix

Why cook slowly? Inexpensive cuts of meat also happen to possess an inordinate amount of flavor, but to enjoy it, you first need to break down all the connective tissue in the meat. Steady low temperatures do it best, which is why slow cookers are so useful: Dump a bunch of inexpensive meat and vegetables into the vessel, cover with your choice of liquid, press on, and disappear for 8 hours. When you come back, a pot filled with tender, flavorful, ready-to-eat meaty goodness will be awaiting.

Four Bold Braises

Slow cookers make culinary geniuses out of people who can't fry an egg. So what are you waiting for? Crock, lock, and load.

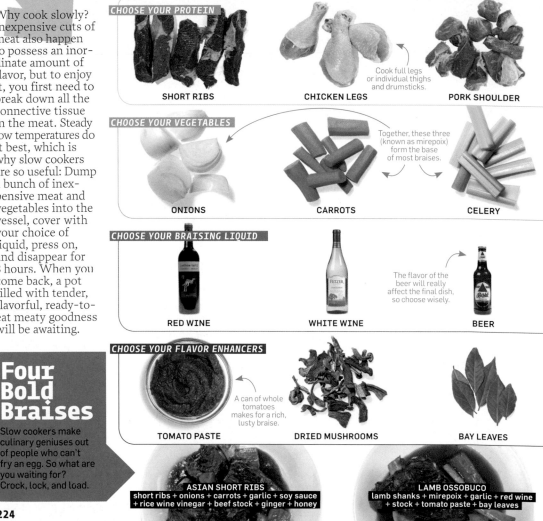

CHOOSE YOUR PROTEIN

SHORT RIBS

CHICKEN LEGS

Cook full legs or individual thighs and drumsticks.

PORK SHOULDER

CHOOSE YOUR VEGETABLES

ONIONS

CARROTS

Together, these three (known as mirepoix) form the base of most braises.

CELERY

CHOOSE YOUR BRAISING LIQUID

RED WINE

WHITE WINE

The flavor of the beer will really affect the final dish, so choose wisely.

BEER

CHOOSE YOUR FLAVOR ENHANCERS

TOMATO PASTE

A can of whole tomatoes makes for a rich, lusty braise.

DRIED MUSHROOMS

BAY LEAVES

ASIAN SHORT RIBS
short ribs + onions + carrots + garlic + soy sauce + rice wine vinegar + beef stock + ginger + honey

LAMB OSSOBUCO
lamb shanks + mirepoix + garlic + red wine + stock + tomato paste + bay leaves

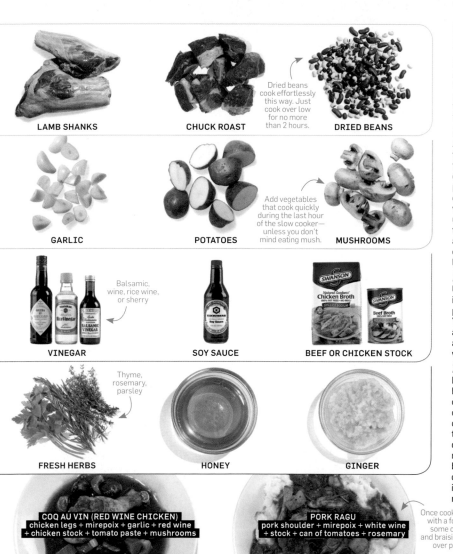

The Rules of the Braise

Step 1

Always fully brown your meat in oil first. The deeper the caramelization, the more flavor the final dish will have.

Step 2

After you've browned the meat and transferred to the slow cooker, deglaze the hot cooking pan by adding wine or other liquid and using a wooden spoon to scrape up any crusty bits stuck to the bottom. This will allow you to extract every last bit of flavor left behind by the meat.

Step 3

Use enough liquid (including the liquid from the pan) to cover the meat. Your best bet is to pair at least half stock with another flavorful liquid—wine, beer, vinegar, soy.

Step 4

Build flavor with vegetables, spices, herbs, and other add-ons. Top and cook on low for 8 hours or on high for 4. All of these recipes (and the other slow cooker recipes in the book) can be done without a slow cooker. Simply place in a 300°F oven until the meat begins to fall apart.

LAMB SHANKS

CHUCK ROAST

Dried beans cook effortlessly this way. Just cook over low for no more than 2 hours.

DRIED BEANS

GARLIC

POTATOES

Add vegetables that cook quickly during the last hour of the slow cooker—unless you don't mind eating mush.

MUSHROOMS

Balsamic, wine, rice wine, or sherry

VINEGAR

SOY SAUCE

BEEF OR CHICKEN STOCK

Thyme, rosemary, parsley

FRESH HERBS

HONEY

GINGER

COQ AU VIN (RED WINE CHICKEN)
chicken legs + mirepoix + garlic + red wine + chicken stock + tomato paste + mushrooms

PORK RAGU
pork shoulder + mirepoix + white wine + stock + can of tomatoes + rosemary

Once cooked, shred the meat with a fork, combine with some of the vegetables and braising liquid, and serve over pasta or polenta.

Cook This!
Chicken Pot Pie

Pot pies may be one of America's favorite comfort foods, but there's nothing comforting about a dish that packs nearly 4 days' worth of trans fat. We clear out the artery-clogging fats, cut the calories by 60 percent, and deliver an easy pot pie you're bound to love.

You'll Need:

- 2 Tbsp butter
- 1 onion, chopped
- 2 carrots, chopped
- 2 cloves garlic, minced
- 2 cups stemmed and quartered white or cremini mushrooms
- 2 cups frozen pearl onions
- 2 cups chopped cooked chicken (leftover or pulled from a store-bought rotisserie chicken)
- ¼ cup flour
- 2 cups low-sodium chicken broth, warmed
- 1 cup 2% or whole milk
- ½ cup half-and-half
- 1½ cups frozen peas

Salt and black pepper to taste
- 1 sheet puff pastry, defrosted
- 2 egg whites, lightly beaten

How to Make It:

- Heat the butter in a large sauté pan or pot over medium heat. When it's melted, add the onion, carrots, and garlic and cook until the onion is translucent and the carrots begin to soften, about 5 minutes. Add the mushrooms and pearl onions and cook, stirring occasionally, for another 5 minutes. Stir in the chicken and the flour, using a wooden spoon to ensure the vegetables and meat are evenly coated with flour.

- Slowly pour in the chicken broth, using a whisk to beat it in to help avoid clumping with the flour (having the broth warm or hot helps smooth out the sauce). Once the broth is incorporated, add the milk and half-and-half and simmer for 10 to 15 minutes, until the sauce has thickened substantially and lightly clings to the vegetables and chicken. Stir in the peas. Season with salt and pepper.

- Preheat the oven to 375°F. Cut the pastry into quarters. Roll out each piece on a floured surface to make a 6" square.

- Divide the chicken mixture among 4 ovenproof bowls. Place a pastry square over the top of each bowl and trim away the excess with a paring knife; pinch the dough around the edges of the bowl to secure it. Brush the tops with the egg whites and bake until golden brown, about 25 minutes.

Makes 4 servings /
Cost per serving: $3.84

> *350 calories*
> *15 g fat (8 g saturated)*
> *650 mg sodium*

Not That!
Boston Market Pastry Top Chicken Pot Pie
Price: $5.00

> *800 calories*
> *48 g fat*
> *(18 g saturated fat,*
> *7 g trans fat)*
> *1,090 mg sodium*

Save!
450 calories
and $1.16!

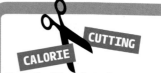

CALORIE CUTTING

The bulk of the calories in pot pies comes from the butter-laden pastry that crowns the bowls. This recipe calls for puff pastry rolled extra thin to minimize the caloric impact—but to further reduce your fat intake, you can make two quick substitutions: **1)** Instead of puff pastry, try a few layers of phyllo dough brushed with a bit of butter. Even then, it's still lighter and less caloric than puff pastry. **2)** Replace the half-and-half with another ½ cup milk.

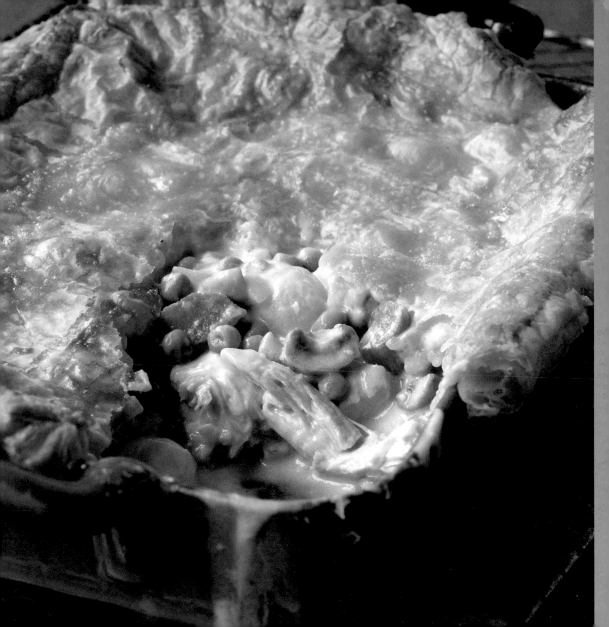

Cook This!
Shrimp and Grits

Most shrimp that shows up on restaurant menus is either breaded and fried or sautéed in a bath of melted butter. Instead, we spike sautéed shrimp with scallions, cayenne, and crispy hunks of kielbasa to keep the calories, amazingly enough, below 400.

You'll Need:

- 1 Tbsp canola oil
- 1 cup diced cooked turkey kielbasa
- 4 scallions, whites and greens separated, chopped
- 1 clove garlic, minced
- 8 oz fresh mushrooms (button, cremini, or shiitake), stems removed, sliced
- 1 pound shrimp, peeled and deveined
- ½ cup low-sodium chicken broth
- Salt and black pepper to taste
- ½ tsp cayenne pepper
- ½ cup quick-cooking grits
- ¼ cup shredded Cheddar cheese

How to Make It:

- Heat the oil in a large cast-iron skillet or sauté pan over medium-high heat until lightly smoking. Add the kielbasa; cook for a few minutes, until lightly browned. Add the scallion whites, garlic, and mushrooms. Cook until the mushrooms are lightly browned, 3 to 4 minutes.

- Add the shrimp and continue cooking until the shrimp are just pink and firm to the touch. Stir in the broth and cook for another 3 minutes, until the liquid has reduced by half and the shrimp are cooked all the way through. Season with salt, pepper, and cayenne.

- While the shrimp are cooking, cook the grits according to the package instructions. When they're thick and creamy, add the cheese and season with salt and pepper.

- Divide the grits and shrimp among 4 bowls and garnish with the scallion greens.

Makes 4 servings / Cost per serving: $3.24

Save!
820 calories and $10.75!

340 calories
10 g fat (4 g saturated)
610 mg sodium

1,160 calories
45 g fat
(12 g saturated)
1,648 mg sodium

Not That!
Red Lobster Parrot Bay Jumbo Coconut Shrimp with Mashed Potatoes
Price: $13.99

STEP-BY-STEP

Deveining shrimp

That vein people always refer to when talking about shrimp? It's actually their digestive tract. You're definitely going to want to cut it out. Here's how.

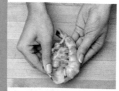

Step 1: *Peel the shell and remove the tail.*

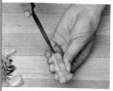

Step 2: *Make a shallow incision along the back.*

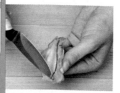

Step 3: *Fish out the vein with the tip of your knife.*

228

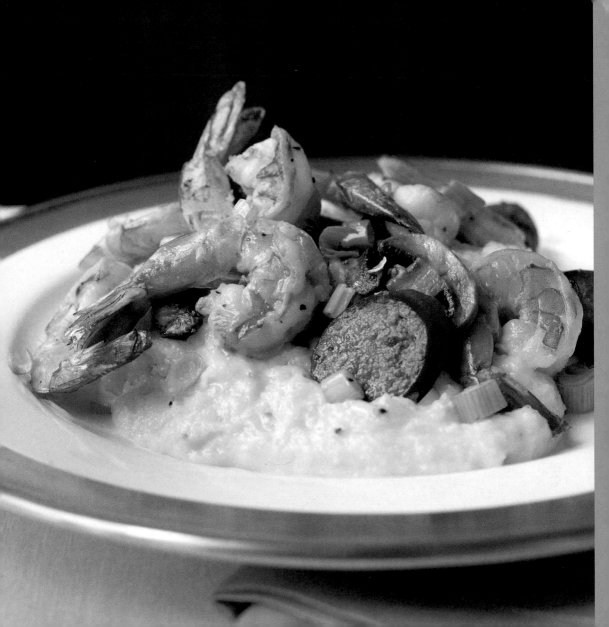

Macaroni & Cheese

Ask Americans what they would eat for their last meal on earth and most would likely tell you mac and cheese. Too bad restaurants and frozen-food purveyors start their macaroni and cheese with a base of cream and butter—a recipe for caloric calamity. This version is based on béchamel—butter, flour, and milk—which helps cut the calories in half. We add jalapeños and prosciutto for some spicy, smoky goodness; feel free to leave them out.

You'll Need:

- 2 Tbsp butter
- ½ yellow onion, minced
- 2 Tbsp flour
- 3 cups milk
- 2 cups shredded extra-sharp Cheddar
- Salt and black pepper to taste
- 1 lb elbow macaroni, penne, or shells
- ¼ cup chopped Pickled Jalapeños (see page 304)
- 2 oz prosciutto or ham, cut into thin strips
- ½ cup panko bread crumbs
- ¼ cup grated Parmesan

How to Make It:

- Preheat the oven to 375°F.

- Melt the butter in a large saucepan over medium heat. Add the onion and cook until soft and translucent (but not browned), about 3 minutes. Add the flour and stir to incorporate into the butter. Pour in the milk a few tablespoons at a time, using a whisk to incorporate the flour and prevent lumps from forming. When all the milk has been added, allow the sauce to simmer for 10 minutes, until it begins to thicken. Stir in the cheese and season with salt and pepper.

- Cook the pasta according to the package instructions until al dente, drain, and return to the pot. Add the cheese sauce, jalapeños, and prosciutto and stir to fully incorporate. Divide the mixture among 6 individual crocks or pour into a large baking dish. Top with the bread crumbs and sprinkle with the Parmesan.

- Bake for 10 minutes. Turn on the broiler and broil until the bread crumbs are golden brown and crispy, about another 3 minutes.

Makes 6 servings /
Cost per serving: $1.03

480 calories
9 g fat (5 g saturated)
450 mg sodium

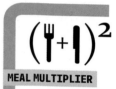

$$(\lmoustache + |)^2$$

MEAL MULTIPLIER

Classic Cheddar-based mac and cheese is tough to beat, but besides having high calorie and fat counts, it also provides little redeeming nutrition. Boost the health profile (and the hunger-squashing potential) of your mac and cheese by adding any of the following to the pasta when you toss it with the cheese sauce.

- 1 cup caramelized onions
- 2 cups roughly chopped or cherry tomatoes
- 6 oz grilled chicken and 1 cup sautéed mushrooms
- 2 cups chopped steamed or sautéed broccoli

Not That!

The Cheescake Factory Macaroni & Cheese
Price: $5.95

1,462 calories
45 g saturated fat
1,330 mg sodium

Save!
982 calories and $4.92!

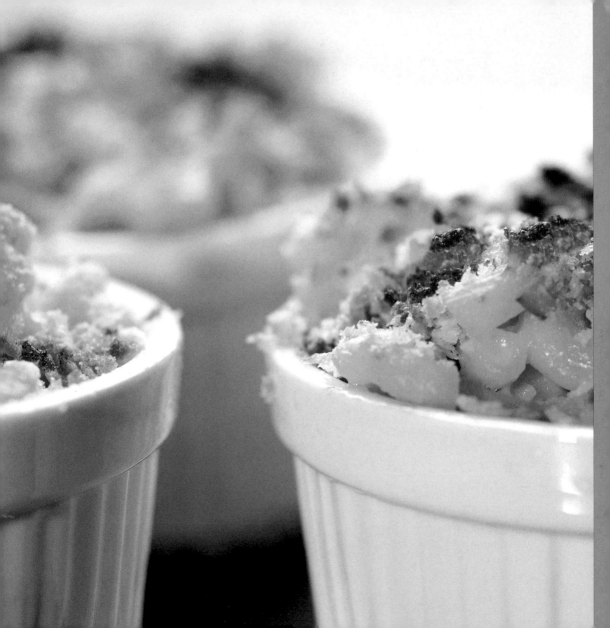

Honey-Mustard Salmon

with Roasted Asparagus

Many Americans view fresh fish as restaurant fare, food best left to professionals to skillfully prepare. But when you leave the fish cooking to "professionals" at places like Outback, Friday's, and Applebee's, your hopes of a healthy dinner may be sunk. Why blow the cash and the heavy caloric toll on a meal you can prepare at home in less time than it takes to order out? Plus, if you ever hope to get a kid to eat fish, this 3-minute sauce (which goes great on shrimp, scallops, and chicken, as well) is the key.

You'll Need:

- 1 Tbsp butter
- 1 Tbsp brown sugar
- 2 Tbsp Dijon mustard
- 1 Tbsp honey
- 1 Tbsp soy sauce
- ½ Tbsp olive oil
- Salt and black pepper to taste
- 4 salmon fillets (6 oz each)
- Roasted Parmesan Asparagus (see page 301)

How to Make It:

- Preheat the oven to 400°F. Combine the butter and brown sugar in a bowl and microwave for 30 seconds, until the butter and sugar have melted together. Stir in the mustard, honey, and soy sauce.

- Heat the oil in an ovenproof skillet over high heat. Season the salmon with salt and pepper and add to the pan flesh-side down. Cook for 3 to 4 minutes until fully browned and flip. Brush with half of the glaze and place the pan in the oven until the salmon is firm and flaky (but before the white fat begins to form on the surface), about 5 minutes. Remove, brush the salmon with more of the honey mustard, and serve with the asparagus.

Makes 4 servings /
Cost per serving: $2.77

370 calories
21 g fat (6 g saturated)
530 mg sodium

Save!
756 calories
and $11.18!

Not That!
Outback
Salmon Griller
Price: $13.95

1,126 calories
25 g saturated
1,567 mg sodium

Pan-searing

This restaurant technique yields incomparably moist flesh with a lovely crust—perfect for fish, beef, and chicken. Here's how to nail it.

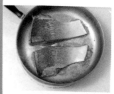

Step 1: *Cook flesh-side down over high heat.*

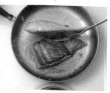

Step 2: *Flip once fully browned, about 4 minutes.*

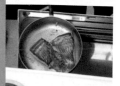

Step 3: *Finish cooking in a 400°F oven for 5 to 7 minutes.*

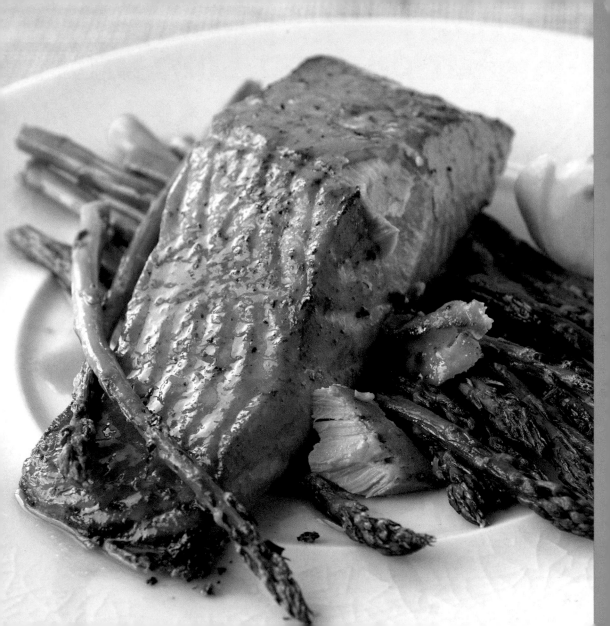

Cook This!
Turkey Meat Loaf with Spicy Tomato Chutney

Did you know it takes Boston Market 55 ingredients to make its meat loaf? Among those ingredients are three different uses of partially hydrogenated cottonseed oil, which gives each slice nearly a day's worth of heart-threatening trans fat. Suffice it to say, it ain't your mother's meat loaf. But neither is our version, since rather than using a deluge of ketchup to keep it from drying out in the oven, we make an antioxidant-packed chunky tomato chutney to keep this meat loaf as tender and moist as any you've ever tasted.

You'll Need:

TOMATO CHUTNEY

- ½ Tbsp olive oil
- 1 medium onion, sliced
- 2 cloves garlic, minced
- 3 large tomatoes, seeded and chopped
- ½ cup roasted red peppers
- ¾ cup ketchup
- ¼ cup Worcestershire sauce

Pinch of red pepper flakes

Salt and black pepper to taste

MEAT LOAF

- 1 Tbsp olive oil
- 1 medium onion, chopped
- 2 cloves garlic, minced
- 2 teaspoons salt
- 1 teaspoon pepper
- ½ tsp dried rosemary
- 3 lb ground turkey
- 1 cup bread crumbs
- 2 eggs, lightly beaten

How to Make It:

- For the chutney, heat the oil in a medium saucepan over medium-high heat. Cook the onion and garlic until translucent, then add the tomatoes and peppers and cook for a few minutes more, until the tomatoes are soft and saucy. Add the ketchup, Worcestershire, and pepper flakes and simmer for 10 to 15 minutes. Season with salt and pepper.

- Preheat the oven to 350°F.

- For the meatloaf, heat the oil in a medium skillet or sauté pan over medium heat. Sauté the onion and garlic until cooked through but not brown. Transfer to a bowl and gently mix in 1 cup of the chutney plus the remaining ingredients. (Don't overmix, unless you like tough meat loaf.)

- Dump the meat loaf out into a baking dish and loosely form into a log. Cover with half of the remaining chutney.

- Bake the meat loaf for 60 to 90 minutes, until an instant-read thermometer inserted into the center reads 160°F. Serve the meat loaf with the remaining tomato chutney.

Makes 8 servings /
Cost per serving: $2.76

330 calories
7 g fat (1 g saturated)
970 mg sodium

520 calories
36 g fat
(16 g saturated,
1.5 g trans)
1,030 mg sodium

Not That!
Boston Market Meatloaf
Price: $4.29

Save!
190 calories
and $1.53!

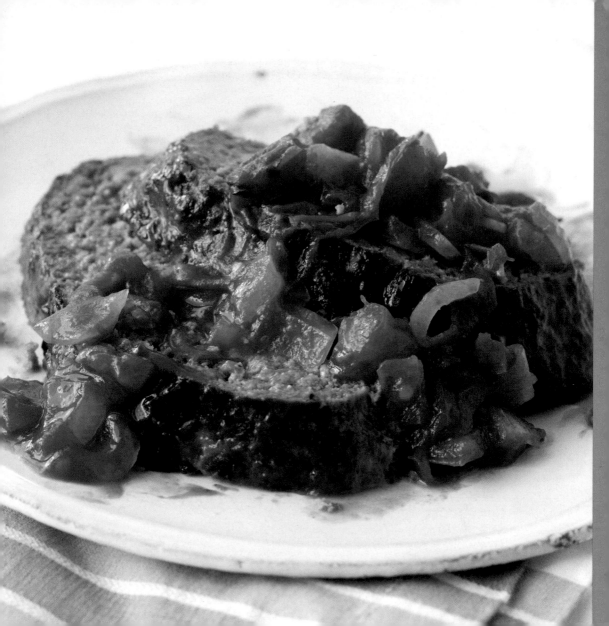

Beer Brisket

Don't mess with Texas, they say, and we try not to. But it's hard not to fall in love with some of their more inspired culinary treasures like fajitas, nachos, and smoked brisket. They all share one thing in common, though: a need for nutritional improvement. We deliver that here with a leaner cut of beef, a light sauce, and a modest portion size.

You'll Need:

- 3–4 lb lean brisket
- 2 Tbsp chili powder
- 1 tsp smoked paprika
- Salt and black pepper to taste
- 1 can or bottle dark beer
- ¼ cup apple cider vinegar
- ½ cup ketchup
- 2 Tbsp honey

While a lean brisket is critical to keep the calories down, you'll want at least a thin layer of milky white fat on top, which helps naturally baste the meat and keep it moist while it cooks.

How to Make It:

- Preheat the oven to 325°F. Rub the brisket all over with the chili powder, paprika, and plenty of salt and pepper. Place the brisket in a baking dish, pour in half of the beer and cover tightly with foil. Bake for 2 hours, until the brisket is very tender.

- At this point, you can eat the brisket and be really happy with the results. But to add that authentic char and smoky flavor, you'll need to heat a gas or charcoal grill (if using charcoal, add a handful of soaked hickory or oak chips for great smoky flavor).

- Combine half of the remaining beer with the vinegar, ketchup, and honey and brush over the brisket. Place on the coolest part of the grill and cook until lightly charred all over, brushing with more of the beer mixture along the way. After the meat rests for 10 minutes, carve and serve with a bit more sauce or on a warm roll for a mean brisket sandwich.

Makes 8 servings / Cost per serving: $2.40

Adds a deep smoky note to the crust of the meat without actually having to fire up the wood chunks.

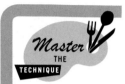

Master THE **TECHNIQUE**

Savvy shortcut

Classic barbecue dishes like pulled pork and brisket taste best when smoked over wood chunks long and slow, but do you have 8 hours to spare to cook dinner? The most efficient way to tenderize a large, tough cut of meat is in the oven. Place the meat in a baking or roasting dish, fill with an inch of liquid (water, beer, wine, etc.), and cover tightly with foil. Cook at 250°F until the meat is pull-apart tender. Finish on the grill to add a great smoky flavor.

470 calories
24 g fat (8 g saturated)
670 mg sodium

1,092 calories
88 g fat
(30 g saturated)

Not That!
Lone Star Steakhouse Texas Ribeye
Price: $19.25

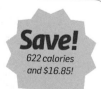

Save!
622 calories and $16.85!

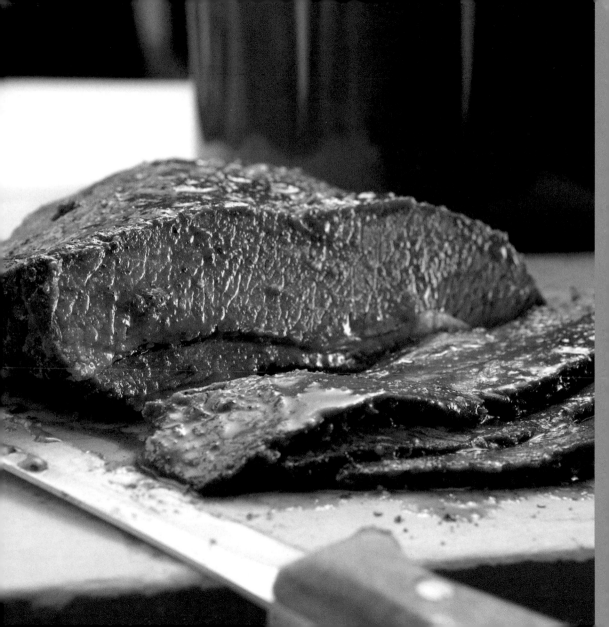

Cook This!
Prime Rib with Italian Herb Sauce

Consider this your ace in the hole for the holiday season. It's an impressive dish that feels incredibly fancy, but requires nothing more than a quick rubdown and a few pulses from the food processor. With the herb-based sauce replacing horseradish cream, this roast outsizzles any prime rib you'd find at a buffet carving table.

You'll Need:

- 1 Tbsp chopped fresh rosemary
- 3 cloves garlic, minced
- 1 Tbsp olive oil
- 1 prime rib roast (3 lb), trimmed of surface fat
- Salt and black pepper to taste

SALSA VERDE

- 2 cups chopped fresh flat-leaf parsley
- ¼ cup fresh mint leaves
- 1 Tbsp Dijon mustard
- 2 Tbsp capers
- 2 or 3 anchovies (optional)
- Juice of 1 lemon
- 2 Tbsp red wine vinegar
- ¼ cup olive oil

How to Make It:

- Preheat the oven to 450°F. Mix the rosemary, garlic, and olive oil. Season the roast all over with salt and pepper, then rub with the rosemary mixture. (For deeper flavor, do this at least 2 hours before cooking.)

- Place the roast in a large roasting pan or baking dish and bake for 20 minutes. Turn the heat down to 350°F and continue cooking until an instant-read thermometer inserted into the center of the roast reads 135°F, 30 to 45 minutes more. Remove from the oven and allow to rest at least 10 minutes before carving.

- While the beef rests, combine the parsley, mint, mustard, capers, anchovies (if using), lemon juice, and vinegar in a food processor. Pulse a few times to begin the chopping, then keep it running while you slowly add the olive oil until the mixture looks just like pesto. Serve slices of prime rib with the sauce drizzled over the top.

Makes 8 servings /
Cost per serving: $3.72

CALORIE CUTTING

Prime rib comes from the same cut of beef used to make rib eye, which tends to be fattier than other popular cuts of beef. Even with a light hand, it's bound to carry close to half a day's saturated fat per serving. Cut that number in half by roasting up a whole tenderloin instead. Sold at most supermarkets (and more inexpensively at clubs like Costco and Sam's Club), beef tenderloins make for easy, but impressive special dinner dishes. Just cut the cooking time down to 25 to 30 minutes total.

450 calories
29 g fat
(10 g saturated)
670 mg sodium

900 calories
42 g fat
(17 g saturated)
2,480 mg sodium

Not That!
Denny's Prime Rib Sizzlin' Skillet Dinner Price: $11.75

Save!
450 calories
and $8.03!

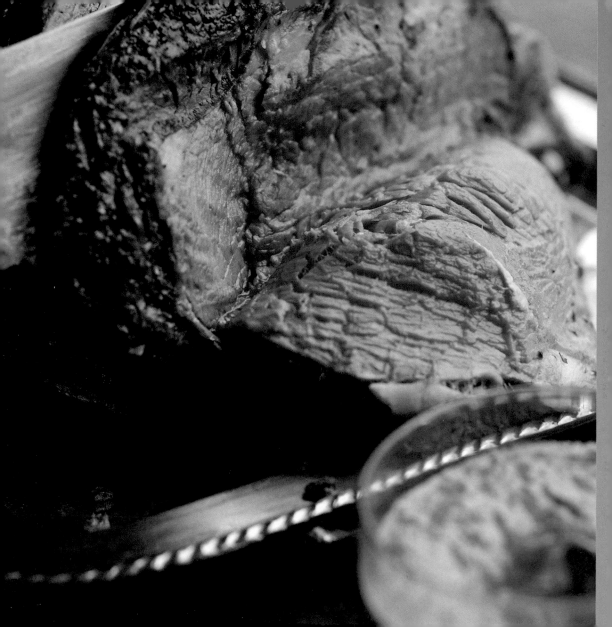

Stuffed Chicken

The cheesy restaurant chicken dish (one likely to involve bacon and ranch dressing as well) will ruin any shot you have at a good day of eating. Apply those same appealing flavors at home to crispy stuffed chicken, though, and you'll escape unscathed.

You'll Need:

- 2 Tbsp olive oil
- 2 oz prosciutto, thinly sliced
- 4 cups baby spinach
- ¼ cup roasted red peppers
- 2 Tbsp pine nuts
- Salt and black pepper to taste
- 4 boneless, skinless chicken breasts (6 oz each), pounded to ½" thickness (many markets sell chicken cutlets already pounded)
- ½ cup shredded fontina or mozzarella cheese
- 2 eggs, lightly beaten
- 2 cups bread crumbs, preferably panko

How to Make It:

- Heat ½ tablespoon olive oil in a sauté pan or cast-iron skillet over medium heat. When hot, add the prosciutto strips. Cook until lightly crisp, about 1 minute. Add the spinach, peppers, and pine nuts. Cook until the spinach is fully wilted, about 2 to 3 minutes. Season with salt and pepper. Reserve.
- Lay the chicken breasts flat on a cutting board. Season lightly with salt and pepper. Divide the spinach mixture and cheese among the breasts, cheating the components toward the top of the chicken. Wrap one end of the chicken around the mix and roll tightly, as if making a burrito. Secure the ends with toothpicks.
- Combine the eggs in a shallow bowl. Mix the bread crumbs on a plate with salt and pepper. Dredge the chicken first in the eggs, then in the crumbs, making sure they're fully coated.
- Wipe out the skillet. Heat the remaining oil in the pan over medium heat. Add the chicken and cook on all sides until the crust is golden brown and the chicken is cooked all the way through, about 10 minutes.

Makes 4 servings /
Cost per serving: $4.00

500 calories
19 g fat
(4.5 g saturated)
790 mg sodium

Stuffing chicken

Why waste cash on overpriced prestuffed chicken at the supermarket when you can do better in minutes at home? Here's how.

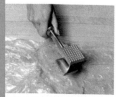

Step 1: *Cover with plastic wrap and pound until thin.*

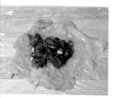

Step 2: *Place your filling toward the top of the meat.*

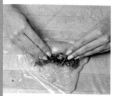

Step 3: *Roll tightly like a sleeping bag; secure.*

Not That!
Outback Steakhouse Alice Springs Chicken
Price: $13.95

1,304 calories
94 g fat
(42.5 g saturated)
2,147 mg sodium

Save!
804 calories
and $9.95!

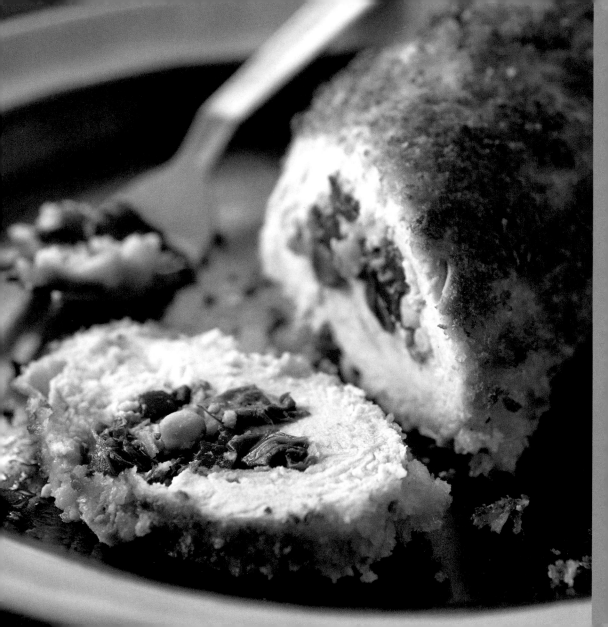

Turkey Chili

Though we've never been shy about professing our undying affection for chili, it's not without its dangers, namely soaring sodium counts and reliance on fatty ground beef. Go lean by using ground turkey and build flavor with spices, beer, and a bit of chocolate.

You'll Need:

- 1 Tbsp canola oil
- 1 large onion, chopped
- 2 cloves garlic, minced
- 1 tsp ground cumin
- ½ tsp dried oregano
- ¼ cup chili powder
- ⅛ tsp ground cinnamon
- 2 bay leaves
- 2 lb lean ground turkey
- 2 Tbsp tomato paste
- 1 piece (1 oz) dark chocolate or 1 Tbsp cocoa powder
- 1 bottle or can (12 oz) dark beer

- 1 Tbsp chopped chipotle pepper
- 1 can (28 oz) whole peeled tomatoes
- 1 can (14 oz) white beans, rinsed and drained
- 1 can (14 oz) pinto beans, rinsed and drained
- Salt and black pepper to taste
- Hot sauce or cayenne (optional) to taste
- Raw onions, shredded cheese, chopped scallions, lime wedges, sour cream (optional)

How to Make It:

- Heat the oil in a large pot over medium heat. Add the onion and garlic and cook until the onion is translucent, about 5 minutes. Add the cumin, oregano, chili powder, cinnamon, and bay leaves and cook for another 2 to 3 minutes, until the spices are very fragrant.

- Add the turkey and tomato paste and stir with a wooden spoon until the turkey is no longer pink. Add the chocolate, beer, chipotle, and tomatoes, squeezing each tomato between your fingers so that it's still chunky but not whole. Turn down the heat and simmer for 45 minutes.

- Add the beans and season with salt and pepper. Taste; if you like your chili hotter, add your favorite hot sauce or a few pinches of cayenne. Cook until the beans are hot. Serve topped with your choice of garnishes.

Makes 6 servings /
Cost per serving: $3.65

330 calories
6 g fat (1 g saturated)
490 mg sodium

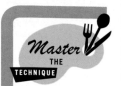

Master **THE** `TECHNIQUE`

Make your own chili powder

What sets competition chili cooks apart from each other isn't meat or beans (almost all of them use chuck and onions and little else), it's the spices. Premade chili powder is great in a pinch, but the fresh stuff is infinitely better. Buy a mix of dried chiles from a Mexican grocer (anchos are mild and fruity, New Mexican chiles are earthy, and chiles de arbol are fiery hot), remove the stems and seeds, toast the peppers briefly in a dry skillet, then grind into powder in a coffee grinder. Your next batch is guaranteed to be competition quality.

Not That!

579 calories
35 g fat
1,655 mg sodium

Red Robin Red's Homemade Chili (Bowl) Price: $4.99

Save!
249 calories
and $1.34!

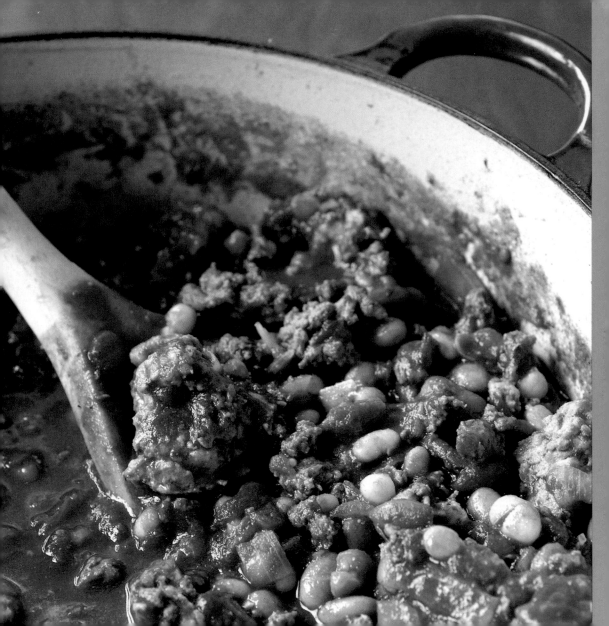

Cornmeal Catfish with Corn Salsa

Nearly all catfish you encounter on restaurant menus has one thing in common: a long soak in hot fat. We've never quite understood the appeal. Once food is battered and fried, doesn't it all start to taste the same? This catfish creation mimics the satisfying crunch of a fried fillet and the corn salsa provides more flavor than you'd ever find in a coat of soybean oil.

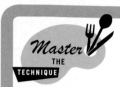

Master THE TECHNIQUE

You'll Need:

- 4 tsp canola oil
- 1 ear corn, kernels removed from the cob
- 1 can (16 oz) black beans, rinsed and drained
- 1 avocado, pitted, and cut into cubes
- Juice of 1 lime, plus wedges for garnish
- 1 jalapeño, minced
- Salt and black pepper
- 1 cup cornmeal
- ⅛ tsp cayenne pepper
- 4 catfish fillets (6 oz each)

How to Make It:

- Heat 1 teaspoon of the oil in a medium saucepan over medium-high heat. Add the corn kernels and cook, stirring occasionally, until they're lightly browned, about 5 minutes. Add the beans and warm through. Transfer to a bowl and stir in the avocado, lime juice, and jalapeño; season with salt and pepper.

- Pour the cornmeal onto a large plate; season with the cayenne, 1 teaspoon salt, and ¼ teaspoon pepper. Dredge the fillets in the cornmeal until evenly coated.

- Heat the remaining 3 teaspoons of oil in a large nonstick skillet or sauté pan over medium heat. When the oil is hot, add the catfish and cook for 4 to 5 minutes per side, until the coating is golden and crispy and the fish flakes easily. Serve the fish topped with the salsa, along with additional lime wedges, if you like.

Makes 4 servings / Cost per serving: $4.14

— *Catfish is affordable and found in most markets, but flounder and tilapia are good substitutes.*

430 calories
20 g fat (4 g saturated)
460 mg sodium

Pan-frying

The virtues of pan-frying are manifold. First, you don't have to spend the money on an entire bottle of oil to fry a few pieces of fish or chicken. Next, you avoid the mess of deep-frying at home. Finally, and most important, pan-frying provides the delicious flavor and crispy texture of deep-frying for a fraction of the calories. Film a pan with ¼ inch of oil (peanut is best, both for its high smoke point and its healthy fat profile) and heat over medium. Lightly flour or bread your chicken, pork, or fish (pounded chicken and pork and thin cuts of fish work best since they cook quickly and evenly) and add one piece at a time to the pan. Don't crowd (!) or the oil temperature will plummet and the crust will be soggy. Cook until a deep golden crust develops on each side, adding more oil if the pan dries up along the way.

Not That!
Red Lobster Fried Catfish with Tartar Sauce
Price: $11.50

570 calories
37 g fat (5 g saturated)
670 mg sodium

Save!
140 calories and $7.36!

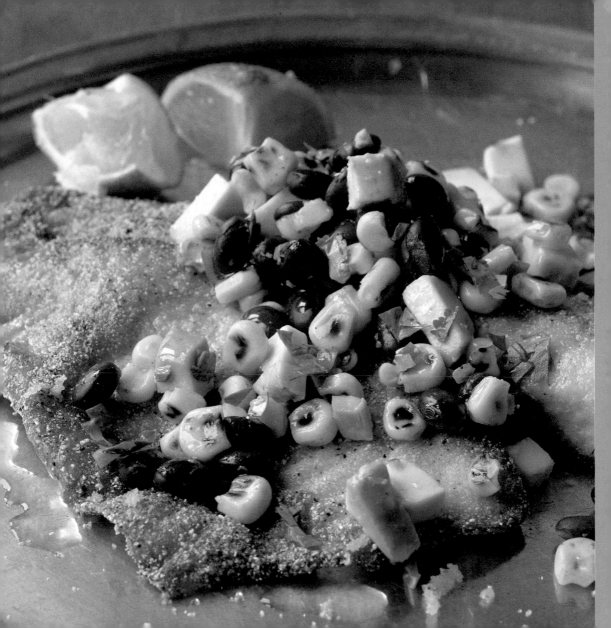

Loaded Pizza

Ordering a supreme pizza for delivery is an open invitation for caloric calamity. Best-case scenario, you're looking at 250 calories a slice; worst case, 500 or more. Here, we use Boboli's whole-wheat thin crust shell as a low-cal, fiber-rich base. We then load the pizza with a team of nutritional all-stars (red peppers, artichokes, fresh basil) and a good amount of turkey pepperoni. Torn deli ham or Canadian bacon would also work great here.

You'll Need:

- 12" Boboli whole-wheat thin pizza crust
- 1 cup tomato-basil pasta sauce (we like Muir Glen)
- 2 cups shredded part-skim mozzarella
- 15 slices turkey pepperoni
- ½ cup sliced onion
- ½ cup chopped roasted red peppers
- ½ cup chopped green olives
- 2 cloves garlic, minced
- ½ tsp red pepper flakes
- 1 jar (6 oz) artichoke hearts, drained
- 1 cup fresh basil leaves (optional)

Fresh basil is a perfect pizza garnish, but unless you have other uses for it, it's probably not worth the extra $2 or $3 price tag.

How to Make It:

- Preheat the oven to 400°F. Cover the crust with sauce and then cheese. Sprinkle with the pepperoni, onion, peppers, olives, garlic, pepper flakes, and artichokes.

- Bake for 12 to 15 minutes, until the cheese is melted and bubbling. Top with the basil (if using) and serve immediately.

Makes 4 servings / Cost per serving: $3.07

300 calories
14 g fat (6 g saturated)
780 mg sodium

Not That!

Pizza Hut Supreme Pan Pizza (2 large slices)
Price: $4.55

800 calories
40 g fat (16 g saturated)
1,780 mg sodium

Save!
500 calories and $1.48!

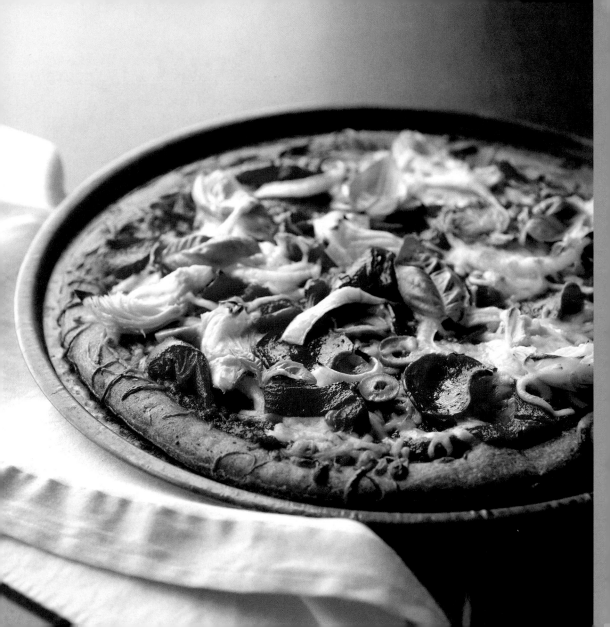

Herb Roast Chicken with Root Vegetables

They say you can judge a cook by how well they roast a chicken. If that's the case, Boston Market's cooks need a little help. (Surprised?) This recipe produces an incomparably moist bird, simple enough to make on a weeknight, but elegant enough to serve to guests.

You'll Need:

- 2 **cloves garlic, minced**
- 1 **Tbsp finely chopped fresh rosemary**
- **Zest and juice of 1 lemon**
- 1 **Tbsp olive oil**
- 1 **chicken (4 lb)**
- **Salt and black pepper to taste**
- 1 **large russet potato, sliced into ⅛" rounds**
- 2 **onions, quartered**
- 4 **large carrots, cut into large chunks**

Almost any herb works here: thyme, parsley, oregano, basil, or sage.

How to Make It:

- Preheat the oven to 450°F. Mix the garlic, rosemary, lemon zest, and half of the olive oil.

- Working on the chicken, gently separate the skin from the flesh at the bottom of the breast and spoon in half of the rosemary mixture; use your hands to spread it around as thoroughly as possible. Spread the remaining half over the top of the chicken and then season with plenty of salt and pepper.

- Mix the potato, onions, carrots, remaining olive oil, and a good pinch of salt and pepper. Arrange the vegetables in the bottom of a roasting pan and place the chicken on top, breast side up. Roast for 20 to 30 minutes, until the skin is lightly browned.

- Reduce the oven temperature to 350°F and roast for another 30 minutes or so. The chicken is done when the juices between the breast and the leg run clear and an instant-read thermometer inserted deep into the thigh reads 155°F.

- Remove from the oven and allow to rest for 10 minutes before carving. Serve with the vegetables.

Makes 4 servings /
Cost per serving: $3.90

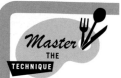

Master THE TECHNIQUE

Presalting

The question of when to salt meat is a subject of much debate in food science circles. Salt draws moisture out, which in theory can dry out a protein. But if you leave it long enough, the moisture will be reabsorbed back into the meat, along with a big shot of seasoning. Rubbing the chicken all over with a teaspoon of kosher salt the night before allows the salt to penetrate all the way to the bone. If you want one way to combat dry, bland chicken, this is it.

420 calories
10 g fat (2 g saturated)
610 mg sodium

880 calories
45.5 g fat (12.5 g saturated)
2,220 mg sodium

Not That!
Boston Market ¼ White BBQ Chicken with Potato Salad
Price: $9.60

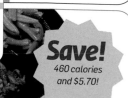

Save!
460 calories and $5.70!

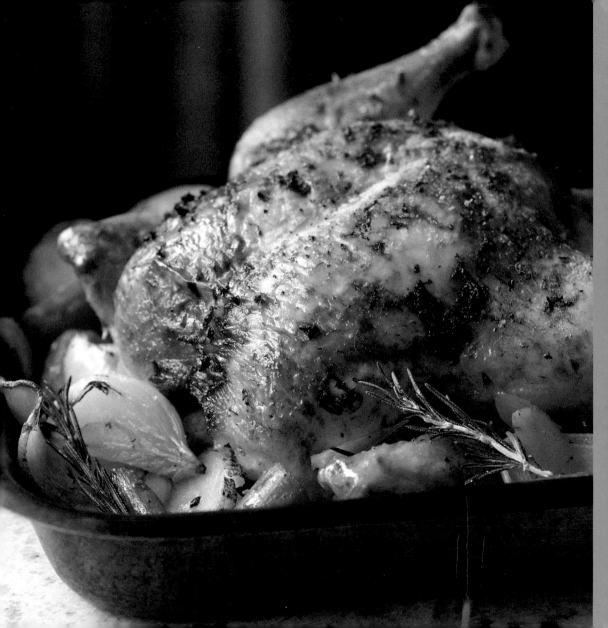

Cook This!

French Pot Roast

Every culture has its version of pot roast, that amazing slow-cooked amalgamation of hearty meat and vegetable chunks and flavorful broth. When it comes to picking the best rendition, we have to side with Julia Child, who believed the French boeuf bourguignonne was the world's finest pot roast. Here's an easy, healthy version to tackle.

You'll Need:

- 2 **strips bacon,** cut into ½" pieces
- ¼ **cup flour**
- **Salt and black pepper** to taste
- 2 **lb chuck roast,** excess fat removed, cut into 1" pieces
- ½ **bottle dry red wine**
- 2 **cups low-sodium beef broth**
- 2 **Tbsp tomato paste**
- 2 **bay leaves**
- 2 **cups frozen pearl onions**
- ½ **lb button mushrooms,** stems removed
- 1 **cup frozen peas**

How to Make It:

- Preheat a large skillet or nonstick sauté pan over medium-high heat. Cook the bacon until the fat is rendered and the bacon is crisp. Remove the bacon with a slotted spoon and drain on paper towels; set aside. Leave the pan on the heat.

- Combine the flour and plenty of salt and pepper in a sealable plastic bag. Working in batches, add the beef and shake until the pieces are lightly covered; remove the beef from the bag and shake off the excess flour. Add the pieces to the hot pan and cook until all sides are golden brown.

- Remove the beef and add to a slow cooker. When all the beef has been browned, add 1 cup wine to the hot pan and scrape up any brown bits from the bottom with a wooden spoon. Pour over the beef, along with the rest of the wine, the broth, the tomato paste, bay leaves, and bacon pieces.

- Set the slow cooker to high and cook for 4 hours, until the beef is tender and

falls apart with pressure from a fork. In the last 30 minutes of cooking, add the pearl onions and mushrooms. Right before serving, add the peas and simmer for a few minutes to cook through. Discard the bay leaves.

- Serve the stew by itself or over mashed potatoes or buttered egg noodles with a good ladle of the cooking broth.

Makes 4 servings / Cost per serving: $4.00

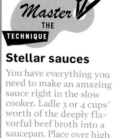

Master THE TECHNIQUE

Stellar sauces

You have everything you need to make an amazing sauce right in the slow cooker. Ladle 3 or 4 cups' worth of the deeply flavorful beef broth into a saucepan. Place over high heat and cook for 7 to 10 minutes until the sauce reduces by about 75 percent, enough to cling to the back of a spoon. Add a pat of cold butter and stir to incorporate. Do this for any braised or slow-cooked dish and your loved ones will think you're going to culinary school in your spare time.

---

500 calories
12 g fat (4 g saturated)
640 mg sodium

727 calories
34 g fat (14 g saturated, 4 g trans fat)
2,900 mg sodium

Not That!

Bob Evans Pot Roast Beef Stew Deep-Dish Dinner
Price: $7.60

Save!
227 calories and $3.60!

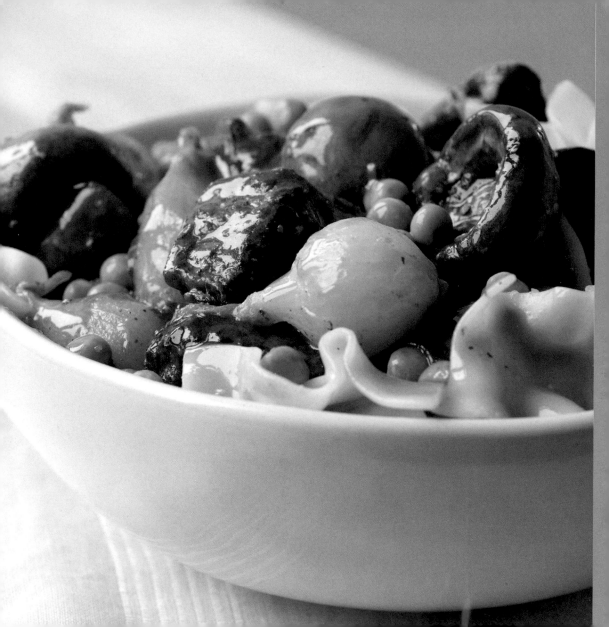

Chapter

Cook This, *Not That!*

Ethnic Dishes

The world's greatest cuisines also happen to be the healthiest. Here's how to capture them in your kitchen.

If you want to know what makes America great, just look at the makeup of the Supreme Court. Here you'll find a Scalia, a Ginsberg, and a Sotomayor serving alongside a Thomas and a Kennedy, and each of these justices got there the same way: Fifty or a hundred or several hundred years ago, somebody came to America, and today their child or grandchild or great grandchild has climbed his or her way up to the highest authority in the land. Pretty great, right?

Lost in Translation

But if you want to know what makes America fat, just look at the menu of any ethnic restaurant. People who are poor, hungry, and yearning to be free hop into America's melting pot and become reborn with unlimited opportunity. But when dishes that make for healthy and nutritious fare in other countries get dumped into America's melting pot, they come out spiked with sugar, fouled by fat, and corrupted by calories.

Indeed, visitors from overseas are often stunned to discover the food that American marketers are selling in their names: You'll never find anything resembling French dressing in France. A native Italian would be utterly confounded by a stuffed-crust pizza. And people in China have never even heard of General Tso or his little chicken friend, either. All of these American corruptions of traditional ethnic cuisines have added fat and calories while taking away the unique flavors—and health benefits—of the foods they were based on. The result: America has a higher obesity rate than any of the countries from which we take our most popular meals.

Cook This, Not That! has set out to correct the corrupted and reboot the nutritionally bankrupt. Our secret weapon (and yours)? The spice rack. Much of the uniqueness of ethnic eats comes from the unexpected spices they carry—and those spices can deliver a serious health benefit as well. For example, a study in the *British Journal of Nutrition* found that capsaicins in red pepper—a staple spice in homes from Korea to Kenya to Cabo—can help you cut calories, without even knowing it. In the study, subjects ate an appetizer before lunch, but only some of those appetizers were made with red pepper. Those in the red pepper group ate 5 percent fewer calories. But what's more shocking is that when given a snack 3 hours later, the red pepper group once again underate their nonpeppered peers, and this time by 22 percent! And what's great is that the fiery spice fits nicely with just about any dish in this book.

The recipes in this chapter hew closely to their original sources, while incorporating a little American pizzazz—but none of the additional calories. Fire them up, and you'll realize that most restaurant chains have about as much ethnic authenticity as a Taco Bell chihauhua.

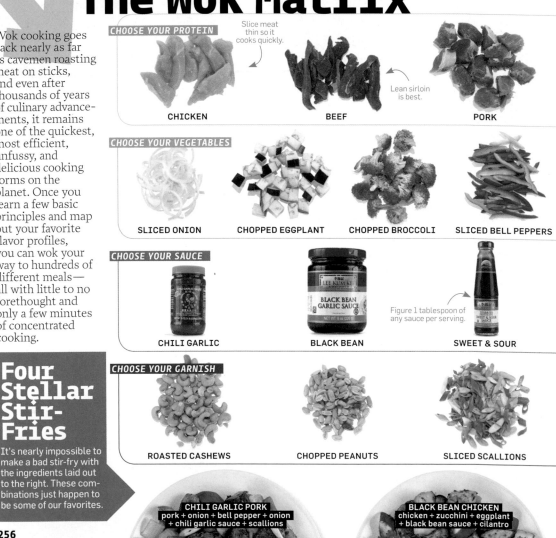

Cook This!
The Wok Matrix

Wok cooking goes back nearly as far as cavemen roasting meat on sticks, and even after thousands of years of culinary advancements, it remains one of the quickest, most efficient, unfussy, and delicious cooking forms on the planet. Once you learn a few basic principles and map out your favorite flavor profiles, you can wok your way to hundreds of different meals—all with little to no forethought and only a few minutes of concentrated cooking.

Four Stellar Stir-Fries

It's nearly impossible to make a bad stir-fry with the ingredients laid out to the right. These combinations just happen to be some of our favorites.

CHOOSE YOUR PROTEIN

Slice meat thin so it cooks quickly.

CHICKEN

BEEF

Lean sirloin is best.

PORK

CHOOSE YOUR VEGETABLES

SLICED ONION

CHOPPED EGGPLANT

CHOPPED BROCCOLI

SLICED BELL PEPPERS

CHOOSE YOUR SAUCE

CHILI GARLIC

LEE KUM KEE
BLACK BEAN
GARLIC SAUCE
NET WT. 8 oz (226g)

BLACK BEAN

Figure 1 tablespoon of any sauce per serving.

SWEET & SOUR

CHOOSE YOUR GARNISH

ROASTED CASHEWS

CHOPPED PEANUTS

SLICED SCALLIONS

CHILI GARLIC PORK
pork + onion + bell pepper + onion + chili garlic sauce + scallions

BLACK BEAN CHICKEN
chicken + zucchini + eggplant + black bean sauce + cilantro

256

The Rules of the Wok

Step 1

Crank the heat and add just enough oil (peanut or canola) to coat the wok—1 to 2 tablespoons. When the oil is hot, add the protein and cook it until it changes color, moving it constantly with a wooden spoon or metal spatula to ensure even cooking. Remove the protein and set it aside.

Step 2

Use a paper towel and tongs to wipe out the wok. Add a touch more oil and when hot, add a teaspoon each of thinly sliced ginger and garlic and cook until fragrant—15 seconds or so.

Step 3

Add your vegetables and cook them for 3 to 4 minutes. Again, it's important to keep things moving with your spoon or spatula. A perfectly stir-fried vegetable is fork tender with a little crunch.

Step 4

Return the protein to the wok. Most Chinese chefs add a ⅓ cup of broth and a pinch of cornstarch. Cook over high heat until the broth thickens, about 1 minute, then stir in your sauce. Cook for another minute, garnish, and eat.

SHRIMP

Cut firm tofu into ½-inch cubes.

TOFU

EGGS

SLICED MUSHROOMS

GREEN BEANS

SLICED CARROTS

DICED ZUCCHINI

HOISIN

Combine with a bit of rice wine vinegar and chili sauce.

SOY

OYSTER SAUCE

Like peanuts and cashews, these add textural contrast.

WATER CHESTNUTS

DRIED CHILES

CILANTRO

BROCCOLI BEEF
beef + broccoli + bell pepper + oyster sauce + water chestnuts

VEGETARIAN FEAST
tofu + eggplant + zucchini + carrots + broccoli + hoisin

Shrimp Lo Mein

Restaurant wok-fried noodle and rice dishes tend to be heavy on starch and oil, with a few token vegetables thrown in for color. We prefer our lo mein long on produce, short on oil, and rich with the flavors that make Asian cuisine one of the world's best.

You'll Need:

12 oz lo mein noodles

1 Tbsp peanut or vegetable oil

2 cloves garlic, minced

1 Tbsp grated fresh ginger

4 scallions, whites and greens separated, chopped

4 oz shiitake mushrooms

2 medium carrots, cut into thin slices

½ red bell pepper, sliced

¾ lb medium shrimp, peeled and deveined

2 Tbsp oyster sauce

2 Tbsp low-sodium soy sauce

How to Make It:

- Prepare the noodles according to the package instructions.
- In a wok or large skillet, heat the oil over high heat. When the oil is lightly smoking, add the garlic, ginger, and scallion whites and stir-fry for 30 seconds, until lightly golden. Add the mushrooms, carrots, and bell pepper, and continue cooking for 3 to 4 minutes, using a metal spatula to keep the vegetables in near-constant motion.
- Toss in the shrimp and cook until just pink and slightly firm. Add the cooked noodles, oyster sauce, and soy sauce to the pan. Cook for 1 to 2 minutes more, until the sauce is thickened and covers the noodles in a light sheen. Divide the mixture among 4 plates and garnish with the scallion greens.

Makes 4 servings / Cost per serving: $4.95

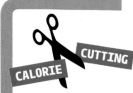

CALORIE CUTTING

Forget the fork

Our brains have nearly as much of an impact on our appetites as our stomachs do, and it's easier than you might think to trick both. One way is to forget the fork and break out the chopsticks instead. Besides being culturally correct, chopsticks make you work for your food, slowing down the eating process just enough for your brain to send signals to your stomach that it's full before you overeat.

490 calories
9 g fat (2 g saturated)
680 mg sodium

1,308 calories
57 g fat (3 g saturated)
4,245 mg sodium

Not That!

P.F. Chang's Shrimp Lo Mein
Price: $8.95

Save!
818 calories and $4.00!

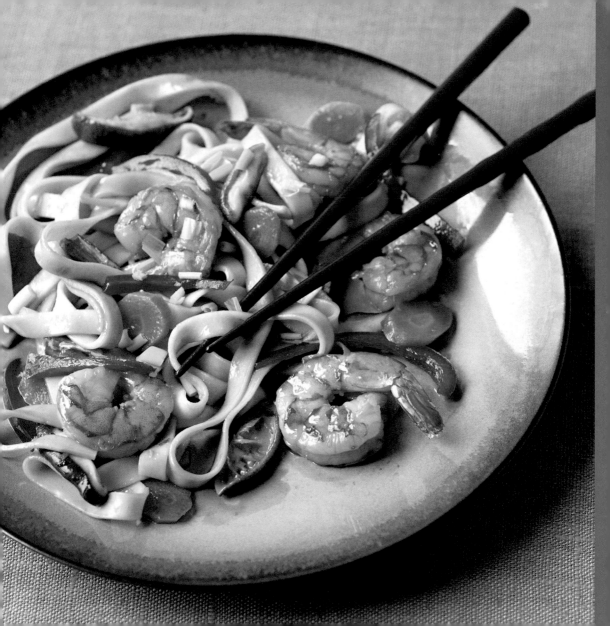

Chicken Cacciatore

In the pantheon of classic Italian-American dishes, chicken cacciatore emerges at the top of the nutritional totem pole. That's because it derives its flavor from a lusty stew of tomatoes, peppers, onions, and wine—not a blanket of cheese or oil-soaked bread crumbs.

You'll Need:

- 2 Tbsp olive oil
- 8 boneless chicken thighs (or a mix of thighs and drumsticks)
- Salt and black pepper to taste
- 1 medium onion, thinly sliced
- 1 red bell pepper, thinly sliced
- 10–12 green or black olives, pitted and roughly chopped
- 4 cloves garlic, minced
- 1 tsp red pepper flakes
- ½ cup dry red wine
- 1½ cups chicken broth
- 1 lb Italian tomatoes, coarsely chopped
- 2 Tbsp chopped flat-leaf parsley

How to Make It:

- Heat the oil in a large cast-iron skillet or sauté pan over high heat. Season the chicken with salt and pepper and add to the skillet, skin side down. Cook 8 to 10 minutes, until lightly browned and crisp on all sides. Transfer to a plate.

- Lower the heat and add the onion, bell pepper, olives, garlic, and pepper flakes. Cook until the vegetables have softened, about 10 minutes. Pour in the wine and simmer, stirring occasionally, until it's nearly evaporated, about 5 minutes.

- Add the broth and tomatoes to the skillet. Return the chicken to the pan, tucking it into the vegetables skin side up, and bring to a simmer. Cook over medium heat for another 20 minutes, until the chicken is extremely tender and the sauce is reduced by half. Sprinkle with the parsley. Serve on soft polenta, quinoa, or a small bed of mashed potatoes.

Makes 4 servings / Cost per serving: $3.80

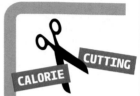

CALORIE CUTTING

Choosing chicken

While boneless, skinless chicken is the leanest protein in the meat case, we leave the skin on here because it helps prevent the chicken from drying out during the cooking process. That doesn't mean you have to eat it, though. Leave the skin on while the chicken simmers to insulate and baste the meat, then simply pull it off before eating. The result? The moistest chicken imaginable for a light caloric toll.

430 calories
13 g fat (2 g saturated)
560 mg sodium

1,020 calories
53 g fat
(22 g saturated)
1,880 mg sodium

Not That

Olive Garden Chicken Scampi
Price: $13.75

Save!
590 calories and $9.95!

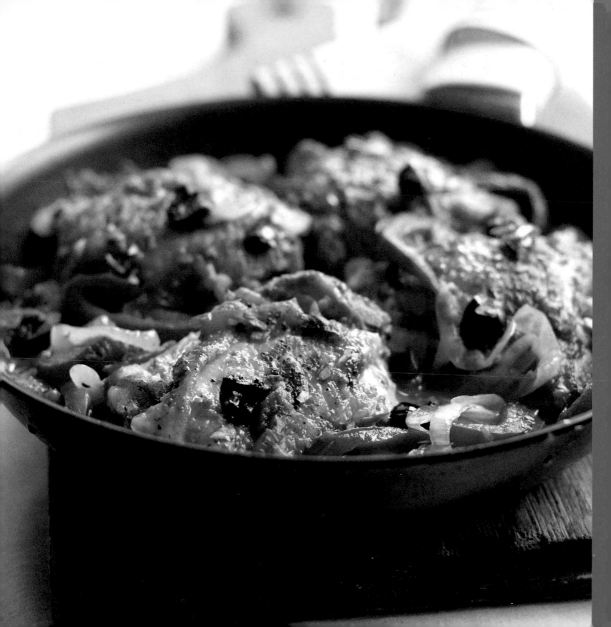

Cook This!
Chicken Mole Enchiladas

Real Mexican food—the way it's cooked in places like Puebla, Oaxaca, and Mexico City—can be incredibly healthy fare, reliant as it is on tons of fresh produce and lean proteins. Problem is, when Mexican food migrated north, it picked up thousands of calories' worth of cheese, sour cream, and oily sauces on the trip. These enchiladas are not only easier to make than the Americanized versions served in most restaurants, they're also tastier and contain just 30 percent of the calories.

You'll Need:

1 bottle (8 oz) mole negro sauce

About 2 cups low-sodium chicken broth

4 cups shredded cooked chicken (store-bought rotisserie chicken works well)

8 corn tortillas

½ cup crumbled queso fresco or feta

½ red onion, sliced into thin rings

How to Make It:

- In a medium saucepan, combine the mole and enough broth to thin it out to the consistency of ranch dressing (bottled moles vary in concentration). Simmer for 10 to 15 minutes, adding more broth as you need it.

- Heat the chicken in the microwave on 50% power for about a minute. Add a few tablespoons of the mole and toss to evenly coat the chicken with a thin layer of the sauce.

- Heat a large cast-iron skillet or sauté pan over medium heat. When hot, toast the tortillas individually until pliable and lightly browned on the surface. Immediately place a scoop of the chicken in the center of each tortilla and roll like a burrito (they should be well filled but not overflowing with chicken). Serve topped with a few tablespoons of mole sauce, a sprinkle of cheese, and onion rings.

Makes 4 servings /
Cost per serving: $2.85

410 calories
15 g fat
(3.5 g saturated)
430 mg sodium

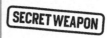
SECRET WEAPON

Mole negro

Mexican mole is one of the world's most delicious and nuanced sauces, made from up to 35 ingredients, including chiles, nuts, spices, and chocolate. Making mole from scratch is a full-day endeavor reserved for special occasions in Mexico; luckily, great bottled mole is sold all over the country. Keep a few jars on hand for instant enchiladas, to punch up the flavor in your next batch of tacos, or to do as the Mexicans do and serve simply with roasted chicken or turkey. The most popular variety is made by Dona Maria and is available in the ethnic sections of major supermarkets or online at mexgrocer.com.

Not That!
On the Border Pepper Jack Chicken Grilled Enchiladas
Price: $9.79

1,210 calories
52 g fat
(16 g saturated)
3,560 mg sodium

Save!
800 calories and $6.94!

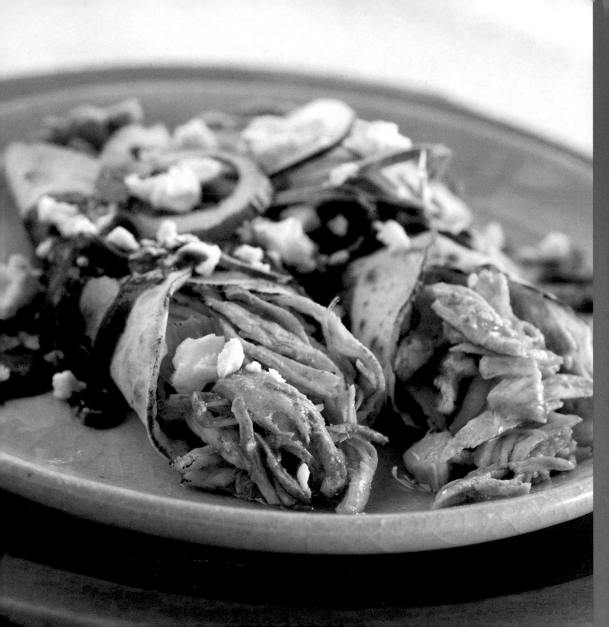

Roast Pork Loin ◆

Porchetta-Style with Lemony White Beans

Pork's role in American chain restaurants is limited to pork chops, ribs, and bacon. The Italian take on the pig is the opposite: They embrace and use the whole animal in a variety of ingenious and economizing ways. And none is more dramatic than porchetta, a whole suckling pig stuffed with fennel and herbs and roasted until crispy on the outside and tender on the inside. We've ditched the whole pig but applied the same flavor-packed treatment to our favorite cut: the lean, meaty loin. Consider this our contribution to pig appreciation.

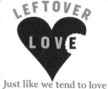

LEFTOVER LOVE

You'll Need:

- 3 cloves garlic, minced
- Grated zest of 2 oranges
- 1 Tbsp fennel seeds
- 1½ Tbsp chopped fresh rosemary
- 1 Tbsp olive oil
- 1 pork loin (2 lb), preferably with a small rim of fat still attached
- Salt and black pepper to taste
- 2 cans (16 oz each) cannellini, Great Northern, or white kidney beans, rinsed and drained
- Juice of 1 lemon

How to Make It:

- Preheat the oven to 450°F. On a cutting board, combine the garlic, orange zest, fennel seeds, and 1 tablespoon of the rosemary. Run your knife repeatedly through the mix until it begins to take on a pastelike consistency. Scoop it up into a bowl and add the olive oil. Season the pork with salt and pepper, then rub it all over with the paste. At this point, you can cook it immediately or marinate the loin for up to 4 hours in the refrigerator for deeper flavor.

- Lay the pork in a roasting pan and roast for 25 to 30 minutes (depending on the thickness of the loin), until an instant-read thermometer inserted into the middle reads 150° to 155°F. Remove from the oven and allow to rest for 10 minutes before slicing.

- While the pork rests, combine the beans, lemon juice, and the remaining ½ tablespoon of rosemary in a saucepan and cook until warm all the way through. Season with salt and pepper. Serve slices of the pork over the beans.

Makes 6 servings / Cost per serving: $3.17

Just like we tend to love the turkey sandwiches as much as the Thanksgiving turkey itself, no sandwich is more prized in Italy than one made with leftover porchetta. See what the fuss is all about: In the oven reheat slices of the pork at 350°F, then serve a few good hunks on a warm crusty roll like ciabatta topped with a pile of spicy sautéed spinach (see page 295).

350 calories
10 g fat (3 g saturated)
410 mg sodium

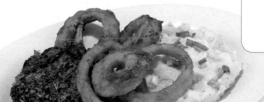

Not That!
IHOP Savory Pork Chops
Price: $8.99

1,500 calories

Save!
1,150 calories and $5.82!

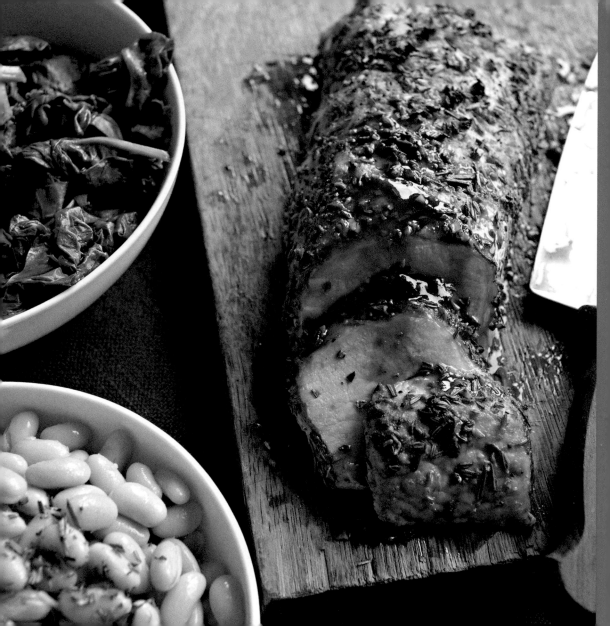

Cook This!
Chicken Fried Rice

The name says it all: One of the most nutritionally dubious staples (white rice) combined with the most treacherous technique (frying). The calorie counts are predictably stratospheric; even a small scoop used as a base for a stir-fry will run around 500 calories. More important, it contains little to no true nutrition. Our recipe turns fried rice on its head, relying on a ton of fresh produce, considerably less rice, and a bit of oil for crisping it up.

You'll Need:

- 1 Tbsp peanut or vegetable oil
- 4 scallions, greens and whites separated, chopped
- 1 Tbsp grated fresh ginger
- 2 cloves garlic, minced
- 1 medium zucchini, diced
- 2 carrots, diced
- 2 cups bite-size broccoli florets
- 2 cups mushrooms (preferably shiitake), stems removed, sliced
- ½ lb boneless, skinless chicken thighs, sliced into thin bite-size pieces
- 4 cups cooked brown rice
- 2 Tbsp low-sodium soy sauce
- 2 eggs, lightly beaten

How to Make It:

- In a wok or a large nonstick skillet, heat the oil over medium-high heat. When the oil is lightly smoking, add the scallion whites, ginger, and garlic and cook for 30 to 45 seconds. Add the zucchini, carrots, broccoli, and mushrooms and cook for 4 to 5 minutes, using a spatula to stir the vegetables throughout. Add the chicken and continue cooking for 2 to 3 minutes, until the pieces are no longer pink.

- Stir in the rice and soy sauce and cook for another 5 minutes, allowing the rice to get crispy on the bottom. Create an empty space in the middle of the pan and add the eggs. Use a spoon or the spatula to quickly scramble the eggs until light and fluffy, then stir them into the rest of the ingredients. Serve garnished with the scallion greens.

Makes 4 servings / Cost per serving: $3.57

Scallion greens are best used for garnish at the end, whereas the whites should be used like onions, to build flavor from the beginning.

390 calories
10 g fat
(2.5 g saturated)
720 mg sodium

1,532 calories
64 g fat
(12 g saturated)
4,548 mg sodium

Master THE TECHNIQUE

Crispy rice
You might not find it at your local Chinese joint, but really well-made fried rice contains grains with a lightly crisp, caramelized exterior, which deepens the flavor and the texture of the dish immensely. To achieve that coveted crisp, you'll need to turn up the heat to high during the final moments of cooking. Don't stir the pan—just let the rice sit there for up to 2 minutes as the heat of the pan does its magic.

Not That!
P.F. Chang's Chicken Fried Rice
Price: $7.50

Save!
1,142 calories and $3.93!

266

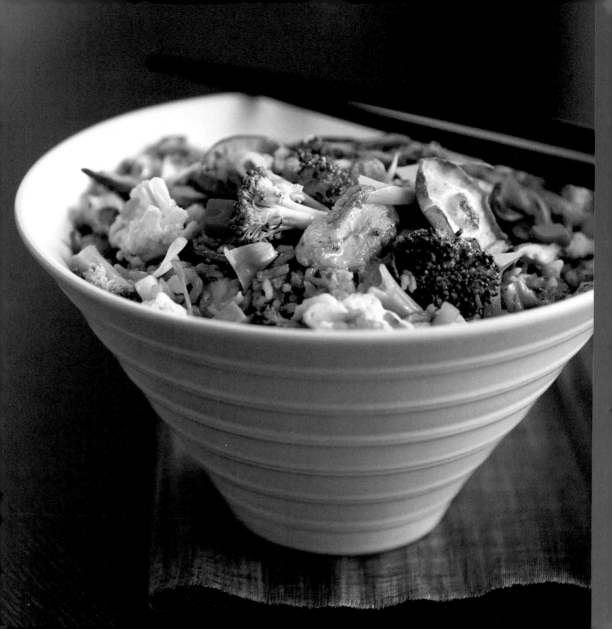

Halibut in a Bag

A hunk of halibut is one of the planet's healthiest foods. A hunk of halibut smothered in butter and half a day's worth of sodium is decidedly not. This recipe uses a simple—but often overlooked—technique and a handful of potent flavor builders to create one of the most perfectly balanced meals in this entire book.

You'll Need:

- 2 fillets of halibut or other firm white fish (5 oz each)
- 1 jar (8 oz) marinated artichoke hearts, drained
- 1 cup cherry tomatoes
- 2 Tbsp chopped kalamata olives
- ½ medium fennel bulb, thinly sliced
- 1 lemon, half cut into thin slices, the other half cut into quarters
- ½ Tbsp olive oil
- ¼ cup dry white wine
- Salt and black pepper to taste

How to Make It:

- Preheat the oven to 400°F.
- Take 2 large sheets of parchment paper or foil, place a fillet in the center of each, and top equally with the artichokes, tomatoes, olives, fennel, and lemon slices. Drizzle with the olive oil and wine; season with salt and pepper. Fold the paper or foil over the fish and seal by tightly rolling up the edges, creating a secure pouch. It's important the packets are fully sealed, so that the steam created inside can't escape.
- Place the pouches on a baking sheet in the center of the oven and bake for 20 to 25 minutes, depending on how thick the fish is. Serve with the remaining lemon wedges.

Makes 2 servings / Cost per serving: $9.50

Fennel is a bulbous vegetable with a cool anise undertone. If you're not a fan of licorice (or don't want to spend $3 on a fennel bulb for this recipe), yellow onion can stand in.

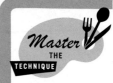

Master THE TECHNIQUE

Cooking in a bag

The French call it *en papillote;* the Italians, *en cartoccio.* Forget about the fancy monikers—just know that cooking in a bag is a technique that combines health, flavor, and convenience as effectively as any cooking method in the kitchen. By adding a bit of liquid (wine, broth, lemon juice), you create a perfect steaming environment for chicken, fish, and seafood. Toss in tomatoes, onions, zucchini—anything that will cook in 15 minutes or less—to bolster the flavor. The best part? No cleanup.

300 calories
8 g fat (1 g saturated)
870 mg sodium

770 calories
34 g fat (11 g saturated)
1,100 mg sodium

Not That!
Romano's Macaroni Grill Grilled Halibut
Price: $16.99

Save!
470 calories and $7.49!

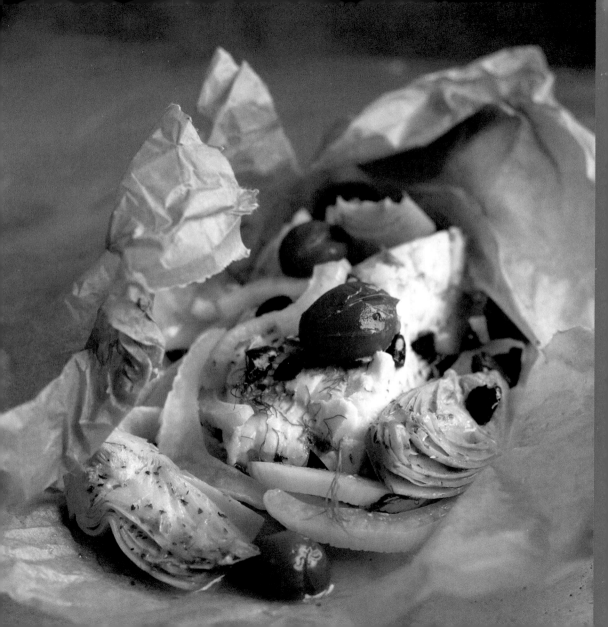

Cook This!
Shrimp Scampi

In restaurant-speak, "scampi" is code for "buckets of butter," a distressing translation for the discerning diner. The rich flavors in this version don't derive from fat; they come from garlic, chiles, and fresh chopped herbs.

You'll Need:

- 1 Tbsp olive oil
- 3 cloves garlic, minced
- Red pepper flakes
- 1 small red onion, thinly sliced
- 1 lb medium shrimp, peeled and deveined
- Salt and black pepper to taste
- Chopped flat-leaf parsley
- Zest and juice from 1 lemon

How to Make It:

- Heat the olive oil in a large skillet or sauté pan over medium heat. Add the garlic and pepper flakes and cook until the garlic is light brown, about 30 seconds. (Careful! Garlic burns and turns bitter easily.) Add the onion and continue cooking until it is translucent.

- Season the shrimp with a pinch of salt and add to the pan. Cook, stirring occasionally, until the shrimp are pink and lightly caramelized. Remove from the heat, stir in the parsley, lemon zest, and lemon juice. Season with salt and pepper. Serve as is or on top of a small portion of buttered linguine, quinoa, or couscous.

Makes 4 servings / Cost per serving: $2.95

Farmed shrimp from Thailand and other parts of Asia are often processed in squalid conditions. Whenever possible, look for shrimp from the Gulf or off the coast of the Carolinas.

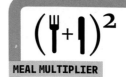

$$(\dagger + \mathbf{l})^2$$

MEAL MULTIPLIER

Scampi need not be confined to shrimp cooked in garlic buter. Consider this version as a base, one that can stand up to a number of tweaks and additions. Here are a few to try.

- ½ lb white or cremini mushrooms, sliced
- 4 cups baby spinach
- ¼ cup chopped sundried tomatoes
- Ground turkey sautéed with ginger, garlic, and soy sauce
- 1 small jar marinated artichoke hearts
- ½ cup roasted red pepper strips

170 calories
6 g fat (1 g saturated)
470 mg sodium

1,670 calories

Not That!
Carrabba's Shrimp Scampi
Price: $10.00

Save!
1,500 calories
and $7.05!

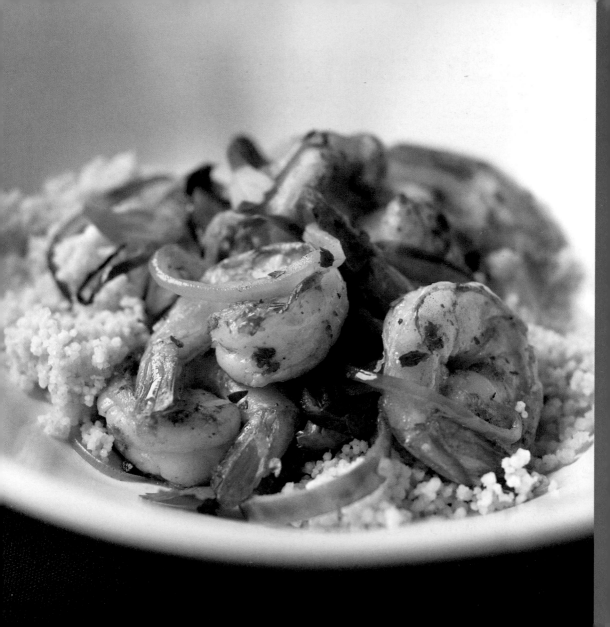

Chicken Marsala

Another delicious Italian creation that has suffered at the hands of the corporate cooks. The idea—chicken smothered in mushrooms and a sweet Marsala wine sauce—is an unassailable one, but the overbuttered, overoiled, overeverything execution by most restaurants drive the dish into the danger zone. This is exactly the type of recipe that's worth mastering at home, not just so you can save 500 or more calories over dinner, but because it's an easy way to show off for your next round of dinner guests.

You'll Need:

- 4 boneless, skinless chicken breasts, pounded to uniform ¼" thickness
- 1 cup flour
- Salt and black pepper to taste
- 1 Tbsp olive oil
- 2 oz prosciutto, sliced into thin strips
- 8 oz cremini mushrooms, stemmed and sliced
- ¾ cup Marsala wine
- ¾ cup low-sodium chicken broth
- ¼ cup chopped fresh parsley

How to Make It:

- Season the chicken with a good pinch of salt and pepper. Place the flour in a shallow bowl and add the chicken; coat evenly, shaking off any excess flour.
- Heat the olive oil in a large nonstick pan or cast-iron skillet over medium heat. Cook the chicken (don't overcrowd the pan; cook in two batches if need be) for 3 to 4 minutes per side, until golden brown on the outside and cooked all the way through. Transfer to a serving platter and keep warm.
- Add additional oil to the pan if needed, then sauté the prosciutto for 1 to 2 minutes, until it starts to crisp up. Add the mushrooms and continue sautéing until well browned. Stir in the Marsala and broth, scraping up any browned bits stuck to the bottom of the pan. Cook until the liquid has reduced to about ½ cup. Season with salt and pepper, add the parsley, and pour over the chicken.

Makes 4 servings /
Cost per serving: $5.20

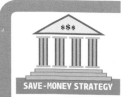

SAVE-MONEY STRATEGY

You'll find a lot of recipes in the book calling for prosciutto. The best imported stuff (labeled Prosciutto di Parma and Prosciutto San Danielle) can cost upward of $20 per pound, and its savory nuances should be appreciated on its own with a glass of wine. For recipes like this, where the prosciutto is cooked, use the cheaper domestic versions found in most deli cases—you'll save about $10 per pound.

390 calories
9 g fat
(2 g saturated)
520 mg sodium

650 calories
12 g saturated fat
1,790 mg sodium

Not That!

Romano's Macaroni Grill Chicken Marsala
Price: $12.99

Save!
260 calories
and $7.79!

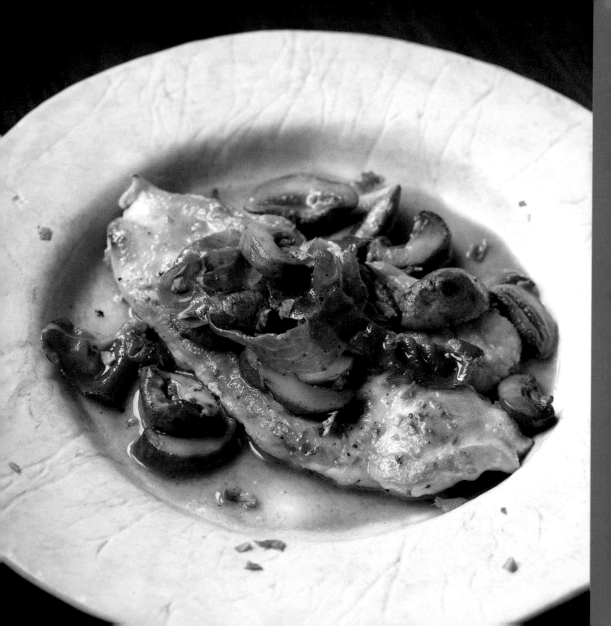

Cook This!
Miso Cod with Spicy Cucumbers

This dish is slightly more elegant (and considerably more nutritious) than the fishy fare you'll encounter at most chain restaurants, but it's just as easy to prepare. The salty-sweetness of the miso marinade pairs perfectly with the quick-pickled cucumbers for a dish that takes no more than 20 minutes of actual cooking time, yet will elevate you to the status of the Iron Chef in the eyes of those you serve it to.

You'll Need:

- 1 cup white miso paste
- ½ cup mirin
- 2 Tbsp brown sugar
- 4 cod fillets (6 oz each)
- 1 large English cucumber, seeded and sliced into half moons
- ¼ cup rice wine vinegar
- 1 Tbsp salt
- 1 Tbsp sugar
- 2 tsp red pepper flakes

How to Make It:

- Combine the miso, mirin, and brown sugar in a bowl. Stir to thoroughly combine. Pour the marinade over the cod and marinate in the fridge for up to 12 hours.

- Mix the cucumber, vinegar, salt, sugar, and pepper flakes in a bowl. Allow the cucumbers to pickle for at least 30 minutes and up to 24 hours in the refrigerator.

- Preheat the broiler. Remove the cod from the marinade and place on a baking sheet. Set the baking sheet 6" below the broiler and cook for 8 to 10 minutes, until the fish is deeply caramelized and flakes with gentle pressure. Serve the cod with the cucumber.

Makes 4 servings / Cost per serving: $4.22

Cod is the traditional go-to with this miso marinade, but sea bass, swordfish, and halibut would all work just as well.

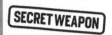

SECRET WEAPON

Miso paste

Pureed fermented soybeans might not sound like good eats, but miso paste is truly one of the world's great flavor enhancers. It's a huge source of umami, the so-called fifth flavor group often described as earthy or savory, and it's loaded with B vitamins to boot. The Japanese, umami addicts that they are, use miso paste for soups, sauces, marinades, and dressings. White works great as a marinade for fish and a base for soups and dressings, while the more intense red miso elevates the intensity of a grilled steak to stratospheric levels. Find it at Asian groceries or at asianfoodgrocer.com.

260 calories
1 g fat (3.5 g saturated)
980 mg sodium

582 calories
30 g fat (8 g saturated)
3,390 mg sodium
40 g protein

Not That!
P.F. Chang's Oolong Marinated Sea Bass
Price: $21.95

Save!
322 calories and $17.73!

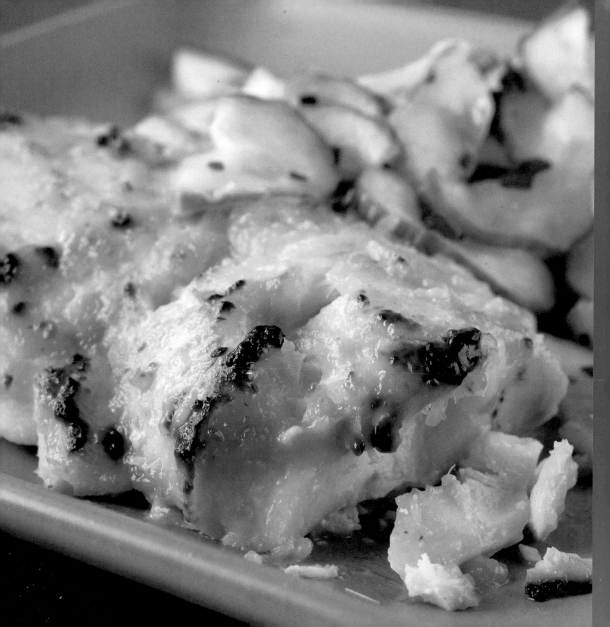

Chicken Parmesan

This Italian-American staple normally suffers from a glut of oil, an excess of cheese, and a huge bed of carb-heavy spaghetti as the base. We shallow-fry a modest portion of chicken to minimize oil soakage, then use fresh mozzarella (which is lower in calories and fat) to top it off. For sides, trade the spaghetti bed for garlicky sautéed spinach.

You'll Need:

- 4 **boneless, skinless chicken breast halves (4–6 oz each)**
- ½ **tsp salt**
- ½ **tsp black pepper**
- 2 **egg whites, lightly beaten**
- 1 **cup bread crumbs, preferably panko**
- 2 **Tbsp grated Parmesan**
- ½ **Tbsp dried Italian seasoning**
- 1 **Tbsp olive oil**
- 1 **cup tomato sauce (we love anything from Muir Glen)**
- 4 **oz shredded part-skim mozzarella**

Fresh basil leaves (optional)

How to Make It:

- Preheat the broiler. Cover the chicken breasts with parchment paper or plastic wrap and, using a meat mallet or a heavy-bottomed pan, pound the chicken until it is uniformly ¼" thick. Season with the salt and pepper.

- Place the egg whites in a shallow bowl. Mix the bread crumbs, Parmesan, and Italian seasoning on a large plate.

- Dip each breast into the egg whites to coat both sides and then into the crumb mixture, patting the crumbs so they fully cover the chicken.

- Heat the oil in a large skillet or sauté pan over medium heat. Cook the chicken for 3 to 4 minutes on the first side before turning. (The crust should be deeply browned and crunchy.) Cook for another 2 to 3 minutes, then transfer the chicken to a baking sheet.

- Spoon the tomato sauce over the chicken pieces, then top with the cheese and place underneath the broiler for 2 to 3 minutes or until the cheese is fully melted and bubbling. Serve garnished with basil (if using).

Makes 4 servings / Cost per serving: $3.79

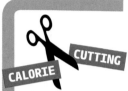

CALORIE CUTTING

Oven frying

Chicken parm is normally made by shallow frying the breaded meat in a pan, which is exactly what we do here. But if you want to save time and calories with only the barest sacrifice in flavor, skip the sauté pan and use the oven instead. Bake the chicken breasts in a 400° F oven until the crust is golden and the meat is firm, about 15 minutes.

340 calories
11 g fat
(4 g saturated)
670 mg sodium

850 calories
11 g saturated fat
1,700 mg sodium

Not That!

Romano's Macaroni Grill Chicken Parmigiana
Price: $13.25

Save!
510 calories and
$9.46!

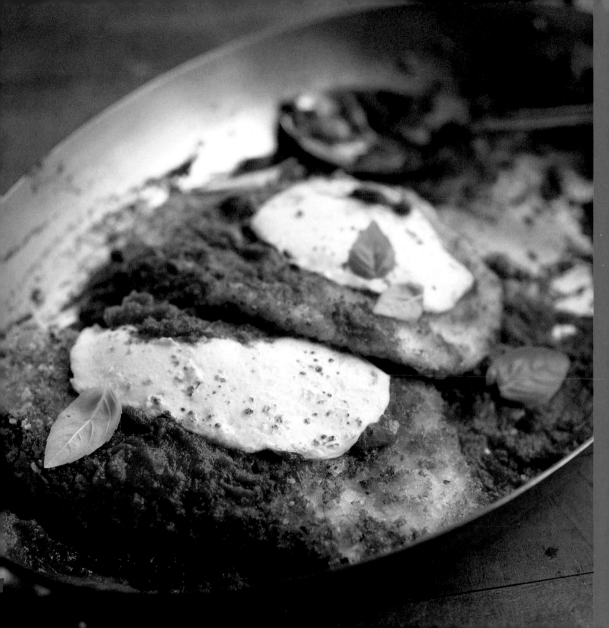

Pork Chile Verde

This isn't a dish that's on most Americans' radar, but it should be. Tender pieces of pork stewed in a lively, slightly spicy broth studded with vegetables. Add a few warm tortillas, a hunk of lime, and a cerveza and you're halfway to Mexico with a huge grin on your face. Just make sure you enjoy this one in the comfort and safety of your own kitchen, okay?

You'll Need:

- 1 Tbsp canola oil
- 2 lb boneless pork shoulder, cut into 1" cubes
- Salt and black pepper to taste
- 1 cup low-sodium chicken broth
- 1 bottle salsa verde (15 oz)
- 1 medium onion, quartered
- 1 large green bell pepper, chopped into big chunks
- 2 cups small marble or fingerling potatoes (optional)
- 8 corn tortillas
- 2 limes, cut into quarters

How to Make It:

- Heat the oil in a large skillet or sauté pan over high heat. Season the pork with salt and pepper. Working in batches, add the pork to the skillet and sear on all sides until caramelized on the outside but still raw in the center (don't overcrowd the pork or it will steam, not brown). Transfer to a slow cooker.

- Add the broth to the hot skillet and use a wooden spoon to scrape up any crispy, flavorful bits of pork. Pour the broth over the pork, along with the salsa verde, onion, and bell pepper. Set the slow cooker to high and cook for 4 hours (or low and cook for 8), until the pork is extremely tender. If using the potatoes, add them to the pot in the final hour of cooking.

- Serve the pork in bowls with the stewed vegetables, along with a ladle of the cooking liquid. Have hot corn tortillas and lime hunks on hand for makeshift tacos.

Makes 6 servings / Cost per serving: $2.90

Salsa verde is a mild salsa made from tangy tomatillos, and onions. Perfect for tacos and eggs.

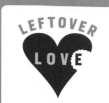

LEFTOVER LOVE

Extra chile verde is an infinite source of inspiration and deliciousness. Start at breakfast: Warm up a small bowl of the leftovers and top with two gently poached eggs. For lunch, serve a scoop over a bowl of black beans and fresh avovado. For dinner, chop the meat and the vegetables and stuff into warm corn tortillas. Top with the stewy liquid, cheese, and raw onion for first-class enchiladas.

460 calories
24 g fat (8 g saturated)
620 mg sodium

1,030 calories
44 g fat
(15 g saturated)
2,510 mg sodium

Not That!
Chevys Fresh Mex Chile Verde
Price: $8.99

Save!
570 calories and $6.09!

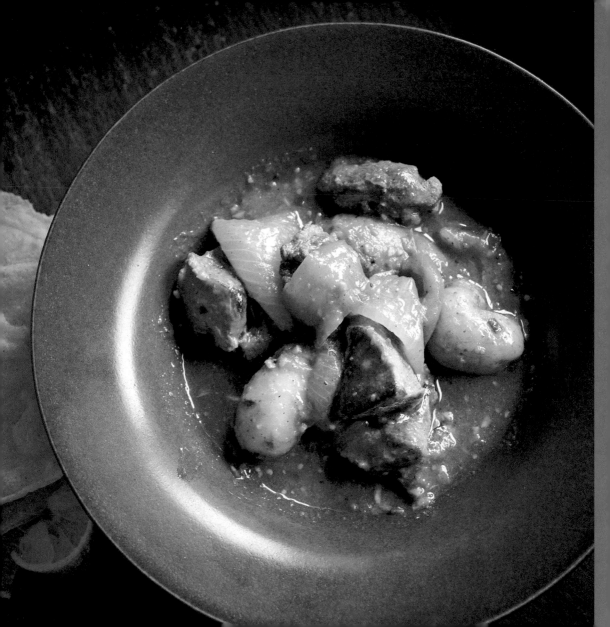

Cook This!

Seared Scallops with White Beans and Spinach

You have to look long and hard to find a scallop on a chain restaurant's menu and we can't quite figure out why. They're a tremendous lean source of protein, supereasy to cook, and stack up well with bold and subtle flavors alike. Learn to properly sear a scallop (hint: Make sure the scallop is very dry and the pan is very hot) and you'll be won over.

You'll Need:

- 2 strips bacon, chopped into small pieces •
- ½ red onion, minced
- 1 clove garlic, minced
- 1½ cans white beans (14 oz each), rinsed and drained
- 4 cups baby spinach
- 1 lb large sea scallops
- Salt and black pepper to taste
- 1 Tbsp butter
- Juice of 1 lemon

There are a lot of different types of white beans sold in cans. All will work, but cannellini beans are best.

How to Make It:

- Heat a medium saucepan over low heat. Cook the bacon until it has begun to crisp. Add the onion and garlic; sauté until the onion is soft and translucent, 2 to 3 minutes. Add the white beans and spinach and simmer until the beans are hot and the spinach is wilted. Keep warm.

- Heat a large cast-iron skillet or sauté pan over medium-high heat. Blot the scallops dry with a paper towel and season with salt and pepper on both sides. Add the butter and the scallops to the pan and sear the scallops for 2 to 3 minutes per side, until deeply caramelized.

- Before serving, add the lemon juice to the beans. Season with salt and pepper. Divide the beans among 4 warm bowls or plates and top with scallops.

Makes 4 servings / Cost per serving: $9.37

Feel free to kill the bacon, but for about 18 calories per serving, it adds a ton of flavor to the overall dish.

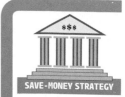

SAVE-MONEY STRATEGY

Sea scallops in the seafood case can be pricey, but scallops—like shrimp—rarely arrive at the market fresh. Instead, they're frozen after catching and defrosted when put on sale. So why pay the extra cash for faux-fresh scallops when you can buy them frozen for a fraction of the price? Grocers like Trader Joe's and Whole Foods sell bags of high-quality frozen scallops and shrimp for about 60 percent of the cost.

280 calories
7 g fat (2.5 g saturated)
360 mg sodium

594 calories
28 g fat (4 g saturated)
3,600 mg sodium

Not That!
P.F. Chang's Cantonese Scallops
Price: $16.04

Save!
314 calories and $6.67!

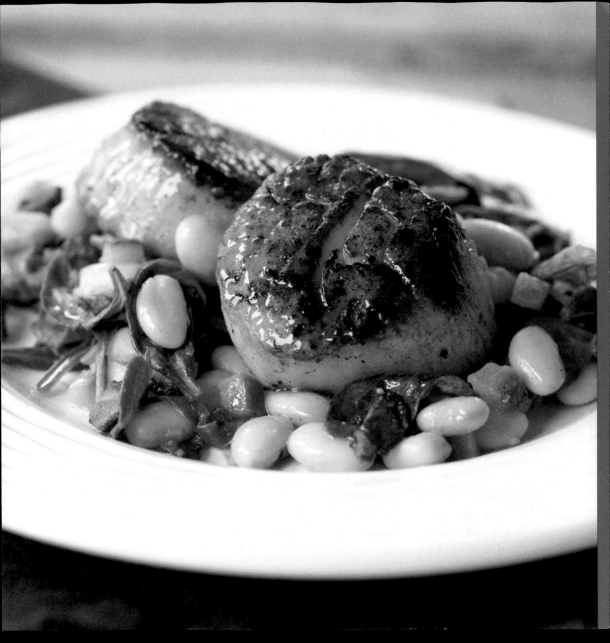

Short Ribs Braised in Guinness

Seems like braised short ribs adorn every French and Italian menu in the country these days. And why not? It's an inexpensive dish that takes minimal effort from the chef but that can still fetch a $20+ price tag wherever it's served. Why pay the money for something you can do just as well at home, especially if you can cut the calories in half?

You'll Need:

- 1 Tbsp canola oil
- 2 lb boneless short ribs
- Salt and black pepper to taste
- 2 cans or bottles (12 oz each) Guinness Draught
- 2 cups low-sodium beef broth
- 3 large carrots, cut into large chunks
- 2 onions, quartered
- 2 stalks celery, cut into large chunks
- 8 cloves garlic, peeled
- 2 bay leaves

GREMOLATA (optional)
- ½ cup chopped parsley
- 2 cloves garlic, minced
- Grated zest of 2 oranges or lemons

How to Make It:

- Heat the oil in a large skillet or sauté pan over high heat. Season all sides of the ribs with salt and pepper. Cook them until a rich brown crust develops on the outside. Remove the ribs and place in a slow cooker. While the pan is still hot, add the beer and scrape up any bits stuck to the bottom with a wooden spoon. Pour the beer over the short ribs.

- Add the broth, carrots, onions, celery, garlic, and bay leaves to the short ribs and set the slow cooker to high. Cook for 4 hours, until the beef is tender and nearly falling apart. Discard the bay leaves.

- If using gremolata, mix the parsley, garlic, and orange zest. Serve the beef (along with some of the reduced sauce) over soft polenta or mashed potatoes. Sprinkle with the gremolata (if using).

Makes 4 servings / Cost per serving: $4.90

540 calories
26 g fat
(9 g saturated)
660 mg sodium

1,060 calories
58 g fat
(26 g saturated)
2,970 mg sodium

Not That!
Olive Garden Chianti Braised Short Ribs
Price: $21.25

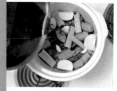

Save!
520 calories
and $16.35!

How to braise anything

Any tough cut of meat can be transformed into a delicious dinner through the alchemy of braising. It's a simple three-step process.

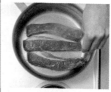

Step 1: *Sear the meat until brown all over.*

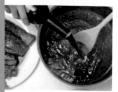

Step 2: *Deglaze the pan with a flavorful liquid.*

Step 3: *Add vegetables and stock to cover; simmer.*

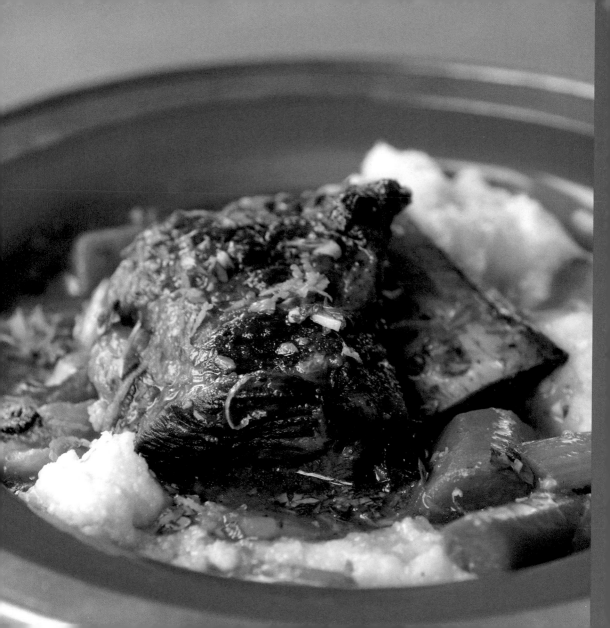

Chapter 11

Cook This, Not That!

Sides, Snacks & Sauces

Supporting cast foods should strengthen your diet, not sabotage it. Here's our blueprint for success.

When you sit down at your local chain restaurant and order something ginormous—a hulking burger, a big, muscular fillet, or cheesy pile of carbs—you pretty much know that you're flirting with disaster. Those entrées are like Dr. Evil. They're bad, and you know they're bad. (He's called "Dr. Evil," after all! What, you couldn't figure that out?) Maybe you're going to split that big dish, or leave a bit behind, or take it home in a doggie bag for tomorrow's lunch. Or maybe you're going to indulge, willfully. As with Dr. Evil, you've been warned.

Remaking the Mini Me's

But the trouble doesn't stop there. The side dishes and sauces taking up valuable plate space at your local restaurant aren't Dr. Evil. They're Mini Me. They're little, they have cute names ("Tots!") and funny shapes ("Rings!")—they even come in the guise of benevolence ("Veggies!"). They couldn't possibly be so bad, right? But like any shagalicious secret agent knows, the sidekicks are often more effective at spreading mischief than the big poobah.

Indeed, sides like Boston Market's potato salad, Cheesecake Factory's sautéed spinach, and Outback's baked sweet potato can add 400 or 500 calories or more to a dish. There are more than a few restaurants and fast-food outlets that fail to offer a single side that hasn't been mugged by a deep fryer. So even if you make the smart choice and go with the grilled salmon, that pile of crispy potatoes erases any chance of you escaping lunch or dinner for less than 800 calories. And the "healthy" options—the ubiquitous mix of broccoli, carrots, and squash—are lifeless medleys of overcooked, under-appealing vegetables, zapped to within an inch of their lives by some kid in a paper hat making $7 an hour.

Condiments don't fare much better. We're not sure when the words sauce and oil became synonymous, but the tough truth is that most things that can be drizzled on top of your steak or your salad will inflate your dish by 150 calories or more. Take the Honey Lime Cilantro dressing at T.G.I. Friday's. Sounds healthy enough, and sure a light sheen on your salad or a drizzle over your grilled chicken can't do much damage, right? At 450 calories for a side container, it packs more calories than a McDonald's Quarter Pounder. Other condiments at the country's largest restaurants don't fare much better.

It's a tragedy, really. Sides and condiments may be just supporting actors, but their performance can absolutely carry a dish. In a perfect world, three or four healthy, flavorful sides make an amazing meal on their own.

That's exactly what we give you in this chapter, a cadre of condiments, sides, and snacks that pack the type of flavor you're normally used to getting from 1,000-calorie entrées. Consider them a forceful rebuttal to the Mini Me's of the restaurant world.

The Snack Matrix

Hundred-calorie snack packs are the hottest thing in the packaged food industry since the hot sauce wars of '87. But while they may provide a decent defense against portion distortion, nearly all of them are total junk. Oreos, Chips Ahoy!, Cheetos—these heavily processed nutritional vortexes do little to stem hunger. Luckily, there are more than a few ways to put a solid snack together. Here, we've created a range of two-piece snack combinations, one part relying on a healthy vehicle like fresh fruit and whole wheat crackers, the other being a tasty topper with real nutritional benefits. Each component adds up to 100 calories, which is ideal since two 200-calorie snacks strategically timed throughout the day are just what your body needs to maximize metabolism and keep you burning calories around the clock. More than anything, you'll see how easy it is to put together a great-tasting combo loaded with the foundations of sound snacking: fiber, lean protein, healthy fat, and a cache of nutrients, or some delicious combination thereof.

KEY:

Fiber
Protein
Healthy fat

If the box is empty, it's because they don't go well together

	PART-SKIM MOZZARELLA CHEESE (1.5 oz)	GUACAMOLE (2 oz)
APPLE SLICES (1 medium apple)	✔✔	✔✔
BABY CARROTS (as many as you want)	✔✔	✔✔
WHOLE WHEAT CRACKERS like Triscuits (5 crackers)	✔✔	✔✔
BLACK BEAN CHIPS (10 chips)	✔✔	✔✔
PEAR SLICES (1 medium pear)	✔✔	✔✔
PRETZELS (1 oz)	✔	✔
WHOLE WHEAT PITA (1 medium pita)	✔✔	✔✔
CELERY STICKS (as many as you want)	✔✔	✔✔

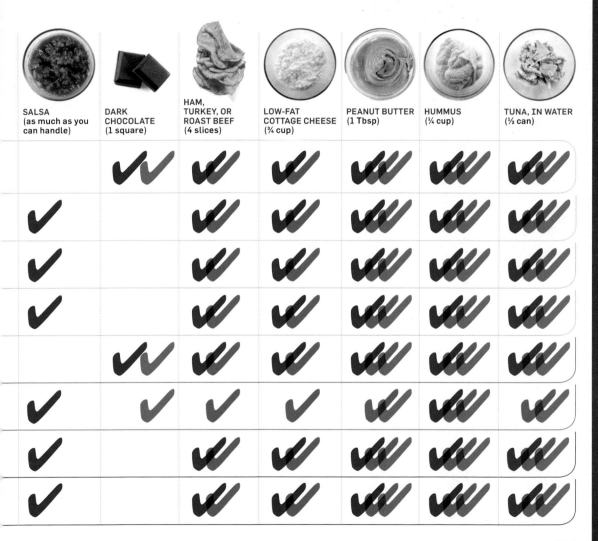

	SALSA (as much as you can handle)	DARK CHOCOLATE (1 square)	HAM, TURKEY, OR ROAST BEEF (4 slices)	LOW-FAT COTTAGE CHEESE (¾ cup)	PEANUT BUTTER (1 Tbsp)	HUMMUS (¼ cup)	TUNA, IN WATER (½ can)
		✔✔	✔✔	✔✔	✔✔✔	✔✔✔	✔✔✔
	✔		✔✔	✔✔	✔✔✔	✔✔✔	✔✔✔
	✔		✔✔	✔✔	✔✔✔	✔✔✔	✔✔✔
	✔		✔✔	✔✔	✔✔✔	✔✔✔	✔✔✔
		✔✔	✔✔	✔✔	✔✔✔	✔✔✔	✔✔✔
	✔	✔	✔	✔	✔✔	✔✔	✔✔
	✔		✔✔	✔✔	✔✔✔	✔✔✔	✔✔✔
	✔		✔✔	✔✔	✔✔✔	✔✔✔	✔✔✔

Cook This!
Seize These Seeds

As much as we love almonds, peanuts, and cashews—America's most popular nuts—there are way too many great nuts to crack to fall back on the same trio time and again. Each of the following nuts not only offers its own diverse package of nutrients, it also infuses snacktime with a diversity of big flavor.

Pistachios (1 oz)

Monounsaturated fat: 7 g

Protein: 6 g

Fiber: 3 g

Phytosterols: 61 mg

What You Need to Know: Phytosterols, a plant cholesterol found in pistachios and hazelnuts, can produce a 10-point drop in your triglycerides and a 16-point decline in your LDL (bad) cholesterol, reports the *Journal of the American College of Nutrition*.

Walnuts (1 oz)

Monounsaturated fat: 2.5 g

Protein: 4 g

Fiber: 2 g

Omega-3 fatty acids: 2,542 mg

What You Need to Know: Walnuts contain 2.5 g omega-3s per 1-ounce serving, and Harvard research shows that getting more omega-3s in your diet may help ward off depression and the ultimate bummer: a heart attack.

Pecans (1 oz)

Monounsaturated fat: 12 g

Protein: 3 g

Fiber: 3 g

Antioxidants: 144 millimoles per ounce

What You Need to Know: Pecans pack the most antioxidants of any nut. Adding them to your diet may reduce your risk of cancer, heart disease, and Alzheimer's disease.

Hazelnuts (1 oz)

Monounsaturated fat: 13 g

Protein: 4 g

Fiber: 3 g

Phytosterols: 27 mg

What You Need to Know: Men who ate a handful of hazelnuts daily boosted their HDL (good) cholesterol levels by 12 percent, according to a study in the *European Journal of Clinical Nutrition*.

Brazil nuts (1 oz)

Monounsaturated fat: 7 g

Protein: 4 g

Fiber: 2 g

Selenium: 544 micrograms

What You Need to Know: No food packs more selenium, a mineral linked to prostate-cancer protection. University of Arizona scientists also found that selenium may prevent colon cancer in men.

The Healthiest Nuts

Over the past decade, nuts have risen to the top of the healthy-snack list. But which one is king? Pecans, according to a USDA study that analyzed 10 popular nuts for their content of antioxidants.

Total Antioxidants
Micromoles per gram

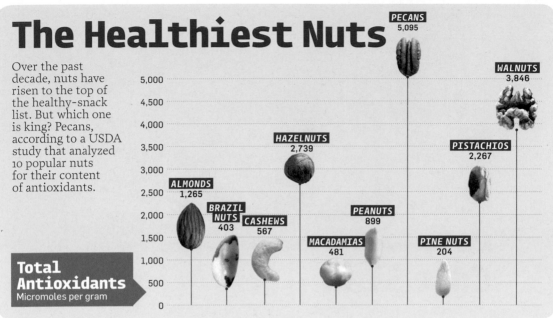

PECANS 5,095
WALNUTS 3,846
HAZELNUTS 2,739
PISTACHIOS 2,267
ALMONDS 1,265
BRAZIL NUTS 403
CASHEWS 567
PEANUTS 899
MACADAMIAS 481
PINE NUTS 204

Spice Roasted Nuts

Toasting nuts awakens and deepens their natural flavor, plus it allows you to customize them with your own favorite spice mixtures. Here are four reliable routes to take.

120 calories
11 g fat (1.5 g saturated)
150 mg sodium

You'll Need:

For Chili Almonds:
1 cup whole unpeeled almonds + ⅛ tsp chili powder + ⅛ tsp cayenne pepper + salt

For Curried Cashews:
1 cup unsalted cashews + 1 tsp curry powder

For Five-Spice Peanuts:
1 cup salted peanuts + ½ tsp Chinese five-spice powder

For Cocoa Pecans:
1 cup pecan halves + ½ Tbsp cocoa powder + ¼ tsp ground cinnamon + 2 Tbsp sugar

How to Make It:

• Preheat the oven to 400°F. Heat 1 tablespoon butter and the appropriate spices in a small saucepan. Stir in the nuts, then spread them on a baking sheet. Roast for 10 to 12 minutes, until very fragrant and warm, but not overly toasted. Each combo makes 8 servings.

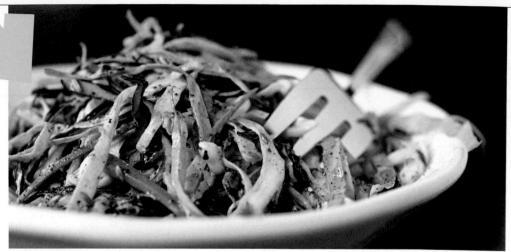

Cole Slaw

Crunchy, cool, and suffused with vinegar tang, this slaw has nothing to do with those soupy, mayo-drenched, oversweetened versions you find in most supermarket deli cases. Great as a side, but also perfect for topping sandwiches.

You'll Need:

- 2 Tbsp Dijon mustard
- 2 Tbsp mayonnaise
- 2 Tbsp vinegar (red wine, white wine, or cider)
- 2 Tbsp canola oil
- Salt and black pepper to taste
- ½ head green cabbage, very thinly sliced
- ½ head red cabbage, very thinly sliced
- 3 carrots, cut into thin strips
- 1 tsp fennel seeds
- Pickled Jalapeños (see page 304), optional

How to Make It:

- Mix the mustard, mayonnaise and vinegar in a bowl. Slowly whisk in the oil. Season with salt and pepper.
- Combine the cabbages, carrots, fennel seeds, jalapeños (if using), and dressing in a large bowl. Toss so that everything is evenly coated and season with more salt and pepper.

Makes 6 servings

> *130 calories*
> *8 g fat (1 g saturated)*
> *200 mg sodium*

Brussels and Bacon

Brussels sprouts are the type of food that strikes horror in the hearts of picky eaters. We promise, the smoke of the bacon, the heat of the red pepper flakes, and the crunch of the almond will win over even the most stubborn veggi-phobe.

You'll Need:

- 4 strips bacon, chopped into small pieces
- 2 cloves garlic, peeled
- 1 tsp red pepper flakes
- 1 lb Brussels sprouts, bottoms trimmed, cut in half
- Salt and black pepper to taste
- 2 Tbsp sliced almonds

How to Make It:

- Heat a large skillet or sauté pan over medium heat. Add the bacon and cook until crispy, about 5 minutes. Remove to a plate lined with paper towels. Discard all but 1 tablespoon of the rendered bacon fat.

- Add the garlic, pepper flakes, Brussels sprouts, and a pinch of salt to the skillet. Sauté until the sprouts are lightly browned on the outside and tender—but still firm—throughout, 10 to 12 minutes. Add the almonds and sauté for another minute or two. Season with salt and pepper.

Makes 4 servings

120 calories
5 g fat (1.5 g saturated)
310 mg sodium

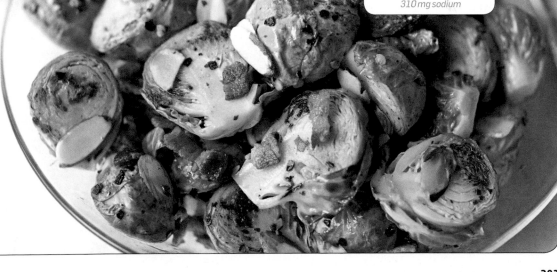

293

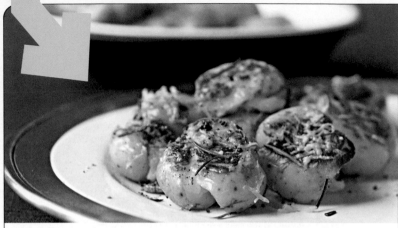

Smashed Potatoes

These potatoes are as good subbing in for greasy French fries at dinner as they are usurping calorie-laden hash browns at breakfast.

You'll Need:

- 2 lb small potatoes, like Yukon Golds
- Salt and black pepper to taste
- 1 Tbsp olive oil
- 2 cloves garlic, peeled
- 1 Tbsp minced fresh rosemary or 1 tsp dried
- 2 Tbsp grated Romano or Parmesan

How to Make It:

- Place the potatoes in a pot and fill with enough cold water to cover. Add 1 teaspoon salt and bring to a boil. Cook the potatoes until just tender all the way through, about 20 minutes. Drain.
- When cool enough to handle, use your palm to carefully smash the spuds just enough to break the skin and flatten the potatoes.
- Heat the oil in a large cast-iron skillet over medium heat. Add the potatoes in a single layer, along with the garlic and rosemary. Cook until the potatoes are deeply browned and crispy on one side, 7 to 10 minutes, then flip and repeat. Add the cheese in the final moments of cooking, so that it melts atop the potatoes. Season with salt and pepper.

Makes 4 servings

210 calories
8 g fat (1.5 g saturated)
380 mg sodium

Quinoa Pilaf

If stuck on a deserted island for the rest of your life with but one food to eat, quinoa may very well be your best option. Its complex carbohydrates, healthy fats, and generous protein profile (quinoa is one of the few vegetarian complete proteins) make it one of the healthiest foods on the planet. It's also mighty tasty—as you'll find with this versatile pilaf.

You'll Need:

- 1 cup quinoa
- ½ Tbsp olive oil
- ½ yellow onion, minced
- 1 carrot, finely chopped
- 3 cups low-sodium chicken broth or water
- 2 Tbsp toasted pine nuts
- ¼ cup golden raisins
- ½ cup chopped fresh parsley
- Salt and black pepper to taste

230 calories
7 g fat
(1 g saturated)
320 mg sodium

How to Make It:

- Place the quinoa in a large bowl and rinse in several changes of cold water. Drain thoroughly.

- Heat the oil in a medium saucepan over medium heat. Cook the onion and carrot until softened, then stir in the quinoa and cook until lightly toasted and giving off a nutty smell, about 3 minutes. Add the broth and bring to a simmer. Reduce the heat to low, cover, and simmer until the liquid is fully absorbed, about 20 minutes.

- Transfer the quinoa to a large bowl and fluff with a fork. Stir in the pine nuts, raisins, and parsley.

Makes 4 servings

Pan-Roasted Mushrooms

Not only do these mushrooms make a fantastic side, but they also can be used to smother a steak, slather a sandwich, or punch up a salad. The greater the variety of mushrooms, the better.

110 calories
7 g fat (2.5 g saturated)
440 mg sodium

You'll Need:

- 2 lb mixed mushrooms
- 1 Tbsp olive oil
- Salt and black pepper to taste
- 2 cloves garlic, minced
- 1 Tbsp butter
- ¼ cup chopped fresh parsley

How to Make It:

- Remove the stems and clean the mushroom caps with a damp paper towel. Cut the mushrooms into large, even-size chunks.

- Heat the oil in a large cast-iron skillet over medium-high heat. When the oil is hot, add the mushrooms in a single layer and season with salt and pepper (work in batches if necessary so the mushrooms brown rather than steam). Cook until they begin to brown, about 5 minutes.

- Stir in the garlic and butter. Cook for a few minutes more—to take the raw edge off the garlic—then remove from the heat and add the parsley.

Makes 4 servings

Sautéed Spinach

60 calories
3.5 g fat
(0 g saturated)
390 mg sodium

You could do a lot worse than eat this side every day for the rest of your life. Spinach is like Mother Nature's multivitamin, housing huge deposits of 22 vital nutrients. Try stirring these greens into scrambled eggs or pile on top of garlic-rubbed crusty bread.

You'll Need:

- 1 Tbsp olive oil
- 2 cloves garlic, thinly sliced
- 1 tsp red pepper flakes
- 1 bunch spinach (about 1½ pounds), rinsed
- Juice of 1 lemon
- Salt and black pepper to taste

How to Make It:

- Heat the olive oil in a large skillet or sauté pan over medium heat. Add the garlic and pepper flakes and cook for 1 minute. Stir in the spinach. Cook until the spinach fully wilts, about 5 minutes. Drain any water that accumulates in the bottom of the pan (since spinach is mostly water, there will be plenty of excess liquid). Add the lemon juice and season with salt and pepper.

Makes 4 servings

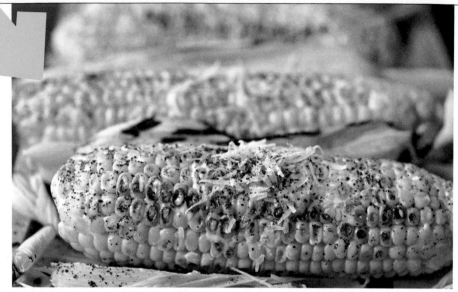

Grilled Mexican-Style Corn

This is how corn is served on the streets of Mexico, robed in a thin sheen of mayo (instead of butter) and topped with a sprinkling of chili powder and cheese. If you want to cut the calories, lime juice and chili powder alone offer a vast improvement over standard boiled corn—but once you try the full package, you'll have a hard time eating it any other way.

You'll Need:

- 4 ears of corn, husked
- 1 tsp salt
- 2 Tbsp mayonnaise
- Juice of 1 lime
- ½ Tbsp chili powder
- Finely grated Parmesan

How to Make It:

- Heat a grill until hot. While the grill is warming up, bring a pot of water to a boil. Add the corn and salt. Boil for 5 to 7 minutes, until the corn until slightly tender, but not cooked all the way through. Drain the corn and transfer to the grill; lightly char the kernels.
- Mix the mayonnaise and lime juice. Remove the corn from the grill, paint with a bit of the citrus mayonnaise, then dust with chili powder and Parmesan.

Makes 4 servings

210 calories
9 g fat
(2 g saturated)
430 mg sodium

Simmered Lentils

160 calories
4.5 g fat
(0.5 g saturated)
540 mg sodium

Loaded with protein, teeming with fiber, and shot through with a massive dose of antioxidants, lentils are a full-blown superfood. Sadly, few people cook them, and fewer restaurants serve them—which is crazy, given how cheap, tasty, and easy to prepare they are. Use this base recipe as a side with grilled or roasted meats and fish (especially salmon). Want more flavor? Start with a hunk of bacon or a ham hock.

You'll Need:

1½ cups lentils

1 Tbsp olive oil

½ onion, chopped

2 carrots, diced

2 cloves garlic, minced

1½ cups low-sodium chicken broth or water

2 bay leaves

½ Tbsp red wine vinegar

Salt and black pepper to taste

How to Make It:

• Rinse the lentils and pick through, discarding any stones.

• Heat the olive oil in a pot over medium heat. Cook the onion, carrots, and garlic until softened, 5 to 7 minutes. Add the lentils, broth, and bay leaves. Simmer until the lentils are just tender, about 20 minutes. Season with the vinegar, salt, and pepper. Discard the bay leaves.

Makes 6 servings

Smoky Baked Beans

170 calories
3 g fat
(1 g saturated)
570 mg sodium

Baked beans, both the type that come in cans and those that come from the kitchens of barbecue shacks, are usually one step away from candy, bombarded as they are with brown sugar, molasses, and honey. Too bad, since beans really are A-list eats. To preserve their health status and maximize deliciousness, we mitigate the sugar surge and build flavor instead with a few of our all-time favorite foods: cayenne, beer, and bacon.

You'll Need:

4 strips bacon, chopped into small pieces

1 medium onion, minced

2 cloves garlic, minced

2 cans (16 oz each) pinto beans, rinsed and drained

1 cup dark beer

¼ cup ketchup

1 Tbsp chili powder

1 Tbsp brown sugar

Pinch of cayenne pepper

How to Make It:

• Heat a large pot or saucepan over medium heat. Add the bacon and cook until it's just turning crispy, 3 to 5 minutes. Add the onion and garlic and sauté until translucent, another 3 minutes. Stir in the beans, beer, ketchup, chili powder, brown sugar, and cayenne. Simmer until the sauce thickens and clings to the beans, about 15 minutes.

Makes 6 servings

Potato Salad

This version is about as classic as potato salad gets, except for the fact that we resist the urge to drown the vegetables in a viscous sea of mayo. Instead, the mayo is bolstered with Dijon and a tangy shot of vinegar. The result: a healthier potato salad that still tastes like the picnic classic we all adore.

You'll Need:

- 3 lb red potatoes, all similar in size
- Salt and black pepper to taste
- 2 stalks celery, chopped
- ¼ cup chopped pickles (preferably gherkins or cornichons)
- 1 small red onion, chopped
- 2 Tbsp Dijon mustard
- ½ cup mayonnaise
- 2 Tbsp white wine vinegar
- 3 hard-boiled eggs, chopped
- Smoked paprika (optional)

How to Make It:

- Place the potatoes in a large pot and fill with enough cold water to easily cover. Season the water with 1 teaspoon salt and bring to a boil. Cook the potatoes until tender all the way through (the tip of a paring knife inserted into a potato will meet little resistance). Drain.
- When cool enough to handle, chop the potatoes into ¾" pieces. Place in a large bowl and add the celery, pickles, onion, mustard, mayonnaise, vinegar, and eggs. Toss to coat. Season with salt and pepper and sprinkle with the paprika (if using).

Makes 10 servings

> 190 calories
> 10 g fat (2 g saturated)
> 320 mg sodium

Homemade Chips

A miniscule 1-ounce portion of potato chips will run you 160 calories and 10 grams of fat. Why settle when you can bake healthier and immensely tastier chips in 20 minutes at home? Customize their flavor depending on your mood.

You'll Need:

- 2 large russet potatoes
- 1 Tbsp olive oil
- Salt and black pepper to taste

OPTIONAL TOPPINGS

- 2 Tbsp finely grated Parmesan
- ½ Tbsp smoked paprika
- 1 Tbsp chopped fresh rosemary
- 1 clove garlic, minced
- ¼ cup chopped parsley and the grated zest of 1 lemon

Sweet Potato Fries

140 calories
3 g fat
(0.5 g saturated)
180 mg sodium

How to Make It:

- Preheat the oven to 400°F. Scrub the potatoes with cold water and cut crosswise into ⅛" thick slices. Toss with the olive oil and season with salt and pepper.

- Spread in a single layer on a baking sheet. (To use the optional toppings: Sprinkle with Parmesan, paprika, or rosemary before baking; add the parsley mixture after baking.) Bake until lightly browned and crispy, about 20 minutes.

Makes 6 servings

Spicy Mashed Sweet Potatoes

Heat and sweet conspire here to make one of our favorite side dishes of all time. Serve these as a bed for Grilled Pork and Peaches (page 176), Turkey Meat Loaf (page 234), or any other grilled or roasted meat.

You'll Need:

2 **large sweet potatoes, peeled and cut into quarters**

Salt and black pepper to taste

1 **cup milk**

2 **Tbsp butter**

1 **Tbsp minced chipotle pepper**

How to Make It:

- Place the sweet potatoes in a pot and fill with enough cold water to cover. Add 1 teaspoon salt and bring to a boil. Cook until the sweet potatoes are tender, but not mushy, about 15 minutes. Drain and return to the pot.

- Heat the milk and butter in a small saucepan. Slowly stir into the sweet potatoes, using a wooden spoon to vigorously incorporate the liquid (this will help create a smooth puree). Stir in the chipotle pepper and season with salt and pepper.

Makes 4 servings

130 calories
6 g fat (4 g saturated)
360 mg sodium

Sweet potatoes have two big nutritional boons that regular potatoes lack: big doses of fiber and vision-strengthening vitamin A. Plus the natural sugars found within them pair perfectly with the fiery cayenne to make fries every bit as enjoyable as the ones that bathe in oil.

70 calories
2 g fat (0 g saturated)
200 mg sodium

You'll Need:

2 **medium sweet potatoes, each peeled and cut into 12 equal wedges**

½ **Tbsp olive oil**

Pinch of cayenne pepper

Salt and black pepper to taste

How to Make It:

- Preheat the oven to 425°F. Combine all the ingredients on a large baking sheet and use your hands to mix them thoroughly. Spread in an even layer. Bake until the sweet potatoes are lightly browned on the outside, crisp to the touch, and tender inside.

Makes 4 servings

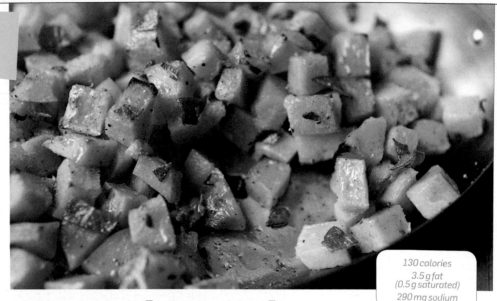

130 calories
3.5 g fat
(0.5 g saturated)
290 mg sodium

Roasted Squash

Butternut squash, especially when roasted, is one of those vegetables that is so delicious you almost feel guilty eating it. Don't—these babies are bursting with A-list nutrients, including cholesterol-fighting, eye-strengthening, anti-inflammatory beta-carotene.

You'll Need:

1 **medium butternut squash**

1 **Tbsp olive oil**

1 **Tbsp maple syrup**

8–10 **fresh sage leaves, chopped (optional)**

Salt and black pepper to taste

How to Make It:

• Preheat the oven to 425°F. Peel the squash with a vegetable peeler or a small paring knife. Slice in half lengthwise and scoop out the seeds; discard the seeds or save for later (see below). Chop the squash into ¾" chunks. Toss with the olive oil, maple syrup, and sage (if using); season with salt and pepper.

• Spread on a baking sheet and roast until lightly browned on the outside and soft and tender all the way through, about 30 minutes. If you like, add the seeds during the last 10 minutes for an extra layer of crunch.

Makes 4 servings

Sweet and Sour Onions

How would you invest 50 calories? On an Oreo cookie? Five or six potato chips? A few sips of Coke? Or, how about a big mound of gooey glazed onions bursting with the yin-yang balance of sugar (most of it natural) and vinegar? Serve a scoop of these brilliant bulbs with your next steak or roast chicken and offer silent thanks to the genius who invented frozen pearl onions.

50 calories
0 g fat
(0 g saturated)
190 mg sodium

You'll Need:

- 1 bag (16 oz) frozen pearl onions
- ¾ cup water
- ¾ cup white or red wine vinegar
- ¼ cup sugar
- Pinch of red pepper flakes
- Salt and black pepper to taste

How to Make It:

- Combine the onions, water, vinegar, sugar, and pepper flakes in a medium saucepan. Place over medium-low heat, cover, and cook for 10 minutes. Remove the lid and cook for another 10 minutes, until the liquid has reduced and begins to cling to the onions. The onions should be tender but not falling apart. Season with salt and pepper.

Makes 4 servings

Roasted Parmesan Asparagus

Asparagus is one of our favorite vegetables, mostly because its sweet, nutty flavor takes well to all sorts of cooking approaches: wrapped in prosciutto and grilled; blanched briefly in boiling water, then topped with a fried egg; shaved raw into a salad. But for a busy night when dinner just needs to appear, you can't beat this approach.

45 calories
4 g fat
(1 g saturated)
330 mg sodium

You'll Need:

- 1 bunch asparagus, about 1½ pounds
- 1 Tbsp olive oil
- 2 Tbsp grated Parmesan
- Salt and black pepper to taste
- Juice of 1 lemon

How to Make It:

- Preheat the oven to 400°F. Hold an asparagus spear at both ends and bend the bottom until the tough, woody section snaps (it will naturally snap off where the tough part of the vegetable ends and the tender part begins). Using that spear as a guide, use a knife to remove the bottoms of the rest of the bunch.
- Place the asparagus in a baking dish. Drizzle with the olive oil, sprinkle with the Parmesan, and season with salt and pepper; toss to coat. Roast until just tender, 10 to 12 minutes. Sprinkle the lemon juice over the asparagus.

Makes 4 servings

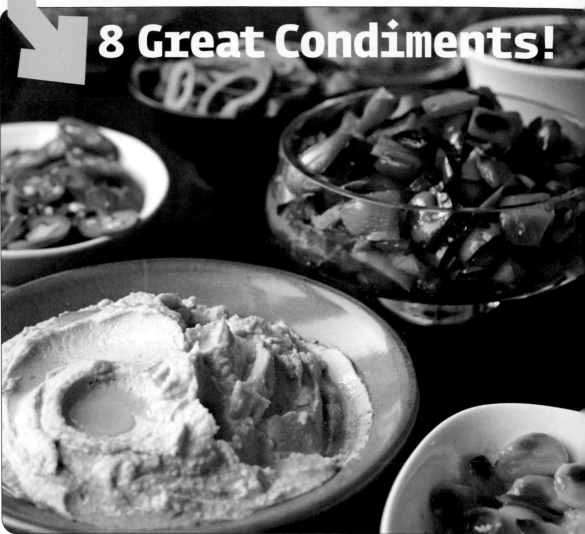

8 Great Condiments!

When it comes down to it, it's the little things that count in the kitchen: when you salt your chicken, where you buy your fish, how long you rest your steak before slicing. Do these simple things correctly and you'll be a better cook on the spot. But, as we've highlighted throughout the book, it also helps to have a few secret weapons up your sleeve. And no weapons can have more of an instant effect on the quality of your food than these eight condiments. They hail from all over the world, but they share one thing in common: They bring maximum flavor impact with minimum effort. Have at least a few of them in the fridge at all times and you can turn even the dullest meal into something memorable.

Pesto

You can buy perfectly fine pesto in the refrigerated section of most supermarkets (we like Cibo), but it will never taste as good as a homemade batch—which, by the way, takes all of 3 minutes to make. This makes enough for a big pasta dish with enough left over to spread on turkey sandwiches and swirl into soups and salad dressing. To keep it extra fresh and green, float a thin layer of oil on top of the pesto before refrigerating—the oil will keep the basil from oxidizing and turning dark.

You'll Need:

2 cloves garlic, chopped

2 Tbsp pine nuts

3 cups fresh basil leaves

¼ cup grated Parmesan

Salt and black pepper to taste

½ cup olive oil

How to Make It:

Place the garlic, pine nuts, basil, and Parmesan, plus a few pinches of salt and pepper, in a food processor. Pulse until the basil is chopped. With the motor running, slowly drizzle in the olive oil until fully incorporated and a paste forms.

Makes about 1 cup

Guacamole

Many American versions of guacamole include ingredients like cumin, scallions, and (gasp!) sour cream. But guac is really at its best with just a few carefully balanced ingredients: garlic (preferably chopped into an oily paste), a good pinch of salt, and a squeeze of lemon or lime. And of course, perfectly ripe Hass avocados. Use that as your base; everything else—onion, jalapeño, cilantro, tomato—is just a bonus.

You'll Need:

2 cloves garlic, peeled

Kosher salt to taste

¼ cup minced red onion

1 Tbsp minced jalapeño

2 ripe avocados, pitted and peeled

Juice of 1 lemon or lime

Chopped fresh cilantro (optional)

How to Make It:

Use the side of a knife to smash the garlic against the cutting board. Finely mince the cloves, then apply a pinch of salt to the garlic and use the side of your knife to work the garlic into a paste (the salt will act as an abrasive). Scoop the garlic into a bowl, then add the onion, jalapeño, and avocado and mash until the avocado is pureed, but still slightly chunky. Stir in the lemon juice, cilantro (if using), and salt to taste.

Makes about 2 cups

Cook This!

Hummus

This punchy puree of chickpeas (aka garbanzo beans), garlic, and olive oil is beloved across much of the Middle East—and increasingly, in restaurants and homes across this country. That's a good thing, since you'd be hard pressed to find a better condiment for dipping (with pitas or fresh vegetables) or spreading. Tahini is a paste made from sesame seeds that tastes a lot like peanut butter; if you can't find any in your local markets, smooth, unsweetened peanut butter will sub in a pinch.

You'll Need:

- 1 can (16 oz) chickpeas, rinsed and drained
- 2 Tbsp tahini
- 1 clove garlic, chopped
- ¼ tsp ground cumin

Juice of 1 lemon

¼ cup olive oil

Salt and black pepper to taste

How to Make It:

Place the chickpeas, tahini, garlic, cumin, and lemon juice in a food processor and pulse a few times. With the motor running, drizzle in the olive oil until a smooth paste forms. Season with salt and pepper.

Makes about 2 cups

Pickled Jalapeños

You can buy jars of pickled jalapeños, but why bother when these take minutes to prep, taste better, and are lighter on the sodium than the store-bought variety? Once you start adding these to sandwiches, eggs, and pretty much any other savory meal, you'll have a hard time stopping. Depending on how hot you like it, you can stop slicing the jalapeños when you reach the serious seed deposits (about three-quarters of the way up on the pepper) or you can cut all the way to the stem.

You'll Need:

- ½ cup apple cider vinegar
- ½ cup water
- 2 Tbsp sugar
- 1 tsp salt

5 or 6 jalapeños, sliced very thinly

How to Make It:

Combine the vinegar, water, sugar, and salt in a small saucepan and heat until the liquid just begins to simmer. Set aside for 5 minutes to cool. Place the jalapeño slices in a sealable jar or container and pour the liquid over the peppers. These are ready to use almost immediately (give them at least 20 minutes of soaking) and keep covered in the fridge for up to 10 days.

Pickled Onions

Raw onions can be harsh and overpowering, but a vinegar solution takes off the edge and replaces it with a lovely sweet-spicy bite. These make one of the best condiments imaginable for sandwiches, tacos, nachos, and burgers alike.

You'll Need:

- ¾ cup white or red wine vinegar
- ¾ cup water
- 2 Tbsp sugar
- 1 tsp salt
- 2 bay leaves

Pinch of red pepper flakes

2 red onions, sliced into thin rings

How to Make It:

Combine the vinegar, water, sugar, salt, bay leaves, and pepper flakes in a small pan and heat until the liquid just begins to simmer. Set aside to cool for 5 minutes. Place the onions in a sealable jar or container and pour the liquid over the onions. These are ready to use almost immediately (give them at least 20 minutes of soaking) and keep covered in the fridge for up to a week.

Caramelized Onions

Sweet, rich caramelized onions have the Midas touch, turning everything they adorn into gastronomic gold. They're the perfect low-calorie flavor builders, working both as a condiment (replacing mayo and spreads on a burger) and as a topping for sandwiches, omelets, or hunks of grilled steak. If you're going to take the time to properly caramelize onions, you might as well make a big batch; they keep in the fridge in a sealed container for 10 days.

You'll Need:

- 1 Tbsp butter
- 4 medium red onions, sliced

Salt and black pepper to taste

- 2 Tbsp balsamic vinegar

How to Make It:

Heat the butter in a large saucepan or pot over medium-low heat. Add the onions and a few pinches of salt and cook, stirring occasionally, until the onions have gone from translucent to a light caramel color, about 20 to 30 minutes. (You can cook these for a shorter time over a higher temperature, but the results won't be quite as good.) Add the vinegar and a few pinches of black pepper and cook for another 3 to 5 minutes.

Makes about 2 cups

Roasted Garlic

Raw garlic can be harsh and overpowering. Overcooked garlic can be acrid and off-putting. But slow-roasted garlic is like savory candy—sweet and inviting with its mellowed garlic flavor. Fold into mashed potatoes or salad dressings (especially Caesar) or simply spread on on a loaf of bread, top with a bit of Parmesan, and bake until brown for heroic garlic bread.

You'll Need:

- 1 head of garlic
- 1 Tbsp olive oil

How to Make It:

Preheat the oven to 325°F. Separate the garlic cloves and peel them. Place in the center of a large piece of aluminum foil and drizzle with the oil. Fold the foil to enclose the garlic. Place on a baking sheet and bake for 35 to 40 minutes, until the garlic is soft enough to spread like warm butter. Transfer to a covered jar or container and store in the fridge for up to 2 weeks.

Pepperonata

This magical pepper trifecta is beloved by Italians. Spicy, tangy, and sweet, it adds pop to pastas, salads, sandwiches—pretty much anything it touches. Use any color pepper but green—ideally one each of red, yellow, and orange.

You'll Need:

- 1 Tbsp olive oil
- 2 cloves garlic
- ½ tsp red pepper flakes
- 3 bell peppers, cut into ½" chunks
- 2 Tbsp red wine vinegar

Salt and black pepper to taste

How to Make It:

Heat the olive oil in a large stainless steel skillet or sauté pan over medium-high heat. Add the garlic cloves and pepper flakes and cook just long enough to infuse the oil, about 1 minute. Toss in the peppers and cook, stirring occasionally, until the peppers are soft and lightly blistered (the best way to do this is with a screaming hot pan). Add the vinegar and cook for a minute. Season with salt and pepper. Store tightly covered in the fridge for up to 1 week.

Makes about 3 cups

Maximum flavor impact for minimum effort

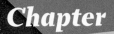

12

Desserts & Drinks

You don't have to give up ice cream, cookies, and apple pie.
You just need to find better versions.

"In all things, moderation," as Aristotle decreed. The great philosopher knew what he was talking about—and not just because it's hard to look lean while wearing a toga. (White just adds on the pounds!) Instinctively, he must have known something about the role of blood sugar in weight management, and how a little dessert is a great thing, and a lot of dessert is something altogether different.

The Anatomy of a Dessert Disaster

See, when we eat a big heaping helping of dessert calories, those calories go rushing into our bloodstream like tweens to a Jonas Brothers concert. That's because desserts are typically packed with refined carbohydrates, which pass through our digestive systems quickly, loading our bloodstreams with sugar in the form of glucose. What our bodies want to do is turn that big surge of glucose into energy and store it in the muscles so we can run and throw and hike and reduce our neighbors to sawdust in a Guitar Hero rematch. But when the calories come too fast, in too concentrated a dose, our bodies get overwhelmed, and we can do only one thing with them—store them in and around our bellies. In fact, a study from Penn State University compared those who eat whole grains to those who eat bloodstream-flooding refined grains, and found that whole-grain eaters lost 2.4 times more belly fat than those who ate refined grains.

So the thing to remember about desserts is that it's not just the fact that you're adding to your daily caloric intake—it's that you're taking those calories in all at once, which means you gain more weight than the next guy, even if the next guy is eating the same amount of calories throughout the day. Dive into, say, a Red Robin Mountain High Mudd Pie, and you've just injected 1,390 calories directly into your bloodstream.

But that doesn't mean you should skip dessert—it just means you need to view dessert not as an indulgence, but as part of your weight-loss arsenal. Indeed, desserts like ice cream are packed with calcium, a mineral that binds to fatty acids in the digestive system, blocking their absorption. Plus, half a cup of vanilla ice cream gives you 19 milligrams of choline, which recent USDA research shows lowers blood levels of homocysteine—an amino acid that can hinder the flow of blood through blood vessels—by 8 percent.

The *Cook This, Not That!* desserts are packed with healthy ingredients that won't flood your bloodstream with a hysterical mob of glucose. Instead, they'll satisfy your cravings and prove that you are nothing if not the master of the sweet science.

The Smoothie Matrix

Of all the staggering stats that accompany this country's obesity crisis, the most telling of all is this: Just 9 percent of Americans eat the daily recommended servings of fruits and vegetables. Cue the smoothie, a beacon of blended hope. For 300 calories or less, you can slurp up two or three servings of belly-filling fruit for breakfast or a midday snack. Plus, they're delicious (need proof? even kids will drink them) and infinitely adaptable. Bottoms up!

The Fantastic Four

To the right are all the ingredients you need to custom blend your smoothies to ensure optimum performance for body and mind. We've started you out with four no-fail concoctions.

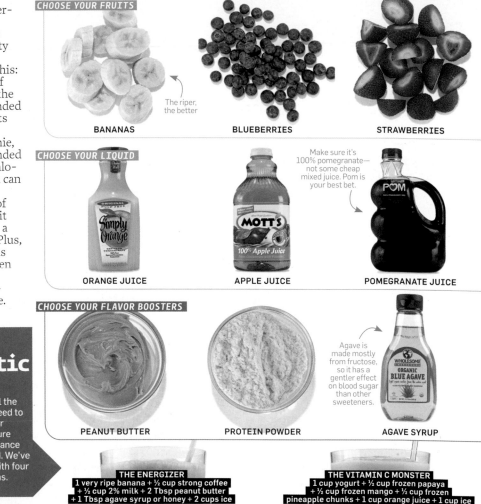

CHOOSE YOUR FRUITS

The riper, the better

BANANAS

BLUEBERRIES

STRAWBERRIES

CHOOSE YOUR LIQUID

Make sure it's 100% pomegranate—not some cheap mixed juice. Pom is your best bet.

ORANGE JUICE

APPLE JUICE

POMEGRANATE JUICE

CHOOSE YOUR FLAVOR BOOSTERS

Agave is made mostly from fructose, so it has a gentler effect on blood sugar than other sweeteners.

PEANUT BUTTER

PROTEIN POWDER

AGAVE SYRUP

THE ENERGIZER
1 very ripe banana + ½ cup strong coffee + ½ cup 2% milk + 2 Tbsp peanut butter + 1 Tbsp agave syrup or honey + 2 cups ice

THE VITAMIN C MONSTER
1 cup yogurt + ½ cup frozen papaya + ½ cup frozen mango + ½ cup frozen pineapple chunks + 1 cup orange juice + 1 cup ice

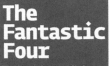

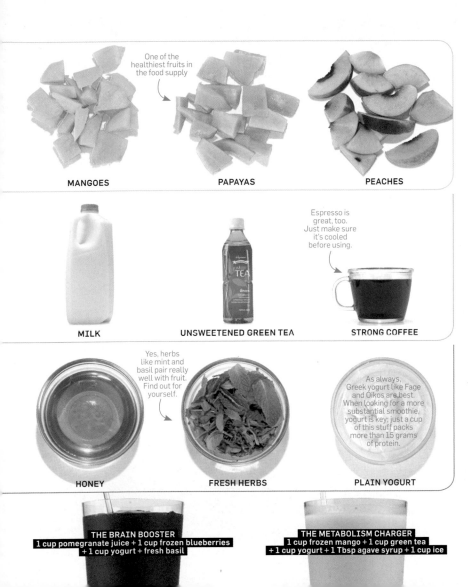

One of the healthiest fruits in the food supply

MANGOES

PAPAYAS

PEACHES

Espresso is great, too. Just make sure it's cooled before using.

MILK

UNSWEETENED GREEN TEA

STRONG COFFEE

Yes, herbs like mint and basil pair really well with fruit. Find out for yourself.

As always, Greek yogurt like Fage and Oikos are best. When looking for a more substantial smoothie, yogurt is key; just a cup of this stuff packs more than 15 grams of protein.

HONEY

FRESH HERBS

PLAIN YOGURT

THE BRAIN BOOSTER
1 cup pomegranate juice + 1 cup frozen blueberries + 1 cup yogurt + fresh basil

THE METABOLISM CHARGER
1 cup frozen mango + 1 cup green tea + 1 cup yogurt + 1 Tbsp agave syrup + 1 cup ice

The Rules of the Smoothie

Step 1
No ice cream. If you want ice cream in your smoothie, call it what it is—a milk shake—and have it for dessert.

Step 2
Use a strong blender. A weak blender won't be able to crush the ice quick enough, which means it melts and ultimately dilutes your precious smoothie, rather than give it that bracing, slushy-like texture you want.

Step 3
Respect the ratio. Once you learn the basic proportions of liquids and solids to toss in the blender, you can turn anything into a pretty drinkable smoothie. For every 3 cups of fruit, you'll need about 1 cup of liquid. Yogurt and ice will both thicken slightly.

Step 4
Ditching ice entirely will give your smoothies a more intense fruit flavor. If you prefer your smoothies sans ice, just make sure the fruit is frozen. (Beyond the bags of frozen fruit, have a few frozen bananas in your freezer at all times.)

Chocolate Chip Cookies

These cookies don't contain applesauce, protein powder, or Splenda—you'll need to find another book for that type of trickery. They're just good, honest, truly delicious chocolate chip cookies. Yes, we've taken it a bit easy on the butter and the chocolate chips for the sake of creating a lighter cookie, but you'll never know the difference.

You'll Need:

- 8 tablespoons butter (1 stick), softened
- ½ cup packed brown sugar
- ½ cup granulated sugar
- 2 eggs
- 1 tsp vanilla extract
- ½ tsp baking soda
- ½ tsp salt
- 2 cups flour
- ½ cup dark chocolate chips
- Flaky sea salt (optional)

How to Make It:

- Preheat the oven to 375°F.
- In a mixing bowl, thoroughly mix the butter, brown sugar, and granulated sugar until creamy. Stir in eggs and vanilla until well incorporated. Add the baking soda, salt, and flour and mix until the dough comes together, being careful not to overmix. Stir in the chocolate chips.
- Drop the dough onto a baking sheet in balls about 3 tablespoons in size, leaving at least 3 inches between cookies.
- Bake until the edges are golden and the middles are just barely set. Remove from the sheet, sprinkle with a bit of sea salt (if using) and cool on a wire rack.

Makes about 12 cookies / Cost per cookie: $0.15

Salt teases out the flavors in any food it touches—even cookies. The crunchy crystals pair beautifully with the warm chocolate.

$$(\P+\P)^2$$

MEAL MULTIPLIER

With this recipe as your base, you can take this crispy yet chewy cookie in all sorts of different directions. Change up the chips by subbing in white or milk chocolate chips, or even peanut butter chips. A handful of dark raisins or a half-cup of shredded coconut bring sweetness of a different, natural variety. And any nuts— especially walnuts and pecans—infuse the cookie with their heart-healthy fats.

190 calories
8 g fat (5 g saturated)
16 g sugars

430 calories
21 g fat
(10 g saturated)
35 g sugar

Not That!
Atlanta Bread Company Chocolate Chunk Cookie
Price: $1.18

Save!
240 calories
and $1.03!

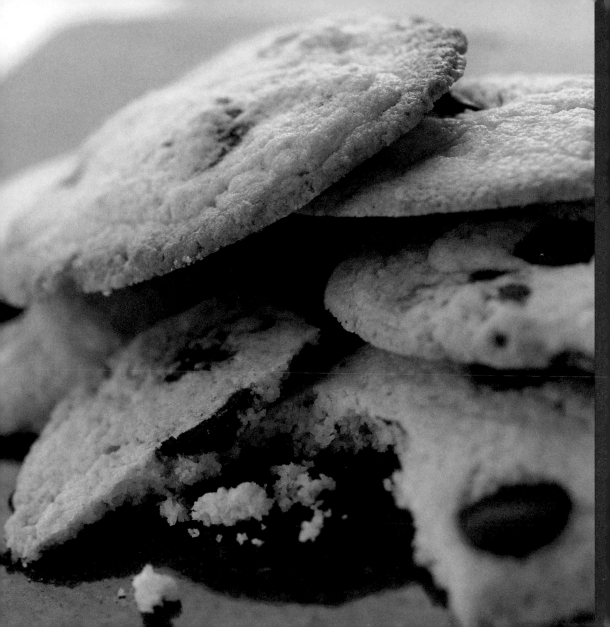

Cook This!
Strawberry Shortcake
with Balsamic

To deliver flavor, the corporate cook relies on hulking scoops of ice cream, oversize brownies, and floods of molten chocolate. The home cook doesn't need such waist-expanding, palate-blunting effects to make dessert memorable. Here, low-calorie angel food cake picks up the smoke and char of the grill and is topped with strawberries soaked in balsamic vinegar and black pepper, an irresistible combination adored throughout northern Italy. Trust us, you'll be hooked.

You'll Need:

- 2 **cups sliced strawberries**
- ¼ **cup balsamic vinegar**
- **Pinch of freshly cracked black pepper**
- 1 **Tbsp butter (optional)**
- 4 **wedges angel food cake, each 1" thick**
- **Whipped cream**

How to Make It:

- Mix the strawberries, vinegar, and pepper and marinate for 10 to 15 minutes.
- Heat a grill, stovetop grill pan, or nonstick sauté pan until hot. (If using the pan, add the butter; if grilling, omit the butter entirely.) Add the cake slices and cook until caramelized and toasted. Transfer to 4 dessert plates. Top with the strawberries, their liquid, and a spoonful of whipped cream.

Makes 4 servings / Cost per serving: $1.70

Research from the USDA shows that strawberries absorb high levels of pesticides when grown conventionally. If ever there were an organic fruit to buy, this is it.

It may seem like a curious addition to this mix, but black pepper brings a subtle heat that pairs well with the fruit and vinegar.

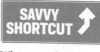

SAVVY SHORTCUT

Why waste time (and calories) baking cakes from home at every grocery store in America sells angel food cake? It's inexpensive, well made, and—at just 72 calories and 0 grams of fat per slice—only marginally worse for you than a rice cake. Plus, it's super versatile, ready in an instant to provide a spongy base for a small ice cream sundae, for dipping into fondue, or for a light rendition of bread pudding. Or top it with grilled fruit (apricots and peaches work best) and crown with a small scoop of vanilla ice cream.

160 calories
6 g fat (3.5 g saturated)
12 g sugars

900 calories
50 g fat
102 g carbohydrates

Not That!
Ruby Tuesday Strawberries & Ice Cream
Price: $4.99

Save!
740 calories and $3.29!

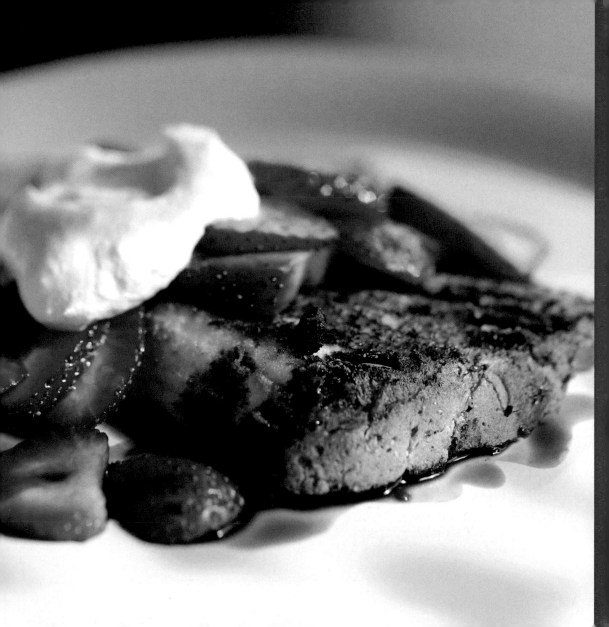

Crispy Apple Turnover

American as it may be, the price of apple pie at a restaurant is a steep one to pay. For that matter, so, too, is the one we pay at Grandma's house when she serves us a warm slice à la mode. But to ditch the dessert over caloric concerns would be downright unpatriotic, so instead we solved apple pie's biggest nutritional setback—serving size—by wrapping up neat little packets of sweetened, spiced apple chunks in flaky puff pastry. The result is a perfectly portioned individual turnover with fewer calories than you'd get from two bites of Cheesecake Factory's Warm Apple Crisp.

You'll Need:

Flour

- 1 sheet puff pastry, defrosted
- 1 cup water
- ½ cup sugar
- 3 Granny Smith apples
- ¼ tsp ground cinnamon
- ⅛ tsp ground ginger
- ⅛ tsp ground nutmeg

Juice of 1 lemon

- 1 egg white, lightly beaten

How to Make It:

- Generously flour a working surface. Roll the puff pastry into a 9" x 15" rectangle. Cut the pastry into 6 equal squares. Refrigerate until needed.

- Bring the water and sugar to a boil in a large saucepan. Peel and core the apples; cut into ½" chunks. Toss the apples with the cinnamon, ginger, nutmeg, and lemon juice, then add to the sugar mixture and simmer until the liquid thickens, 5 to 7 minutes. Set aside to cool.

- Preheat the oven to 425°F. When the apple mixture cools, spoon 2 to 3 tablespoons of apples onto the puff pastry squares, off center. Fold the pastry over the apple filling to make a triangle and seal the perimeter by pinching the edges or pressing the tines of a fork into the dough.

- Place the turnovers on a baking sheet and brush with the egg white. Bake until the dough is crispy and golden brown, 12 to 15 minutes.

Makes 6 servings /
Cost per serving: $1.05

200 calories
8 g fat (1 g saturated)
32 g carbohydrates

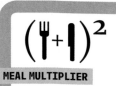

MEAL MULTIPLIER

Puff pastry—made mostly with butter and flour—isn't exactly light fare. But if you roll out a sheet until thin and cut it into six squares, you have a 150-calorie wrap that you can use to house a variety of sweet and savory combinations. Swap out the chunky apple filling for any of the following:

- Shredded chicken, sautéed onions and peppers, Monterey Jack cheese
- Leftover Guinness-Braised Short Ribs (see page 282) and sautéed mushrooms
- Sautéed spinach and onions tossed with feta cheese
- Bourbon-spiked bananas and crushed walnuts (see page 46)

Not That!
Cheesecake Factory Warm Apple Crisp
Price: $6.95

1,355 calories
28 g saturated fat
207 g carbohydrates

Save!
1,155 calories and $5.90!

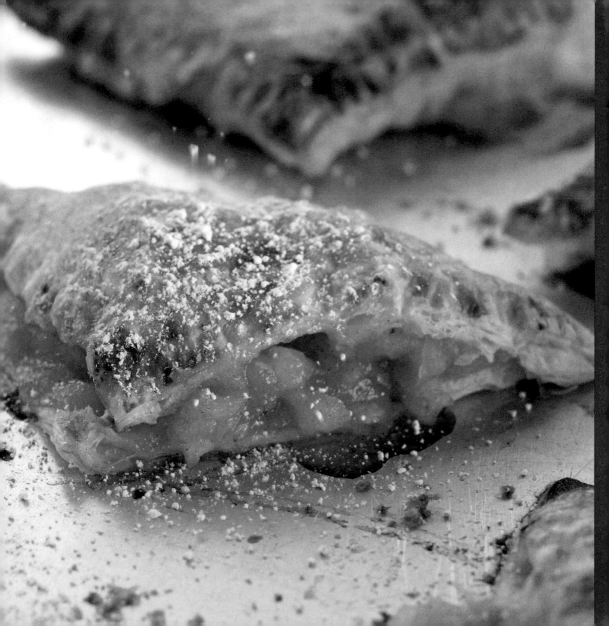

Cook This!
Ricotta Cheesecake with Warm Blueberries

The name says it all: a sugary, fat-laden slice of cake made almost entirely of cheese that we just can't get enough of. Go figure. This version is cut with ricotta for a light, creamy texture, and the warm blueberries lend a delicious dose of brain-boosting anthocyanins.

You'll Need:

- 8 oz graham crackers
- 6 Tbsp (¾ stick) butter, melted
- 1 container (12 oz) part-skim ricotta, drained
- 2 packages (8 oz each) light cream cheese, softened
- ¾ cup + 2 Tbsp sugar
- Grated zest and juice of 1 lemon
- 3 eggs
- 1 bag (16 oz) frozen blueberries

How to Make It:

- Preheat the oven to 350°F. Cover the outside of a 9" springform pan with a layer of aluminum foil.
- Grind the graham crackers in a food processor (or by hand in a plastic bag). Add the melted butter and whiz again for a few seconds. Pour the crumb mixture over the bottom (not the sides) of the pan and use a measuring cup to press them firmly into the pan. Bake for about 15 minutes, until the crust is a deep brown shade.
- Blend the ricotta, cream cheese, ¾ cup sugar, and lemon zest in the (clean) food processor until smooth, stopping occasionally to scrape down the sides of the bowl. Add the eggs and pulse just until blended.
- Pour the cheese mixture over the crust in the pan. Place the springform pan in a baking dish. Pour enough hot water into the dish to come halfway up the sides of the springform pan.
- Bake until the cheesecake is golden and the center of the cake moves slightly when the pan is gently shaken, about 1 hour.

Cool for an hour on the counter, then refrigerate until the cheesecake is cold, at least 4 hours.

- When the cheesecake is ready to be cut, combine the blueberries, lemon juice, and 2 tablespoons sugar in a saucepan. Simmer 5 to 7 minutes, until the blueberries begin to pop and become syrupy. Cut the cake into wedges and serve with a generous scoop of the blueberries over the top.

Makes 10 servings / Cost per serving: $1.96

360 calories
19 g fat
(8 g saturated)
40 g carbohydrates

704 calories
25 g saturated fat
67 g carbohydrates

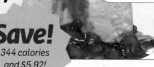

Not That!
Cheesecake Factory Fresh Strawberry Cheesecake
Price: $7.88

Save!
344 calories and $5.92!

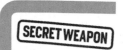

SECRET WEAPON

Citrus zest

The juice inside lemons, limes, and oranges isn't the fruits' only prized possession. The fragrant rind is home to the most intense citrus flavor of all and works great when stirred into everything from borscht to brownies. The best way to get it off is with a microplane, but the fine side of a cheese grater also works. Just be sure to stop as soon as you see the white pith emerge—its bitter notes can sink an otherwise tasty dish.

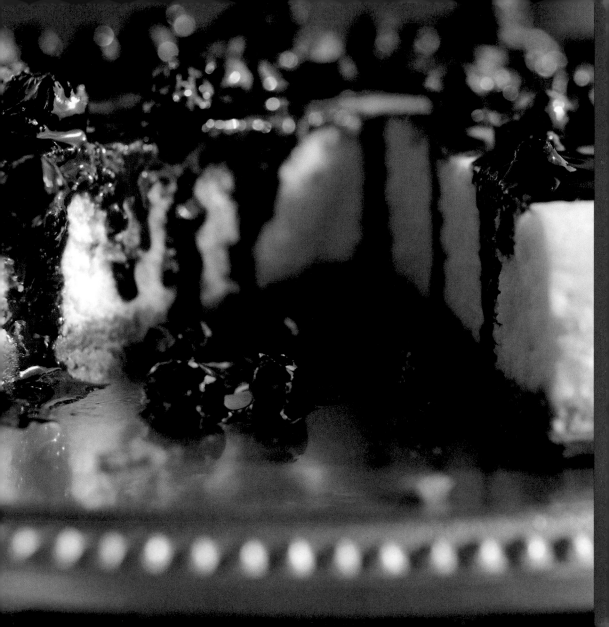

Cook This!
Espresso Granita

A trip to the ice cream parlor used to mean a single scoop of ice cream atop a sugar cone, a perfect little 200-calorie treat. Now, at places like Häagen-Dazs, Baskin-Robbins, and Cold Stone, where serving sizes have grown out of control and high-calorie add-ins are the standard, that same trip to the scoop shop may set you back 1,000 calories. When it comes to dessert, it's best to stay in—especially if you learn to make granitas, frozen desserts that are every bit as satisfying as ice cream and easy enough for a 6-year-old to make.

You'll Need:

- 2 **cups espresso or very strong brewed coffee, warmed**
- ½ **cup sugar**
- **Light whipped topping**
- ½ **cup shaved dark chocolate**

If you have the time and don't mind the extra 50 calories, fresh whipped cream is best. Beat a cup of heavy cream in a cold metal mixing bowl with a tablespoon of sugar until soft peaks form.

How to Make It:

- Combine the espresso with the sugar and stir until the sugar dissolves (if the espresso has cooled, you may need to microwave it for 45 seconds to help the sugar dissolve). Pour the mixture into a shallow metal baking pan (there should be about an inch of liquid) and place in the freezer.

- After 15 to 20 minutes, just as the mix has begun to freeze, remove the dish from the freezer and use a fork to scrape the ice crystals developing on the surface. Careful scraping will help you achieve a light, almost creamy granita, rather than a chunky, icy one. Repeat this step once every 30 to 45 minutes until the granita is entirely frozen.

- For each serving, place a small scoop of the granita in a chilled wine glass, top with a spoonful of whipped topping and a bit of the chocolate, then repeat with a second layer.

Makes 4 servings /
Cost per serving: $0.72

$$(\text{\textbf{\texttt{¶}}}+\text{\texttt{l}})^2$$

MEAL MULTIPLIER

The same granita technique can be applied to dozens of different products with amazing results. Try these, too.

- **Lemon or lime:** Blend 2 cups water, ¾ cup sugar, ½ cup fresh lemon or lime juice
- **Blueberry ginger:** Blend 2 cups blueberries, ¾ cup water, ¼ cup sugar, 1 Tbsp minced ginger
- **Watermelon basil:** Blend 4 cups watermelon chunks, ½ cup sugar, juice of 1 lemon, 8 basil leaves

170 calories
8 g fat (5 g saturated)
28 g sugars

910 calories
54 g fat
(34.5 g saturated)
83 g sugars

Not That!
Cold Stone Creamery Gotta Have It Coffee Ice Cream with Chocolate Chips Price: $4.49

Save!
740 calories
and $3.77!

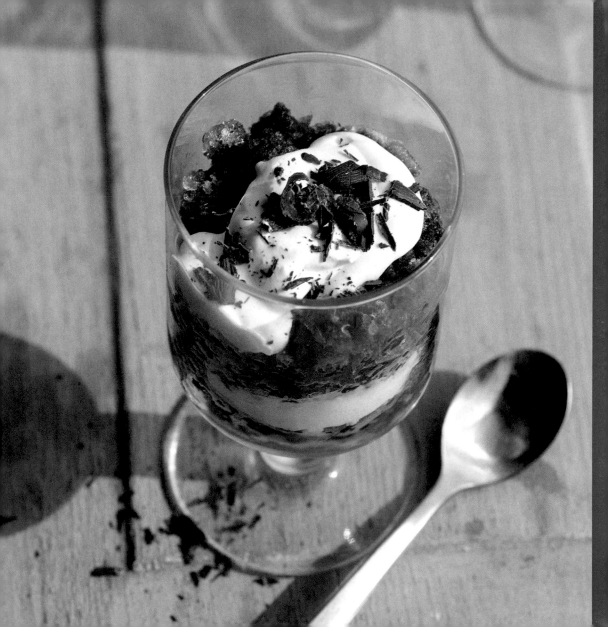

Cook This!
Grilled Apricots

In countries around the world, dessert is often as simple and satisfying as a single piece of perfect fruit. We've followed their lead but gussied it up a bit with yogurt, toasted nuts, and a bit of maple syrup. The result—a warm, cool, and crunchy bowl filled with fiber, protein, and healthy fat—is about as good as dessert ever gets. (In fact, this is so healthy, we almost filed it in the breakfast chapter, which you can certainly do.)

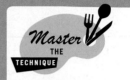

Master THE TECHNIQUE

Grilling fruit

Trapped inside every piece of fruit is a bounty of natural sugars. By applying heat to the surface of the fruit—whether from grilling, sautéing, or broiling—you concentrate those sugars. The result: a luscious, intensely sweet piece of fruit that—with a bit of whipped cream or, in this case, yogurt—stands alone as a healthy dessert. Among the best fruits for cooking are figs, peaches, apricots, nectarines, and apples. Choose ripe but firm fruit that will hold its shape after cooking. Most fruit needs no more than 5 minutes on a grill, under a broiler, or in a sauté pan with a bit of butter.

You'll Need:

- **2** apricots or peaches, halved and pitted
- **2** cups plain Greek-style yogurt (we like Fage 2%)
- **4** Tbsp chopped toasted walnuts
- **4** Tbsp maple syrup

How to Make It:

- Heat a grill, stovetop grill pan, or broiler until hot. Cook the fruit until nicely caramelized on the outside, about 5 minutes. The fruit should be softened but still maintain its shape. Top each fruit half with ½ cup yogurt, 1 tablespoon walnuts, and 1 tablespoon maple syrup.

Makes 4 servings / Cost per serving: $2.23

If you don't have real maple syrup, you're better off with honey or agave syrup than Aunt Jemima.

The easiest way to toast nuts is to roast them in a dry pan set over medium heat for about 5 minutes, stirring once or twice as they toast.

170 calories
7 g fat (2 g saturated)
18 g sugars

770 calories
54 g fat (20 g saturated, 1 g trans)
61 g sugars

Not That!
Cold Stone Creamery Love It Vanilla Bean Ice Cream with Peach Pie Filling and Walnuts Price: $4.68

Save!
600 calories and $2.45!

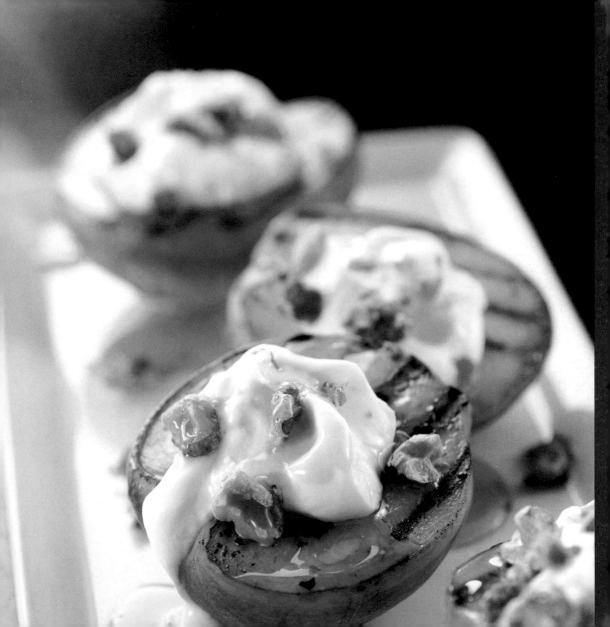

Banana-Rum Splits

The banana split has never been mistaken for health food, but at least there used to be a certain honesty to it: a sliced banana topped with ice cream, nuts, and whipped cream. Now, a banana split is more science experiment than real food. Take the most popular split in the country, the one from Baskin-Robbins. It has no fewer than 50 ingredients, including food dyes, locust gum, and polysorbate 80. It also has as many calories as you should consume in two full meals. Our split, on the other hand, boasts a third of the calories, a hit of booze, and an honesty that harkens to the food days of yore.

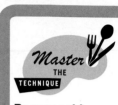

Master THE TECHNIQUE

Boozy cooking

The point of adding booze to a recipe is not to give you a buzz; it's to add rich, complex notes to your food. Dark rum and bourbon, redolent of vanilla and caramel, pair perfectly with sweet foods; red wine and beer add nuance to savory stews and braises. In both cases, the heat burns off most of the alcohol itself, leaving just the concentrated flavors behind. When cooking with high-proof alcohol, take a few precautionary steps: Always add liquor to pans off the heat, and always keep a fire extinguisher in the kitchen.

You'll Need:

½ Tbsp butter

2 bananas

1 Tbsp brown sugar

2 Tbsp dark rum or bourbon (optional)

4 large scoops vanilla ice cream (preferably Breyers All Natural)

¼ cup pecans, toasted and chopped

4 Tbsp dark chocolate syrup or hot fudge sauce

Light whipped topping

How to Make It:

- Heat the butter in a large skillet over medium heat. Slice the bananas in half crosswise, then lengthwise. Place the banana quarters in the hot pan with the brown sugar and cook on one side until deeply caramelized, about 2 minutes. Turn the bananas over and cook for another 30 seconds. Remove from the heat and add the rum. Be careful—even when the pan is removed from the heat, the alcohol can still ignite.

- Place 2 banana quarters and any accumulated liquid in each of 4 bowls. Top with the ice cream, nuts, chocolate, and whipped topping.

Makes 4 servings / Cost per serving: $1.15

You want ripe but firm bananas that will still hold their shape after being hit with the heat of the pan.

350 calories
17 g fat (6 g saturated)
26 g sugars

1,010 calories
34 g fat
(20 g saturated, 1 g trans)
125 g sugars

Not That!
Baskin-Robbins Classic Banana Split
Price: $6.35

Save!
660 calories and $5.20!

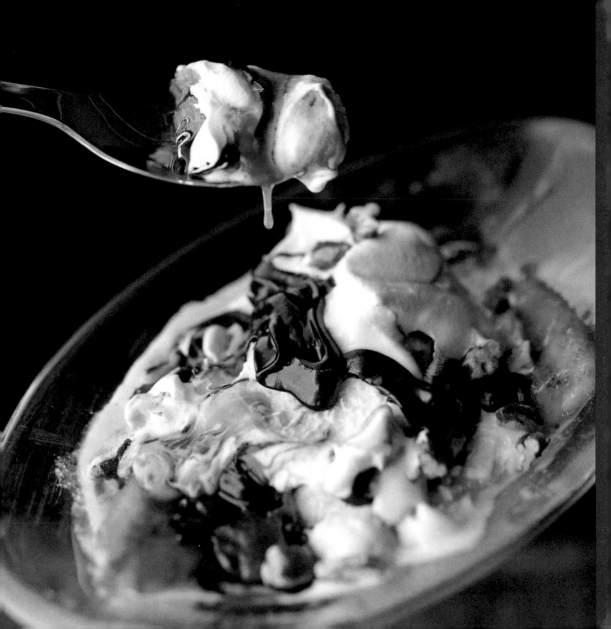

Olive Oil Ice Cream

Studies show that a variety of taste sensations (salty, sweet, spicy) better satisfy the appetite than a single dominant flavor. Maybe that explains just how easy it is to spoon your way mindlessly through a pint of super sweet Ben & Jerry's. This dish (inspired by Iron Chef Mario Batali and his New York restaurant Babbo) taps into that principle, contrasting the smooth sweetness of vanilla ice cream with the flaky crunch of sea salt and the rich, spicy notes of extra-virgin olive oil. The combination is elegant and strangely addictive—and a small bowl will squash your sweet tooth for less than 300 calories.

SECRET WEAPON

Breyers All Natural Ice Cream

The first ingredient in most American ice creams is heavy cream, which is why an average scoop of plain vanilla packs about 200 calories and 13 grams of fat. Breyers All Natural, though, starts with milk, which makes for a lighter scoop; Breyers French Vanilla has just 140 calories and 7 grams of fat. And unlike additive-laden low-fat ice creams, this one has just six ingredients. Make Breyers your go-to brand for all your ice cream needs.

You'll Need:

- 4 large scoops vanilla ice cream (we like Breyers All Natural)
- 2 Tbsp extra-virgin olive oil
- Flaky sea salt
- Cashews (optional)

How to Make It:

- Divide the ice cream among 4 cold bowls. Drizzle with the olive oil and a generous pinch of salt. Scatter a handful of cashews (if using) over the top.

Makes 4 servings / Cost per serving: $0.70

Our favorite sea salt is called Malton sea salt. Skimmed from a saltwater river in England, these delicate crystals provide amazing crunch and a burst of briny joy.

240 calories
18 g fat (6 g saturated)
15 g sugars

380 calories
24 g fat (16 g saturated)
32 g sugars

Not That!

2 scoops Ben & Jerry's Vanilla Ice Cream
Price: $1.95

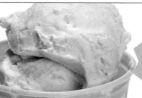

Save!
140 calories
and $1.25!

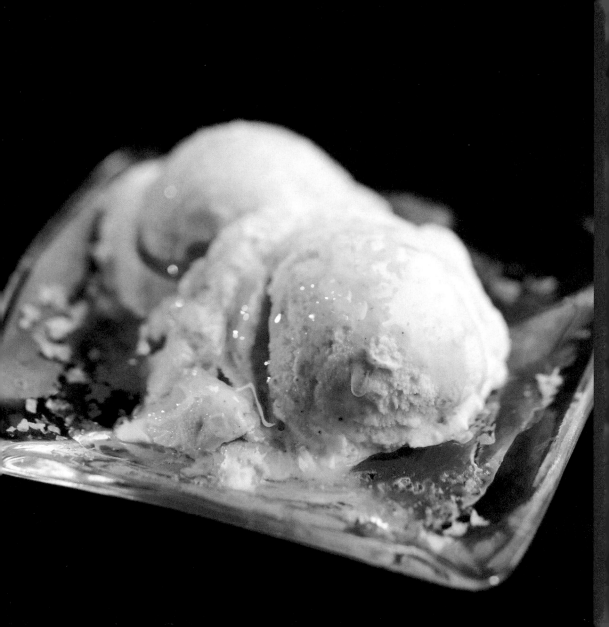

Ice Cream Sandwiches

Food should be fun. If you ever want to encourage a child to learn the importance of feeding him- or herself well, this is the first lesson you need to impart. And what better way to do it than by setting up an ice cream sandwich station? Keep the cookies small and thin, the ice cream light (preferably Breyers All Natural), and the toppings relatively healthy (more fruits and nuts than candy and marshmallows) and you can create a vast array of 200-calorie sandwiches. Our favorite combination? Genevas and coffee ice cream layered with banana slices and crusted in pistachios. The damage? Just 220 calories.

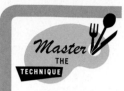

Master **THE TECHNIQUE**

Get kids cooking

No single strategy can better ensure a lifetime of happy, healthy eating habits than bringing kids into the kitchen to pitch in with the cooking. Not only does it familiarize them with basic techniques and safety issues, it exposes them to a world of brand new flavor combinations and foreign ingredients. A picky 8-year-old is more likely to eat that roasted broccoli if he had a hand in its cooking. It's best to start with something easy and fun, and nothing is simpler or more enjoyable than making ice cream sandwiches with a kitchen full of happy, hungry children.

You'll Need:

Ice cream

Graham crackers

Pepperidge Farm cookies (Chessmen and Genevas work best)

Ginger snaps

Sliced bananas

Sliced strawberries

Maraschino cherries

Chopped nuts (walnuts, pecans, pistachios)

Dark chocolate sauce (optional)

The darker the sauce, the less sugar and the more antioxidants it contains.

How to Make It:

- Allow the ice cream to soften on the counter for about 10 minutes. In the meantime, lay out your ingredients of choice on the counter, on plates, or in individual bowls. Allow people to construct their own sandwiches, layering cookies with fruit and ice cream, then rolling the sides of the sandwiches in crushed nuts. If you're looking to gild the lily, drizzle a bit of chocolate syrup over the top.

- Make them quickly, as the ice cream will melt, and arrange on a baking sheet. Place the sandwiches in the freezer for 20 to 30 minutes to firm up, then dig in.

Makes 1 serving / Average cost per serving: $0.81

Varies, but on average:
200 calories
11 g fat (4 g saturated)
19 g sugars

480 calories
31 g fat
(15 g saturated)
35 g sugars

Not That!
Dairy Queen Buster Bar Treat
Price: $1.84

Save!
280 calories
and $1.03!

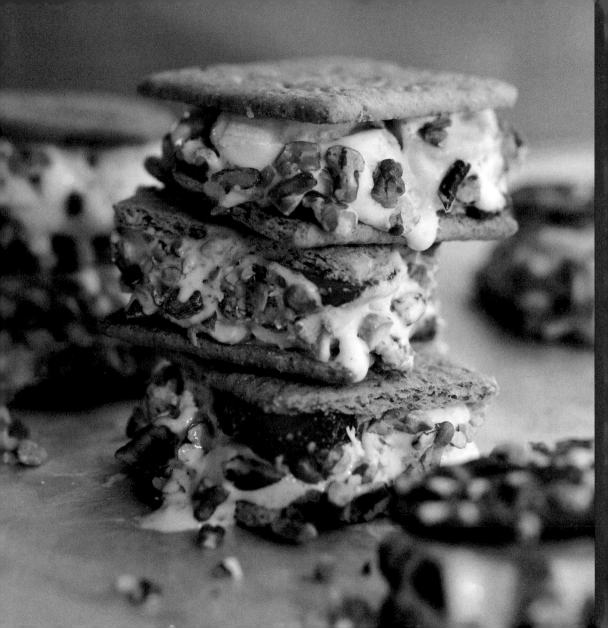

Index